Neighborhoods and Health

Neighborhoods and Health

Edited by

ICHIRO KAWACHI

LISA F. BERKMAN

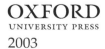

OXFORD
UNIVERSITY PRESS
2003

OXFORD
UNIVERSITY PRESS

Oxford   New York
Auckland   Bangkok   Buenos Aires   Cape Town   Chennai
Dar es Salaam   Delhi   Hong Kong   Istanbul   Karachi   Kolkata
Kuala Lumpur   Madrid   Melbourne   Mexico City   Mumbai
Nairobi   São Paulo   Shanghai   Taipei   Tokyo   Toronto

Published by Oxford University Press, Inc.
198 Madison Avenue, New York, New York, 10016
http://www.oup-usa.org

Oxford is a registered trademark of Oxford University Press

Library of Congress Cataloging-in-Publication Data
Neighborhoods and health /
edited by Ichiro Kawachi, Lisa F. Berkman.
p. ; cm. Includes bibliographical references and index.
ISBN 0-19-513838-4 (cloth)
1. Community health services. 2. Health services accessibility.
3. Medical care—Social aspects. 4. Medical care—Utilization.
I. Kawachi, Ichiro. II. Berkman, Lisa F.
[DNLM: 1. Health Services Accessibility. 2. Community Health Services.
3. Socioeconomic Factors.
W 76 N397 2003]   RA427 .N454 2003   362.1'2—dc21   2002029287

9 8 7 6 5 4 3

Printed in the United States of America
on acid-free paper

Preface

The search for the effects of neighborhoods on health has moved much closer to the center stage of the public health and social sciences research agenda. Researchers have long suspected that where one lives makes a difference to health in addition to who one is. Almost everyone now understands that smoking cigarettes, eating fast foods, and being sedentary can compromise longevity and chances of good health, but can a person's ability to maintain a healthy lifestyle be affected by the smoking habits of other people living in proximity to them, or by access to local grocery stores selling fresh fruit and vegetables, or by the existence of safe parks and recreational spaces in their communities? In other words, can certain social and physical characteristics of residential neighborhoods make a difference to a person's well-being, over and above an individual's intentions and actions to maintain healthy habits? The answer to that question requires new ways of thinking about the determinants of health as well as new analytical methods to test these ideas. If the characteristics of neighborhoods make a difference to health beyond the characteristics of the individuals who live in them, then policy-makers should take heed of the new opportunities to develop health promotion interventions directed at places as well as people.

There are clear signals to indicate that researchers in public health and allied social sciences are converging on the search for place-based influences on health. Even a cursory search of the major professional journals in public health reveals dozens of relevant studies published just in the past few years. Research funding bodies, including the U.S. National Institutes of Health, have assigned priority to the search for neighborhood effects, especially in the context of explaining social inequalities in health. Even so, despite the interest in this subject, we are unaware of any comprehensive text that surveys the theoretical and methodological challenges involved in conducting research in this area.

This book was conceived as a response to that vacuum. We have gathered together contributions from leading international investigators on neighborhoods and health. The contributors represent the diversity of disciplines that have advanced theory, methodology, and empirical evidence in this field of research. Gathered together in this volume are state-of-the-art reflections from social epidemiologists, sociologists, demographers, statisticians, clinicians, and medical geographers.

The book is organized into four parts. The first two chapters provide an overview of research on neighborhoods and health. These chapters lay out the historical motivation behind focusing on neighborhood contexts as determinants of population and individual health. They summarize the major conceptual and theoretical issues that have emerged over two decades of research on neighborhoods and health.

Part I (Chapters 3–8) deals with the methodological complexities of undertaking neighborhood research. The chapters focus on the meaning and interpretation of ecological data (including a discussion of the ecological fallacy—Chapter 3), the analytical potential of multilevel statistical methodology (Chapter 4), the emerging science of "ecometrics" (Chapter 5), and the contributions of sociological theory to characterizing neighborhood contexts (Chapter 6). Chapters 7 and 8 introduce the techniques of geocoding and the construction of area-level indexes of socioeconomic position and deprivation, from U.S. and U.K. perspectives, respectively.

The chapters in Part II showcase the empirical evidence linking neighborhood conditions to health outcomes: infectious disease (Chapter 9), infant health (Chapter 10), and asthma (Chapter 11). These examples were singled out on the basis of their promise for demonstrating the utility of extending etiological hypotheses to the ecological level. Examples of other health outcomes, such as total mortality, cardiovascular disease, and functional limitations in old age, are brought up elsewhere in the volume.

The final section tackles some of the major cross-cutting themes in contemporary neighborhood research. Chapter 12 describes the measurement and health consequences of residential segregation by race and class. Chapter 13 extends the theme of an earlier chapter (6) by focusing on neighborhood context as the basis of social interactions. Chapter 14 is an extended reflection on the interaction between neighborhood research and aging. Finally, Chapter 15 discusses the relevance of studying neighborhoods for social policy.

We feel confident that the material presented in this volume will prove useful to a broad audience, ranging from those who are just beginning to wet their feet in this field of inquiry to experienced practitioners. In addition to providing guidance on methodology and practice, the authors introduce alternative models of neighborhood effects on health (e.g., Chapters 2 and 14) as well as detailed examples of community interventions to improve population health outcomes (e.g., Chapter 11). The potential influence of neighborhood conditions on health is described throughout the life course, from birth and infancy to old age. If the chapters that follow inspire researchers and policy-makers to move the field ahead by refining the methodology, adding to new evidence, or devising novel policy approaches to improve the health of populations, then we will have accomplished our goal in organizing this book.

Boston, Massachusetts   I. K.
                                                                         L. F. B.

Contents

Contributors

DOLORES ACEVEDO-GARCIA,
    PhD, MPA-URP
*Department of Health and Social
    Behavior*
Harvard School of Public Health
Boston, Massachusetts

JENNIFER L. BALFOUR, PhD,
    MPH
*Department of Epidemiology and the
    Center for Social Epidemiology and
    Population Health*
University of Michigan
Ann Arbor, Michigan

LISA F. BERKMAN, PhD
Harvard Center for Society and Health
*Department of Health and Social
    Behavior*
Harvard School of Public Health
Boston Massachusetts

JARVIS CHEN, ScD
*Department of Health and Social
    Behavior*
Harvard School of Public Health
Boston Massachusetts

CHERYL CLARK, MS
*Department of Health and Social
    Behavior*
Harvard School of Public Health
Boston, Massachusetts

JAMES W. COLLINS, JR, MD
Division of Neonatology
Children's Memorial Hospital
Chicago, Illinois

ANA V. DIEZ-ROUX, MD, PhD
Division of General Medicine
*Columbia College of Physicians and
    Surgeons*
Division of Epidemiology
*Joseph P. Mailman School of Public
    Health*
Columbia University
New York, New York

CRAIG DUNCAN, PhD
Population Estimates Office
Office for National Statistics
Southampton, U.K.

ANNE ELLAWAY, PhD
*MRC, Social and Public Health Sciences
    Unit*
University of Glasgow
Glasgow, Scotland

ARON FISCHER, BA
*Department of Health and Social
    Behavior*
Harvard School of Public Health
Boston, Massachusetts

EDWIN B. FISHER, PhD
Department of Psychology
Washington University
Division of Health Behavior Research
Departments of Medicine and Pediatrics
Washington University School of
    Medicine
St. Louis, Missouri

MINDY THOMPSON FULLILOVE,
    MD
The Community Research Group
New York Psychiatric Institute
New York, New York

ANNIE GJELSVIK, MS
Department of Community Health
Brown University
Providence, R.I.

THOMAS A. GLASS, PhD
Department of Epidemiology and the
    Center on Aging and Health
Johns Hopkins Bloomberg School of
    Hygiene and Public Health
Baltimore, Maryland

DAVID GORDON, PhD
Head of the Centre for the Study of
    Poverty and Social Justice
School for Policy Studies
University of Bristol
Bristol, U.K.

JODY HEYMANN, MD, PhD
Department of Health and Social
    Behavior
Harvard School of Public Health
Boston, Massachusetts

JOSEPH W. HOGAN
Center for Statistical Sciences
Brown University
Providence, Rhode Island

ICHIRO KAWACHI, MD, PhD
Harvard Center for Society and Health
Department of Health and Social
    Behavior
Harvard School of Public Health
Boston, Massachusetts

KELVYN JONES, PhD
Department of Geography
University of Bristol
Bristol, U.K.

NANCY KRIEGER, PH.D.
Department of Health and Social
    Behavior
Harvard School of Public Health
Boston, Massachusetts

KERRY LEMIEUX, MS
Department of Health and Social
    Behavior
Harvard School of Public Health
Boston, Massachusetts

KIMBERLY A. LOCHNER, ScD
The Robert Wood Johnson Foundation
Princeton, New Jersey

SALLY MACINTYRE, PhD
MRC, Social and Public Health Sciences
    Unit
University of Glasgow
Glasgow, Scotland

STEPHEN W. RAUDENBUSH, PhD
School of Education
University of Michigan
Ann Arbor, Michigan

ROBERT J. SAMPSON, PhD
Department of Sociology
University of Chicago
Chicago, Illinois

NANCY FISHER SCHULTE, BS
Division of Neonatology
Children's Memorial Hospital
Chicago, Illinois

S. V. SUBRAMANIAN, PHD
Department of Health and Social Behavior
Harvard School of Public Health
Boston, Massachusetts

PAMELA WATERMAN, MPH
Department of Health and Social Behavior
Harvard School of Public Health
Boston, Massachusetts

ROSALIND J. WRIGHT, MD, MPH
Department of Pulmonary and Critical
  Care Medicine
Beth Israel Deaconess Medical Center
Harvard Medical School
Channing Laboratory
Brigham & Women's Hospital
Boston, Massachusetts

SALLY ZIERLER, PHD
Department of Community Health
Brown University
Providence, Rhode Island

Neighborhoods and Health

1
Introduction

Ichiro Kawachi
Lisa F. Berkman

Why Study Neighborhoods?

The insight that where one lives makes a difference to one's health is not new. Such observations have been made since at least the eighteenth century (see, for example, Chapters 2 and 8). What is new is the cross-disciplinary dialogue on concepts, methods, and evidence about the influence of neighborhoods on health. This mix is captured by the authors of the following chapters, who come from backgrounds as diverse as social epidemiology, medical geography, clinical medicine, demography, criminology, educational statistics, urban sociology, and policy studies. Besides the novelty of interdisciplinary exchange, this book was motivated by several other noteworthy trends. Foremost among them is the trend toward rising residential segregation, whether by class or race–ethnicity. As Douglas Massey noted in his 1996 presidential address to the Population Association of America, "urbanization, rising income inequality, and increasing class segregation have produced a geographic concentration of affluence and poverty throughout the world, creating a radical change in the geographic basis of human society" (Massey, 1996, p. 395).

The widening gulf between the rich and poor is mirrored by a growing divergence of their residential environments, such that affluent people are increasingly living and interacting with other affluent people, while the poor increasingly live and interact with other poor people. (See Chapter 12 for an extended discussion of these trends.) Contrary to the claim that places no longer matter, the trends in residential segregation as well as legislative developments (e.g., the devolution of welfare) will continue to ensure that neighborhoods remain relevant to addressing health disparities.

A second noteworthy development has been the emergence of new concepts and methods to analyze neighborhood variations in health. Concepts such as "social capital" and "collective efficacy" in sociology (Chapter 6), as well as novel "exposures" such as witnessing acts of violence as a trigger for asthma (Chapter 11), have spurred researchers to take a fresh look at the influence of places on people's health. In the realm of statistics, the methods to analyze multilevel and hierarchical data have existed for some years (Bryk and Raudenbush, 1995; see Chapter 4), but their application to the study of neighborhoods and health is still very new. As Diez-Roux argues in Chapter 3, our fascination with these methods poses the danger of outpacing our conceptual thinking about how neighborhoods influence health. This book is timely in that it takes stock of both what we know and what we need to know in order to advance to the next stage of evidence and policy.

A final impetus for the preparation of this book was the launching of new initiatives and studies with neighborhoods as their focus. This is true of the Social Science Research Council's research program on the influence of neighborhoods on the development of poor children and adolescents, published in 1997 as a two-volume report edited by Brooks-Gunn, Duncan, and Aber (1997). Closer to the realm of public health, the Project on Human Development in Chicago Neighborhoods was launched in 1995 among 343 Chicago neighborhoods as a prospective, multilevel study of juvenile delinquency and crime (Chapters 5 and 6). After decades of comparative neglect in the health sciences, social scientists have reason to crow about the return of the ecological perspective (Macintyre and Ellaway, 2000).

What, then, is the present state of evidence on neighborhood effects on health outcomes? Individual chapters in Part II of this book will describe the state of the evidence linking neighborhood conditions to selected health outcomes, including infectious diseases (Chapter 9), infant mortality and low birthweight (Chapter 10), and asthma (Chapter 11). In addition, multilevel studies have been published linking various indices of neighborhood deprivation and poverty to individual risks of cigarette smoking (Kleinschmidt et al., 1995; Diez-Roux et al., 1997; Duncan et al., 1999), higher body mass index (Ellaway et al., 1997), depressive symptoms (Aneshensel and Sucoff, 1996; Yen and Kaplan, 1999), lower quality diet (Diez-Roux et al., 1999), poor self-rated health (Humphreys and Carr-Hill, 1991; Robert, 1998), as well as intimate partner violence (O'Campo et al., 1995).

To illustrate the methodological challenges and representative findings of neighborhood research, in the next section we review the multilevel evidence on one of the most common health outcomes studies so far—the risk of dying from any cause. We have chosen to summarize the studies of mortality because death is the final common endpoint of a diverse set of neighborhood influences, including differential access to health services, as well as differential exposures to stressors (e.g., exposure to tobacco advertising, lack of access to fresh foods in retail outlets) and resources (e.g., availability of social support). Besides, everybody would agree that death is a serious outcome, especially if it is premature. Focusing on mortality risk also provides a uniform endpoint against which we can summarize and contrast the studies that have been carried out in diverse countries and settings, using different definitions of "neighborhoods" and neighborhood exposures. Following the overview of the multilevel studies of neighborhood effects on mortality risks, we then turn to discuss a set of emerging conceptual and methodological challenges in neighborhood research.

Neighborhood Effects on Mortality

To date, eight multilevel studies of small-area influences on mortality have been published (Table 1–1). Haan, Kaplan, and Camacho (1987) reported perhaps the earliest such study of all-cause mortality. With the Alameda County Study as a model, they prospectively followed 1,811 adults for a period of nine years. The neighborhood variable of interest was whether the individuals in the study resided in one of the 37 census tracts in Oakland that were federally designated poverty areas. As shown in Table 1–1, the federal designation of a "poverty area" is constructed from census variables, including the percentage of low income families, the percentage of substandard housing, the percentage of adults with low educational attainment, the percentage of unemployed, the percentage of unskilled male laborers, and the percentage of children in homes with a single parent. Haan et al. (1987) reported that the age-, race-, and sex-adjusted mortality risk of living in a poverty area compared to all other areas was 1.71 (95% CI: 1.20 to 2.44). The excess risk of death persisted after adjustment for individual income, employment status, access to medical care, smoking, drinking, exercise, body mass index, and social ties.

Sloggett and Joshi (1994) carried out a nine-year follow-up study of nearly 300,000 adults in the Office of National Statistics Longitudinal Study. This study is a 1% sample of the population of England and Wales administered by the U.K. Office of Population Censuses and Surveys. The area variable of interest in Sloggett and Joshi's analysis was the extent of material deprivation within the electoral wards in which the study subjects lived. Material deprivation was assessed with the Townsend and

TABLE 1–1. Multilevel Studies of Neighborhood Characteristics in Relation to Mortality

Study	Population	Geographic Areas	Neighborhood Measure	Adjusted Relative Risk of Mortality
Haan et al., 1987	Residents of Oakland, CA (Alameda County Study)	Federally designated poverty area of Oakland (37 census tracts)	Federal criteria for poverty area: % low income adjustment, % low education, % unemployed, % substandard housing, % unskilled male laborer, % children in homes with single parent	Between 1.47 and 1.60, depending on covariate adjustment
Sloggett and Joshi, 1998	Residents of U.K. in 1981 (ONS Longitudinal Study)	Electoral wards	Townsend and Carstairs Deprivation Index score: % unemployed, % without access to car, % households not owner occupied, % employed men and women in two lowest classes	1.02 (1.00 to 1.03) for men, 1.04 (1.02 to 1.06) for women
Ecob and Jones, 1998	Residents of U.K. in 1971 (ONS Longitudinal Study)	Electoral wards	Craig-Webber classification of neighborhoods (36 types), e.g., "modern high-status housing," "Mock Tudor areas," "inner-city council estates," "poor quality housing in areas of economic decline."	Odds ratios ranging from 0.87 to 1.38 in women and 0.79 to 1.22 in men, depending on place.

Study	Unit	Socioeconomic characteristic	Result
Anderson et al., 1997	Census tracts	Median family income: low (<$16,200) vs. high (>$22,900)	Between 1.16 (white women), and 1.49 (black men)
Waitzman and Smith, 1998	Census tracts	Federal criteria for poverty area (same as Haan et al., 1987)	1.78 for 25–54 year olds, 0.78 for 55–74 year olds
LeClere et al., 1997	Census tracts	% African-American: highest (>17%) vs. lowest (0.5%)	1.22 for men, 1.17 for women
LeClere et al., 1998	Census tracts	% female-headed families: highest (>24%) vs. lowest (≤9.9%)	1.85 for women [<\#93>65, 1.23 for women ≥65 (cardiovascular mortality)
Yen and Kaplan, 1999	Census tracts	Neighborhood social environment score comprised of 3 subscales: population socioeconomic status, commercial stores, and environment/housing	1.58

Adjusted for individual-level socioeconomic characteristics (and other variables where indicated in text).

Carstairs Index, composed of the percentage of unemployed in the area, the percentage without access to a car, the percentage of houses not owner-occupied, and so on (see Chapter 8 for an extended discussion of this and other indexes of area deprivation). *Before* adjustment for individual socioeconomic disadvantage, the authors found a clear relationship between area-level deprivation and risk of premature death. However, the excess risk of mortality was completely explained away in men once adjustment was made for individual socioeconomic circumstances, while in women the risk was heavily attenuated. The authors concluded that their study did not suggest "any social miasma whereby the shorter life expectancy of disadvantaged people is further reduced if they live in close proximity to other disadvantaged people."

In 1998 the same authors published an update and extension of their ONS analysis, and this is the version summarized in Table 1–1. The Townsend and Carstairs Index was used again to characterize deprivation within wards. With longer followup (1981–1992) the authors reported that area deprivation was now related to both male and female mortality, even after adjustment for individual socioeconomic characteristics. Contextual effects were similarly demonstrated for other health outcomes, such as self-reported long-term limiting illness, low birthweight, and teenage births. Although the updated evidence appeared to overturn their earlier findings, the authors nonetheless concluded that "the role of area in the explanation of outcomes varies but is, at best, secondary. The role of personal circumstances is overriding."

Ecob and Jones (1998) published an independent analysis of the ONS Longitudinal Study that used a different measure of ward-level social circumstances—the Craig-Webber classification of neighborhood types. This was developed from a hierarchical cluster analysis of wards in the United Kingdom using 40 variables derived from the 1971 census. The cluster analysis produces 36 neighborhood types, with descriptions ranging from "modern, low cost owner-occupied housing" to "poor quality housing in areas of economic decline." Arguing that a single index of area deprivation (such as the Townsend Index) may be too restrictive, the authors carried out a multilevel analysis of mortality using the neighborhood types derived from the Craig-Webber classification. Aside from individual socioeconomic circumstances, the authors found evidence for a range of neighborhood contextual effects on mortality risk, from protective effects (e.g., odds ratio = 0.87 for females living in "modern high-status housing") to excess risks (e.g., odds ratio = 1.38 for females living in "inner-city council estates").

Anderson et al. (1997) published an analysis of 239,187 adults who were followed for a period of 11 years in the National Longitudinal Mortality Study. The area variable in this study consisted of median family income at the U.S. Census tract level. Analyses were stratified into two age groups: 25–64 years and 65 or older. Among younger subjects, residing in areas of low median income (<$16,200) compared to high income (>$22,900) was associated with relative risks of all-cause mortality ranging from 1.16 (white women) to 1.49 (black men), *after* controlling for personal income. As might be expected, the strength of association between median income in the neighborhood and risk of death was weaker than the association of low personal income with mortality, which ranged between 1.7 (white women) to 2.3 (black men). Nonetheless, between a quarter and a third of the mortality associated with residence in low income areas was independent of the level of personal income.

Waitzman and Smith (1998) carried out a multilevel study of 10,101 adults in the National Health and Nutrition Examination Survey (NHANES I) during 1971 to 1974 who were followed through to 1987. The area variable of interest in this study was the same as in the study by Haan et al. (1987): federally designated poverty areas (census tracts). Individual-level covariates included (among others) household income, years of formal education, smoking, drinking, exercise, and marital status. The authors split the analyses into two age groups: 25–54 years and ≥55 years. Among the younger subjects the relative risk of all-cause mortality from living in a poverty area, adjusted for individual characteristics, was 1.78 (95% CI: 1.33 to 2.38). Excess risks of death were also present for cardiovascular disease (RR 1.90, 95% CI: 1.24 to 2.90) and cancer (RR 1.95, 95% CI: 1.28 to 2.95).

LeClere et al. (1997, 1998) published two studies linking the 1986–1990 National Health Interview Survey to the National Death Index. A total of 346,917 adults living in 5,919 census tracts throughout the United States were followed to the end of December 1991. In the first study (LeClere et al. 1997) the authors were interested in explicitly testing the ability of neighborhood variables to account for the black–white gap in all-cause mortality. The primary neighborhood variable of interest in this study was the percentage of African-American residents in a census tract, which the authors used as a surrogate for residential segregation. Compared to white men and women, black men and women had age-adjusted relative risks of mortality of 1.45 and 1.35, respectively. Adjusting for individual socioeconomic characteristics (income and education) attenuated these relative risks to 1.19 and 1.13. Further addition of the neighborhood-level variable (percentage of African Americans) to the regression models completely removed the black–white mortality gap (RRs of 1.06 and 1.04 for men and women, respectively). On the basis of these findings, the authors concluded that, over and above the effects of individual socioeconomic characteristics, neighborhood variables could explain part of the excess risk of death experienced by African Americans. Compared to neighborhoods containing few African Americans (= 0.5%), residents of census tracts where more than 17 percent of the population were African Americans had a 22% excess risk of mortality, no matter what their race.

In a second study the same authors (LeClere et al., 1998) investigated the influence of neighborhood variables on the black–white disparity in female cardiovascular disease (CVD) mortality. Specifically, they set out to test whether the neighborhood characteristic "percent single female-headed households" contributed to the black–white differential in CVD mortality. They reasoned that "neighborhoods where a large proportion of families with dependent children are headed by women may contribute to increased financial, physical, and emotional stress both for individual women and for communities in general." Thus, in contrast to most of the studies summarized above, this one begins to formulate and test specific mechanisms by which areas per se affect individual health. Adjusting for individual socioeconomic status, living in neighborhoods where more than a quarter of the households were headed by a single female was associated with relative risks of CVD mortality of 1.85 for women less than 65 and 1.23 for women 65 years old or older. Black women had a higher CVD mortality rate compared to white women (RR = 2.21 for women less than 65 and 1.38 for women 65 or older), but this excess was completely explained by individual socioeconomic status and the percentage of female-headed households in the neighborhood.

Finally, Yen and Kaplan (1999) carried out an eleven-year follow-up study of 996 participants in the Alameda County Study. In common with other studies cited in this section, the authors used the census tract as a proxy for neighborhood. In a departure from the approach used in other studies, however, the authors attempted to construct their own index of neighborhood quality. Neighborhood-level data were compiled from a variety of sources and factor-analyzed to create three subscales of neighborhood social environment: (1) neighborhood socioeconomic status (per capita income, percentage of white collar, percentage of crowding), (2) presence or lack of commercial stores (pharmacies, beauty parlors, barbershops, laundromats, and supermarkets per 1,000 population), and (3) housing and population (percentage of renters, percentage of single-unit dwellings, population size, and area of census tract). All three subscales as well as the overall combined index predicted mortality rates exclusive of individual variables (which included race, income, education, smoking, drinking, body mass index, and perceived health). For example, living in a neighborhood in the bottom third of quality compared to the top was associated with an age- and sex-adjusted relative risk of mortality of 1.58 (95% CI: 1.15 to 2.18). After adjusting for all individual characteristics, the relative risk was still 1.58 (95% CI: 1.13 to 2.24). An interaction between neighborhood quality and personal income was found whereby low-income individuals were more adversely affected by *high* quality neighborhoods, suggesting differential access to resources.

COMMENTARY

In summary, the bulk of evidence from the studies listed in Table 1–1 seems to indicate a moderate (statistically significant relative risks between 1.1 and 1.8) association between neighborhood environment and health, controlling for individual socioeconomic and other characteristics. Nevertheless, several data gaps are revealed by our review of mortality studies.

First, most studies have relied on cross-sections. Even when the design was prospective, investigators have generally neglected to address the issue of residential mobility, and in particular the issue of residential selection as distinct from social causation.

Second, despite moderate contextual effects, the influence of local area on individual health is weak compared to the more powerful effects of proximal individual and household circumstances (Sloggett and Joshi, 1994), leading some investigators to conclude that the most direct way to improve health is to improve individual and family-level socioeconomic circumstances rather than targeting resources to poor areas (Robert, 1998). There are, nonetheless, important theoretical grounds for believing that neighborhood effects may have been under-estimated, chief among them the procedure to adjust neighborhood effects for individual socioeconomic status. To the extent that neighborhood processes affect individual health *via* individual socioeconomic achievement, then controlling for individual socioeconomic status in multilevel models will adjust away the variation of interest (more on this issue later).

Third, most studies have relied on the use of routinely available, census-derived, aggregated information to characterize neighborhood environments. Few attempts have been made to "unpack" the relevant dimensions of neighborhood deprivation on mortality risk. Elsewhere in this volume (Chapters 2 and 6), the authors describe alternative approaches to characterizing neighborhoods, such as through interviews of residents and direct social observation. Alternative approaches to measuring neighborhood conditions raise additional debates about the relative merits of subjective versus objective approaches. We will return to this issue below.

Fourth, census-derived measures are crude in that they seldom permit the investigator to separate out the specific dimensions of neighborhoods that matter for health. Macintyre (Chapter 2) lists four such dimensions, including services and amenities, the social environment, physical aspects of neighborhoods, and the reputation of a neighborhood. Even a measure such as the percentage of single female-headed households (used by LeClere et al. to tap into stressful social obligations and role strain) is confounded by other processes, such as resource deprivation and low levels of "social capital."

Finally, the practice of adopting administrative definitions of neighborhoods (census tracts in U.S. research, electoral wards in U.K. research) inevitably results in exposure misclassification unless the boundaries of relevant neighborhood dimensions (e.g., service delivery, social networks) happen to coincide exactly with them. To the extent that the misclassification is nondifferential with respect to the outcomes, true neighborhood effects will be underestimated. From the foregoing discussion several lessons may be drawn for the future conduct of multilevel studies of area and health.

EMERGING ISSUES IN NEIGHBORHOOD RESEARCH

Despite rapidly converging views from different disciplines about the importance and promise of studying neighborhoods, tensions continue on matters of both theory and methodology. We characterize these tensions as a set of forced dichotomies: social selection versus social causation; contextual versus compositional effects; psychosocial versus material explanations; subjective versus objective assessment of neighborhoods; qualitative versus quantitative approaches to study design and analysis; and the relative importance of neighborhoods versus other "communities." These issues are sufficiently important to warrant separate discussion.

Social Selection versus Social Causation

Economists, especially of the rational choice school of thought, commonly point to the role of residential preference in accounting for area variations in health. For example, poor people choose to move to low-income neighborhoods because of the availability of cheap and affordable housing, and people of minority ethnic groups prefer to move to neighborhoods where lots of other people of the same group live.

Although some of the geographic patterning of health undoubtedly reflects these kinds of residential preferences, it is also overwhelmingly true that many people have no choice about where to live. It has been joked that economics is the study of how people make choices, whereas sociology studies how people often have no choices to make at all (a remark attributed to James Duesenberry in a review of a paper by Gary Becker). Thus, banks have been documented to refuse mortgage loans to minority applicants wishing to purchase new homes, and homeowner associations in gated communities routinely exercise their veto power to prevent families from moving into their neighborhoods on class, color, or other discriminatory grounds. In other words, context determines people's choices. The phenomenon of middle-class flight from urban areas of the United States demonstrates how the quality of neighborhoods can deteriorate over time based on decisions made by *other* people. For families caught in the process of depopulation and "hollowing out" that has characterized many U.S. metropolitan areas during the past two decades, it would be adding insult to injury to claim that they "choose" to live in areas of concentrated poverty. At the affluent end of the socioeconomic scale, very seldom do people with means deliberately "choose" to move into disadvantaged neighborhoods, as is amply demonstrated by trends in rising economic segregation.

That said, research is also needed to document the benefits, if any, of residential choice. Acevedo-Garcia and Lochner (Chapter 12) raise the intriguing possibility of the benefits of race–ethnic and immigrant "enclaves" for their residents' mental health, cultural identity, and political empowerment.

Contextual versus Compositional Effects

A canonical distinction that recurs throughout the chapters in this book is the need to distinguish the contextual effects of neighborhoods from compositional effects. The issue arises because of the need to convince decision makers that the characteristics of places where people live have an influence on health independent of the characteristics of the people in them. (This issue is partly related to the issue of residential selection mentioned above.) If variations in the health achievement of neighborhoods can be entirely explained by the personal characteristics of people who choose to live together, then policy makers need not act beyond improving the circumstances of individuals. Improving the neighborhood environment need lay no additional claim on decision makers as a strategy of population health improvement.

Yet, as Macintyre and Ellaway (Chapter 2) and Diez-Roux (Chapter 3) point out, the compositional–contextual distinction is in many ways an oversimplification. People are not simply parachuted into different neighborhoods. Few personal characteristics are truly exogenous to the social environment. To take a simple example, many researchers have controlled for personal income when looking for the contextual effect of neighborhood income on mortality risk. If a residual and statistically significant effect of neighborhood income persists after such a procedure, then it can be concluded that area-level income exerts an independent "contextual" effect on individual mortality risk. However, the procedure just described overlooks the fact that residential segregation is a powerful *mechanism* by which individuals end up being sorted into low and high incomes. Where one lives affects both the quality of one's education (as human capital investment) as well as access to labor markets and high-paying jobs. Conversely, living in the same neighborhood with lots of other low-income residents affects the level of wages that workers can command. To quote Macintyre, "people make places and places make people." Given these complex interdependencies, the contextual–compositional distinction that researchers strive for begins to seem quite artificial.

The type of statistical overadjustment just described applies also to multilevel analyses that attempt to control for a host of individual-level risk factors as confounders of neighborhood–disease associations; they may actually represent variables lying on the causal pathway between neighborhood exposures and health outcomes. Take, for instance, the practice of controlling for personal behaviors like smoking, lack of exercise, and diet quality when examining the association between neighborhood environment and mortality risk. Only the most ardent proponent of the rational choice school would insist that poor people freely choose to behave poorly. A low-quality diet is often the consequence of limited food choices available in poor neighborhoods (Macintyre and Ellaway, 2000). It may be retorted that grocery owners stock a limited range of foods in response to limited local demand for healthy foods, but even if that is the case, an individual resident expressing a preference to eat a healthy diet is nonetheless denied the opportunity to eat well because of the decisions made by others (a contextual effect). The point is that an analytical contradiction exists in the attempt by investigators to forcibly partition the variance between compositional and contextual effects. While policy makers may wish to know whether they should intervene on people *or* the places where they live, very likely the correct answer is: both.

Psychosocial versus Material Explanations

In common with wider debates in the field of health inequalities (Lynch et al., 1998), some researchers tend to polarize explanations for neighborhood effects on health according to whether they operate through psychosocial *or* material pathways. Clearly, both mechanisms can occur.

Moreover, material circumstances can have psychosocial consequences and vice versa. Broken windows and abandoned vehicles can lead to crime, exposure to crime (a trigger of asthma—see Chapter 11), the loss of the reputation of a neighborhood, despair, and a loss of self-esteem. In turn, crime and social disorder can lead to the flight of commercial facilities and banks. It does not help to advance science, much less policy, to take a polarized stance on these mechanisms.

It has been retorted that an undue focus on psychosocial mechanisms could lead to victim blaming (or in this case, community blaming) as well as the wrong kinds of policies, such as mass psychotherapy to alleviate psychological distress. However, a more nuanced understanding of neighborhood effects would help both researchers and policy makers to identify which mechanisms (and which policies) would more effectively address specific problems. Some problems, such as cognitive impairment due to lead-contaminated housing, have everything to do with material living conditions and nothing to do with psychosocial mechanisms. Other problems, such as the "contagion" effects of high smoking prevalence within an area on smoking initiation among adolescents, have a significant psychosocial component. In the latter case, a successful neighborhood-based intervention might involve networks of peer counselors to help boost levels of self-efficacy to resist peer pressure. To ensure the successful translation of knowledge into action, we must remain cognizant of the full range of mechanisms by which neighborhood environments— both physical and psychosocial—can influence health.

We also need to be clear about the specific mechanisms by which neighborhood characteristics affect specific health outcomes. More than one mechanism may be involved for any given health outcome (see, for example, Chapters 10 and 11, on infant health and asthma, respectively). The important issue for etiological research is to move beyond routinely available aggregate measures of neighborhoods (like percentage of poverty or median income) toward gathering information on specific characteristics of neighborhoods through primary data collection. We need also to move beyond studying all-cause mortality toward examining not only cause-specific mortality, but also distinguishing disease incidence from prevalence–mortality as well as collecting measures of mental health and physiological change.

Subjective versus Objective Assessments

Related to the material circumstances versus psychosocial dichotomy is the distinction commonly drawn between subjective versus objective approaches to characterizing the neighborhood environment. As Macintyre notes in Chapter 2, residents' self-reports of their neighborhood environment frequently display less variation than do objective assessments. For example, asking residents to rate the adequacy of services within their neighborhoods can result in a misleading impression of sameness, leading researchers to falsely conclude that services do not matter in terms of explaining between-place variations in health outcomes. However, an objective count of the same services (e.g., number of local transport services, range of foods available in local grocers) often provides a picture of much wider, and telling, variations.

Undoubtedly, part of the reason for this subjective–objective discrepancy is rooted in the well-known phenomenon of psychological adjustment. Similar to the familiar conundrum of assessing subjective well-being among destitute individuals (about which Amartya Sen has written eloquently), asking residents to rate the quality of their own neighborhoods can be seriously misleading. As Sen (1992) explains, downward leveling of aspirations is a natural protective mechanism against permanent despair. Lessons from educational psychology have similarly taught us to be wary of parental assessments of the quality of their children's day care (in the sense that few parents would admit to sending their children to substandard day care).

On the other hand, it would be a mistake to conclude from the foregoing that researchers should abandon attempts to measure subjective ratings of neighborhood environments. Subjective rating of crime (and fear of crime) is a stronger predictor of behavior (e.g., reluctance to go outdoors to exercise) than are actual crime rates. Subjective assessments therefore tell use something over and above objective data. Clearly, we need both.

A separate problem of endogeneity arises when residents' subjective ratings of their environments are used to predict health outcomes, particularly subjective well-being and mental health. In such cases, the extent to which the respondents' own personality and mental health status may contaminate the ratings of their neighborhood is unknown and unobservable. Independent sources of assessment would be helpful.

Quantitative versus Qualitative Approaches

Following on the theme of subjective versus objective ways of "knowing," a further tension in neighborhood research arises between qualitative versus quantitative approaches to study design and analysis. A valid criticism of this book might be that we have tended to emphasize research carried out in the quantitative realms of social epidemiology, demography, sociology, and medical geography. This peculiar focus is not intended to convey the message that qualitative approaches have less to offer. In fact, the methods of ethnography (and other qualitative approaches to analysis) are considerably more well established than are the canons of quantitative investigation. As Chapter 5 suggests, the benchmarks for assessing the validity and reliability of quantitative assessments of neighborhood characteristics (or what Raudenbush terms "ecometrics") are only now being established. By contrast, ethnographic studies of neighborhoods have a long and distinguished pedigree, led by influential works such as those by Herbert Gans (1962), Elliot Liebow (1967), Carol Stack (1974), William Foote Whyte (1955), and Elijah Anderson (1978, 1990). It hardly needs to be pointed out that qualitative and quantitative approaches offer complementary insights into neighborhood processes and how they affect health. The best studies, such as the Project on Human Development in Chicago Neighborhoods (highlighted by both Raudenbush and Sampson in Chapters 5 and 6, respectively) combine the two approaches.

Qualitative approaches to studying neighborhoods offer the advantage of grounding neighborhood processes within a historical context. They often provide insights that elude statistical measurement. This is perhaps best illustrated by Fullilove (Chapter 9), who traces the spread of the HIV epidemic in the South Bronx. It is virtually impossible to understand the geographic patterning of the HIV epidemic without paying heed to the history of "planned shrinkage" and deliberate decisions made by city planners. "Thick" descriptions of neighborhoods are also uniquely suited for providing in-depth, contextual portraits of the realities of people's daily lives. Ethnographic portraits are "aimed specifically at eliciting the perspective, understanding, and experience of those being studied" (Korbin and Coulton, 1997). Above all, qualitative approaches are singularly effective in communicating to decision makers a coherent and convincing story about how places can affect people's hopes, aspirations, opportunities, and misery, as well as levels of well-being.

Nevertheless, qualitative approaches are rarely sufficient by themselves to produce action because they are limited to observations of a relatively small number of individuals within a circumscribed geographic location. Thick ethnographic descriptions come at the expense of generalizability, and here quantitative approaches help to point to more generalized phenomena. Absent the resources to send an ethnographer into every neighborhood, we need quantitative approaches to abstract and document the influence of neighborhood environments on the health of populations and individuals.

Neighborhoods versus Communities

A final, and possibly most challenging, question concerns the distinction between neighborhoods and other forms of "community." Hillery (1955) observed more than 50 years ago that there were as many definitions of *community* as there were community theorists—about 94 at that time. It is a peculiarly North American phenomenon that *community* has come to be identified in researchers' minds with geographically bounded neighborhoods. However, as we enter the age of globalization, increasing separation of residences and workplaces via long-distance commuting, decreasing dependence on local areas for the necessities of life, the decline of local patterns of social affiliation (Putnam, 2000), and emerging virtual communities exemplified by the spread of the Internet, researchers must seriously question the relevance of geographically defined neighborhoods as an influence on health.

Is the neighborhood dead, as declared by Naisbitt (1982)? Is the focus on neighborhoods based on an overly romanticized notion of the urban village? Is it misguided, possibly even reactionary, to focus on improving neighborhood environments as a means of population health improvement? These are the kinds of inevitable questions that confront any investigator about to launch a study of neighborhood influences on health. Once again, however, we need to steer clear of the pitfall of false dichotomies. The question is not whether neighborhoods *or* communities (however defined) matter. After all, the real estate business would not continue to be as profitable as it is unless location mattered in some real sense. As Chapter 4 by Subramanian, Jones, and Duncan argues, the most promising way forward is actually to go out and collect the data on different contexts (e.g., residential location, workplaces, schools, virtual communities, etc.). Armed with the statistical methods that now exist to handle these complex realities, the onus is then on the investigator to recognize and analyze the contributions of overlapping and interacting contexts. Some years hence it may indeed turn out to be the case that neighborhoods explain rather less of the variations in health than do other contexts. Even so, we need to start somewhere, and by turning to neighborhoods we will have learned something valuable in the process.

Related to the need to study multiple contexts, the discipline of medical geography points us in the direction of simultaneously considering multiple scales of aggregation. Neighborhoods are nested within counties that are themselves nested within metropolitan areas nested within states, nations, trading blocs, and so on. It is crucial to recall that neighborhood characteristics do not occur in a vacuum, that their physical and social environments are shaped by macroeconomic forces, political decisions, and patterns of migration, history, and culture. Some types of exposures, such as the degree of income inequality, may exhibit scant variation at smaller units of aggregation, given the fact of economic segregation (a point emphasized by Krieger and colleagues in Chapter 7).

Specific health outcomes, such as the spread of HIV, may be more meaningfully analyzed by taking into consideration the transport routes and patterns of social networks that connect geographically remote communities (a lesson raised in Chapter 9 by Fullilove). In either case, the conceptual and methodological armamentarium is now available to investigators to undertake studies at more than one, or even two, levels of aggregation.

CONCLUSION

Margaret Thatcher once remarked that "there is no such thing as society. There are only individuals and families." The evidence gathered together in this book surely contradicts this truncated view of modern society. However, as enthusiasm grows for studying the influence of places on people's health, it is the responsibility of investigators to proceed with a high standard of analytical and conceptual rigor. Unbridled enthusiasm all too often can be followed by backlash. We need to be cautious by not promising too much. We hope that the contributions to this book will nudge researchers in a fruitful direction.

REFERENCES

Anderson E (1978). *A Place on the Corner*. Chicago: University of Chicago Press.

Anderson E (1990). *Street Wise: Race, Class, and Change in an Urban Community*. Chicago: University of Chicago Press.

Anderson RT, Sorlie P, Backlund, Johnson N, Kaplan GA (1997). Mortality effects of community socioeconomic status. *Epidemiology* 8: 42–47.

Aneshensel CS, Sucoff CA (1996). The neighborhood context of adolescent mental health. *J Health and Social Behav* 37: 293–310.

Brooks-Gunn J, Duncan GJ, Aber JL, eds. (1997). *Neighborhood Poverty*, vols. 1 and 2. New York: Russell Sage Foundation.

Bryk AS and Raudenbush SW (1992). *Hierarchical Linear Models in Social and Behavioral Science Research: Applications and Data Analysis Methods*. Newbury Park, Calif: Sage Publications.

Diez-Roux AV, Nieto FJ, Muntaner C, Tyroler HA, Comstock GW, Shahar E, Cooper LS, Watson RL, Szklo M (1997). Neighborhood environments and coronary heart disease: A multilevel analysis. *Am J Epidemiol* 146: 48–63.

Diez-Roux AV, Nieto FJ, Caulfield L, Tyroler HA, Watson RL, Szklo M (1999). Neighbourhood differences in diet: The Atherosclerosis Risk in Communities (ARIC) Study. *J Epidemiol Comm Health* 53(1): 55–63.

Duncan C, Jones K, Moon G (1999). Smoking and deprivation: are there neighbourhood effects? *Social Sci Med* 48: 497–505.

Ecob R and Jones K (1998). Mortality variations in England and Wales between types of place: An analysis of the ONS Longitudinal Study. *Soc Sci Med* 47: 2055–2066.

Ellaway A, Anderson A, Macintyre S (1997). Does area of residence affect body size and shape? *Int J Obesity* 21: 304–308.

Gans HJ (1962). *The Urban Villagers*. New York: Free Press.

Goldstein H (1995). *Multilevel Statistical Models*, 2nd ed. London: Arnold.

Haan M, Kaplan GA, Camacho T (1987). Poverty and health. Prospective evidence from the Alameda County Study. *Am J Epidemiol* 125: 989–998.

Hillery GA Jr (1955). Definitions of community: Areas of agreement. *Rural Sociology* 20: 111–123.

Humphreys K and Carr-Hill R (1991). Area variations in health outcomes: Artefact or ecology. *Int J Epidemiol* 20: 251–258.

Kleinschmidt I, Hills M, Elliott P (1995). Smoking behavior can be predicted by neighborhood deprivation measures. *J Epidemiol Comm Health* 49(Suppl 2): S72–S77.

Korbin JE and Coulton CJ. Understanding the neighborhood context for children and families: Combining epidemiological and ethnographic approaches. In Brooks-Gunn J, Duncan GJ, Aber JL, eds. (1997): *Neighborhood Poverty*, vol. 2. New York: Russell Sage Foundation, pp. 65–79.

LeClere FB, Rogers RG, Peters K (1997). Ethnicity and mortality in the United States: individual and community correlates. *Social Forces* 76: 169–198.

LeClere FB, Rogers RG, Peters K (1998). Neighborhood social context and racial differences in women's heart disease mortality. *J Health Soc Behav* 39: 91–107.

Liebow E (1966). *Talley's Corner*. Boston: Little, Brown.

Lynch JW, Davey Smith G, Kaplan GA, House JS (2000). Income inequality and health: Importance to health of individual income, psychosocial environment, or material conditions. *BMJ* 320: 1200–1204.

Macintyre S, Ellaway A (2000). Ecological approaches: Rediscovering the role of the physical and social environment. In Berkman LF and Kawachi I, eds.: *Social Epidemiology*. New York: Oxford University Press, pp. 332–348.

Massey DS (1996). The age of extremes: Concentrated affluence and poverty in the twenty-first century. *Demography* 33: 395–412.

Naisbitt J (1982). *Megatrends: Ten New Directions Transforming Our Lives*. New York: Warner Books.

O'Campo P, Gielen AC, Faden RR, Xue X, Kass N, Wang M-C (1995). Violence by male partners against women during the childbearing year: a contextual analysis. *Am J Public Health* 85: 1092–1097.

Putnam RD (2000). *Bowling Alone: The Collapse and Revival of American Community*. New York: Simon & Schuster.

Robert SA (1998). Community-level socioeconomic status effects on adult health. *J Health Soc Behav* 39: 18–37.

Sen, Amartya (1992). *Inequality Re-examined*. Cambridge, Mass: Harvard University Press.

Sloggett A and Joshi H (1994). Higher mortality in deprived areas: Community or personal disadvantage? *BMJ* 309: 1470–1474.

Sloggett A and Joshi H (1998). Deprivation indicators as predictors of life events 1981–1992 based on the UK ONS longitudinal study. *J Epidemiol Comm Health* 52: 228–233.

Stack CB (1974). *All Our Kin: Strategies for Survival in a Black Community*. New York: Harper & Row.

Waitzman NJ and Smith KR (1998). Phantom of the area: Poverty-area residence and mortality in the United States. *Am J Public Health* 88: 973–976.

Whyte WF (1955). *Street Corner Society*, 2nd ed. Chicago: University of Chicago Press.

Yen IH, Kaplan GA (1999). Neighborhood social environment and risk of death: Multilevel evidence from the Alameda County Study. *Am J Epidemiol* 149(10): 898–907.

Yen IH, Kaplan GA (1999). Poverty area residence and changes in depression and perceived health status: Evidence from the Alameda County Study. *Int J Epidemiol* 28(1): 90–94.

2
Neighborhoods and Health: An Overview

SALLY MACINTYRE
ANNE ELLAWAY

The seminal text on the influence of the environment on health is *Airs, Waters, Places*, written in the fifth century BCE as part of the Hippocratic medical corpus. It is believed that it was intended to help Greek travelling physicians anticipate what diseases they were likely to encounter when beginning practice in new, unfamiliar towns. The three elements in the title referred to features of climate and topography that were believed to influence the prevalence and types of diseases likely to be found in different places, and they illustrated the Greeks' promotion of natural (rather than supernatural) explanations for observed phenomena (Hannaway, 1993).

Increasing urbanization triggered special interest in the relationship between environment and health in seventeenth century England. In Britain "political arithmetic" was first applied systematically to the study of social regularities in death rates in the seventeenth century by William Petty (1623–1687) and John Graunt, whose *Natural and Political Observations upon the Bills of Mortality* was published in 1662. This was based on a quantitative analysis of the weekly bills of mortality compiled in London by parish clerks, which gave numbers and causes of death. Cities in Germany and France also began keeping data on population and causes of death, and Sweden set up a census in 1748.

A common observation in this period was the greater healthiness of country versus city dwelling. John Graunt noted that, "as for unhealthiness, it may well be supposed, that although seasoned bodies may, and do live near as long in London, as elsewhere, yet newcomers and children do not: for the *Smoaks, Stinks* and close *Air*, are less healthful than that of the country; otherwise why do sickly persons remove into the Country Air? And why are there more old men in the country than in

London, per rata?" (quoted in Wear, 1992, p. 130). The explanations given for greater mortality in the towns compared to the countryside included not only physical and topographical features, particularly the quality of the air, but also psychological and moral features. (Graunt, for example, believed that adultery and fornication and anxieties resulting from concern with business were more prevalent in London than in the country [Wear, 1992]).

The British perspective on the relationship of the environment and health was also influenced by the experience of foreign travel and colonization, which exposed people to different environments and different diseases and thus "forced people to articulate their ideas of how to judge whether places were healthy or not" (Wear, 1992, p. 127). Military and naval medicine generated empirical evidence and theories about how to ensure health in different environments, either by choosing the best location for settlements, trying to control the physical environment (for example, draining marshes and house design), or through changing personal habits and practices (Hannaway, 1993, p. 304).

In the mid-eighteenth century the study of medical topography began to flourish widely in Europe and in European colonies overseas. For example, in the 1770s and 1780s an attempt was made to develop medical topographies of the whole of France (more than 225 were produced, covering most regions), and a series of topographies of individual German towns was compiled from the 1750s onward (Hannaway, 1993, p. 301). However, one of the things thwarting a better understanding of the relationship between environment and health was the lack of mathematical tools to analyze the copious data collected in such topographies.

Fee and Porter have noted that "public health in England and America began as response to social and health problems of rapid industrialisation" (Fee & Porter, 1992, p. 249). More robust data about the social and geographical patterning of health became available in the mid nineteenth century in Britain from both specially conducted inquiries into the health of the population, particularly the urban population, and improved official statistics. (The civil registration of births and deaths was introduced in England and Wales in 1837 and made compulsory in 1874; the first census of the entire population was taken in 1851.)

Much information about the social distribution of health and life expectancy came from Edwin Chadwick's *Sanitary Conditions of the Labouring Poor in Great Britain*, which was published in 1842 and collated information from a number of sources including reports sent in by Medical Officers of Health in a wide range of areas (Chadwick, 1842). Table 2–1, based on material presented in the report, shows variations in longevity both among social categories and among areas.

TABLE 2–1. Longevity of Families Belonging to Various Classes:
Average Age at Death

District	Gentry and Professionals	Farmers and Tradesmen	Laborers and Artisans
Rutland	52	41	38
Bath	55	37	25
Leeds	44	27	19
Bethnal Green	45	26	16
Manchester	38	20	17
Liverpool	35	22	15

Source: Wohl, 1983, p. 5.

In each of these areas of the country, the top social stratum (gentry and professionals) lived, on average, longer than the middle social stratum (farmers and tradesmen), who, in turn, lived much longer than did the bottom social stratum (laborers and artisans). However, the average age of death among all three groups differed among these districts; gentry and professionals in Liverpool died earlier than did even laborers and artisans in Rutland. The gentry did best in Bath, whereas laborers and artisans did best in Rutland. The worst place for the top and bottom social groups was Liverpool, but the worst for the middle social group was Manchester.

Chadwick also used maps relating mortality to the social composition of different areas. These showed deaths distributed according to poverty, as is rather elegantly illustrated in his account of a mapping exercise in Scotland:

> To obtain the means of judging of the references to the localities in the sanitary returns from Aberdeen, the reporters were requested to mark on a map the places where the disease fell, and to distinguish with a deeper tint those places on which it fell with the greatest intensity. They were also requested to distinguish by different colours the streets inhabited by the higher, middle and lower classes of society. They returned a map so marked as to disease, but stated that it had been thought unnecessary to distinguish the streets inhabited by the different orders of society, as that was done with sufficient accuracy by the different tints representing the degrees of the prevalence of fever. (Flinn, 1965, pp. 225–226)

The picture painted by these within-city maps in Britain confirms data from a slightly earlier period in Paris. Villerme arranged arrondissements (neighborhoods) in Paris according to the percentages of houses that were exempt from taxation on the grounds of the poverty of the inhabitants, and he related this to the death rate, with the results shown in Table 2–2.

This showed the lowest mortality rates in the three richest ar-rondissements, where fewer than 12% of households were exempt from taxation on grounds of poverty; the highest rates in the three poorest, where more than 30% of households were exempt; and intermediate levels in between.

The linking of birth and death registration data to census data in the middle of the century provided the means for larger-scale and more systematic analyses of mortality. The occupation, address, age, and cause of death of the deceased were recorded on death certificates, and once the whole population was enumerated in a national census, it was possible to calculate death rates for specific occupations, districts, ages, and causes of death using death certificate data as the numerator and census data as the denominator. William Farr, the British registrar-general, examined the social patterning of mortality by comparing the death rates of different localities. Life tables were drawn up for "healthy districts," which could be used as a gold standard against which the rates for other districts could be compared and as a basis for inferring that much premature mortality was due to environmental conditions and was therefore preventable (Farr, 1975; Szreter, 1984).

TABLE 2–2. Mortality Rates in 1817–1821 in Arrondissements in Paris Ranked by Percentage of Properties Exempt from Taxation; Deaths Occurring in Private Houses

Arrondissement	Percentage Exempt	Deaths at Home
Montmartre (richest)	0.07	62
Chausse d'Antin	0.11	60
Roule, Tuileries	0.11	58
Luxembourg	0.15	51
Pt St. Denis	0.19	54
Faubourg St. Denis	0.22	53
St. Avoie	0.22	52
Monnaie, Invalides	0.23	50
Ile St. Louis	0.31	44
Ste. Antoine	0.32	43
Jardin du Roi (poorest)	0.38	43

Source: based on Flinn, 1965, p. 237.

The response of public health reformers to data such as these was to tackle the harmful aspects of the physical and social environment that most damaged the vulnerable by attempting to provide clean water and air, proper drainage and sewerage, adequate housing and education for the working classes, and regulation of working conditions. However, the response of hereditarians to the same data was to argue that they demonstrated not that the poor were ill because of environmental conditions, but that they were ill because of their own fecklessness or moral weakness (Szreter, 1984; Krieger et al., 1993). Although these arguments took place in a context in which mortality was dominated by infectious diseases, similar arguments are apparent 150 years later in a context in which mortality is dominated by chronic and degenerative diseases. To caricature the modern debate, is the poor health of people living in deprived areas due to their own characteristics or behaviors or to features of the local environment?

COMPOSITION OR CONTEXT?

Small-area variations in morbidity, mortality, and health related behavior have been documented consistently during the last 150 years in many countries. It has often been suggested that there are two possible explanations for these geographical variations: compositional and contextual. If we observe differences in health between places, these differences could be because of differences in the kinds of people who live in these places (a compositional explanation), or because of differences between the places (a contextual explanation). For example, the data from Paris or Aberdeen described above might reflect the composition of the population in different areas (poor people die earlier, so areas with lots of poor people will have high death rates), or something to do with the physical and social context (the areas in which poor people are concentrated might, for example, have worse housing, sanitation, or transport facilities and more exposure to physical and social threats to health).

One implication of a compositional explanation is that poor people will have the same death rates wherever they live, whereas an implication of a contextual explanation is that the death rates of poor or affluent individuals will vary depending on what sort of area they live in. A mainly compositional explanation for geographical differences might tend to direct research and policy toward individuals, while a contextual explanation might direct attention toward health-damaging and health-promoting features of neighborhoods (Macintyre, 1997b; Macintyre and Ellaway, 1999).

Within both epidemiology and geography there has been a tendency to ascribe much within-country geographical variation to compositional differences, and until recently there has been an apparent resistance to any role for contextual explanations. It has almost been an article of faith that differences between places are reducible to differences between the types of people living there. For example, it has been argued that mortality differences between people in the west of Scotland and members of the civil service in London, England, are not because of differences between living conditions in the west of Scotland and southeast England, but because of differences in the distribution of deprivation between these two groups (Davey Smith et al., 1995). Similarly, an influential paper that examined the impact on mortality of area-level deprivation markers controlling for equivalent individual markers of deprivation in England and Wales suggested that:

> The evidence does not confirm any social miasma whereby the shorter life expectancy of disadvantaged people is further reduced if they live in close proximity to other disadvantaged people. . . . Deprivation appears to be adequately assessed by personal and household circumstances. Area based measures of deprivation are not efficient substitutes. For maximum effectiveness, health policy needs to target people as well as places. (Sloggett and Joshi, 1994, pp. 1473–1474)

Often, if area differences remained after controlling for individual level characteristics, the response would be: "You can't have controlled for enough individual characteristics."

One reason for the frequent rejection of any idea that context influences health was fear of falling prey to the ecological fallacy. Schwarz noted in 1994 that "epidemiology texts offer a consistent appraisal of ecological studies: they are crude attempts to ascertain individual level correlations. The problems are generally attributed to the ecological fallacy, a logical fallacy inherent in making causal inferences from group data to individual behaviours" (Schwartz, 1994). The ecological fallacy is the incorrect inference that relationships observed at an aggregate level (for example, between the percentage of black people in a community and the literacy rate) will be observed in the same direction and magnitude at an individual level (for example, the likelihood of black people being illiterate) (Robinson, 1950). Concern with the ecological fallacy has led to the avoidance of ecological analysis in health sociology as well as epidemiology. However, as we have argued previously (Macintyre and Ellaway, 2000), it is important to distinguish between the improper use of aggregate data as proxy for individual data (the ecological fallacy) and the analysis of the effects of the social and physical environment on the health of individuals or populations (an ecological perspective).

Another possible reason for the tendency to reject the idea that places themselves influence health has been the concern of many researchers and practitioners in this field to highlight the importance of poverty in causing ill health and disease. The association between places where the poor are concentrated and high rates of ill health, repeatedly demonstrated in both developed and developing countries, is a powerful illustration of the role of poverty and the physical consequences of structured social inequalities. Some of those concerned with issues of equity may have been worried that a place-based focus might divert attention from welfare issues such as redistributive policies. However, a concern for equity could equally be expressed in the demand that all citizens have similar access to decent and health-promoting local environments.

Recent research has tended to show that although "who you are" explains a lot of geographical variation in health outcomes, there is also an effect of "where you are." This has been found for mortality, long-standing illness, perceived general health, low birthweight, health-related behaviors, and cardiovascular risk factors, and much of this work is described in the ensuing chapters of this book.

The identification of contextual effects has occurred despite what might appear to be "over-control" for individual characteristics. For example, Yen and Kaplan controlled for individual level income, education, race–ethnicity, perceived health status, smoking status, body mass index, and alcohol consumption when examining the relationship between neighborhood environment and mortality (Yen and Kaplan, 1999). It could be argued that many of these control variables may actually be on the pathways between area and health; cultural or supply side features of the local area might well influence smoking rates, diet, exercise, and alcohol consumption, thus forming part of the explanation for neighborhood variations in health. It is therefore remarkable that area differences remained once all these variables had been entered into the model.

Which particular features of context influence health, and how, have been neglected issues. Contextual influences tend to be seen as a residual category, a black box or contentless miasma of unspecified influences on health that appear to remain when one controls for whatever individual characteristics one can imagine.

A FALSE DISTINCTION?

We will argue that the distinction between people and places, composition and context, is somewhat artificial. People create places, and places create people.

In much research on socioeconomic inequalities in health, the unit of analysis is the individual or household. Individuals or households are ascribed socioeconomic characteristics based on indicators such as occupation, housing tenure, education, income, and car access (depending on the availability of data in the country), and these indicators are then examined in relation to health. These measures are usually treated as though they were properties of the individuals or households. However, these indicators can be conceived of as determined as much by the place as by the person or family. Occupation, for example, may be determined by the local labor market; housing tenure by the local housing market; education by the available educational system and local provision; income by the prevailing labor market conditions; and car ownership by the density of population, distance to facilities, and local transport networks. Hence, rather than seeing occupation, housing tenure, education, income, and car ownership as properties of individuals, we could perhaps as appropriately see them as reflecting features of the local environment, place characteristics creating people characteristics.

Thus, it may not be appropriate to ask about the effects of living in southeast England compared with the Scottish Highlands while controlling for individual characteristics such as housing tenure or car access, because there is a much smaller rental housing sector in southeast England than elsewhere in the United Kingdom, and car ownership or lack thereof may have an entirely different significance in a remote rural area compared to the center of London. Similarly, comparing the health or health-related behaviors of people living in Silicon Valley with those of residents of the rural Midwest United States, controlling for occupation and income, may miss the point that the industrial and agricultural contexts of these places will influence individual occupation and income levels.

Contextual explanations are perhaps most intuitively plausible when we compare countries: cultural differences in attitudes to smoking may, in large part, be the reason why middle-class professional men are far more likely to smoke in Paris than in San Francisco, and people in California and in countries bordering the Mediterranean may be more likely to eat fresh fruit and salads year round than are those in Russia or Scotland, because of easier access (Ecob and Macintyre, 2000). Income levels for physicians differ markedly between the United States and countries of the former Soviet Union, so we would not think it sensible to ask whether the longevity of physicians differs between the former and the latter while controlling for income.

Contextual explanations are also more intuitively plausible when we look at historical change. For example, the city of Glasgow, in the West of Scotland, was once characterised by heavy manufacturing industry (e.g., the building of locomotives, which were then shipped out to the Indian subcontinent) and shipbuilding. These industries generated apprenticeship schemes and the development of a male skilled manual workforce, so the local occupational class distribution contained a high percentage of men who would be classified as "social class three manual" using the British registrar general's occupational classification of social class. Since World War II a marked decline in heavy industry and shipbuilding has occurred, and an increase in service industries (e.g., telephone call centers and tourism) has arisen as a consequence of global economic trends. Far fewer men are employed in skilled manual occupations, and far more women work in part-time service occupations than did so 30 years ago. This illustrates the point that the social class composition of the Glasgow area is not an intrinsic feature of the locally resident individuals but is, instead, a property of the economic and culturally acceptable occupational opportunities available locally, that is, features of the place.

Between-country and historical differences in health and health-related behavior seem obvious and suggest the role of the social and physical environment in shaping human health. However, the question of whether such cultural, industrial, or ease-of-access explanations might also apply to variations in health or health-related behaviors within countries, whether by region, district, or neighborhood, is more contested and has been less often addressed.

In addition to being wary of the ecological fallacy, we need to be wary of the atomistic fallacy (Riley, 1963). This fallacy involves incorrectly inferring ecological characteristics or associations from individual data (for example, that the combination of many decided electors will produce a decisive election result). An illustration of an atomistic fallacy in the field of neighborhoods and health might be to assume that because all residents in an area are highly socially active, are religiously observant, and have close family and friendship ties, the locality will be characterized by harmony, collective efficacy, and good mental and physical health; the experiences of intergang, interethnic, and interreligious conflicts in Northern Ireland, Bosnia, South Africa, and Glasgow suggest that, sadly, high levels of social capital among individuals can coexist with a conflict-ridden local environment (Portes and Landolt, 1996). However, many so-called descriptions of areas are actually descriptions of the aggregate properties of individuals (for example, the percentage of unemployed, the proportion of home owners to renters, or the percentage of residents participating in religious activities), rather than of properties of the area (for example, job opportunities and the number of vacancies, the size and price of housing units, or the amount of sectarian graffiti or of incidents of interreligious violence or name calling).

It has also been suggested that an approach that statistically controls for the effects of income and other known correlates with health and then examines the residuals for the influence of environment may suffer from the "partialling" fallacy (Halpern, 1995). Thus, the extent of the effect of the environment on health may be hidden by inappropriate control for other known correlates, such as income. Moreover, it is plausible that the influence of income is itself mediated by the environment made possible by that income.

Contextual Explanations (Or the Lack of Them)

The study of geographical variations in health has tended to have one of two purposes: to assist in health service or other types of local planning, particularly in welfare state societies in which there is a desire to match expenditures to some notion of "need" (Fox et al., 1984); or to develop understanding of disease etiology by using ecological, or area, data as a surrogate for unavailable individual-level data (for example, on socioeconomic resources or exposure to environmental pathogens) (Gardner, 1973; Macintyre, Maciver, and Sooman, 1993). Much less work has been done on the etiological significance of place itself for health or disease. As Jones and Moon have argued: "Seldom, however, does location itself play a real part in the analysis; it is the canvas on which events happen but the nature of the locality and its role in structuring health status and health-related behaviour is neglected" (Jones and Moon, 1993, p. 515).

There are a few exceptions. The work of David Barker, an epidemiologist who has focused attention on the role of intrauterine and early life influences on later health, is unusual in searching for a chain of explanations for adult health that includes the physical and social geography of real and historically situated places. For example, an analysis of differences in disease-specific death rates among adults in the late 1960s and early 1970s in three small towns in England (Nelson, Colne, and Burnley) focused on housing and working conditions in these towns at the beginning of the twentieth century. Standardized mortality ratios for all-cause mortality and for ischemic heart disease and cerebrovascular disease were close to the English average in Nelson, and 20% above average in Burnley with Colne lying in between (Barker and Osmond, 1987). Barker notes that

Most of Burnley is in the valley where the Rivers Brun and Calder meet. Nelson and Colne lie above it on the western slopes of the Pennines. The climate is cold and damp, and rainfall is above average. . . . Low lying areas of Burnley were persistently damp, especially those below the high embankment that carries the Leeds–Liverpool canal through the town. During the early 1800s there was extensive housebuilding on land near Burnley town centre that was so marshy that it was unfit for farming. . . . Most houses in the towns were similarly built of stone. In Nelson, however, houses were newer and tended to be more spacious. Mean family size in the towns was similar. The worst houses were the back to back houses in the oldest parts of Burnley and Colne. These were small, had no means of ventilation to the outside air, and lacked facilities for the storage of food and milk. Infant mortality was much higher in such houses. . . . Resettlement of families from back to back houses to "through" houses was accompanied by a fall in infant mortality to around the average for "through" houses, showing that high mortality was a consequence of the structure of back to back houses rather than of the habits of those who occupied them. There were 2,371 of these houses in Burnley and 1,000 in Colne but only 52 in Nelson. . . . In Nelson, communal pits, used for disposal of household refuse, were small and were covered and were in striking contrast to the large open pits in Burnley and Colne, which favoured breeding of flies. . . . Sanitary regulations that were related to the production and sale of milk were more strictly enforced in Nelson. (Barker and Osmond, 1987, p. 751)

Barker concludes by suggesting that specific explanations for differences in adult mortality may be found "in the environmental influences that determined past differences in child development" (Barker and Osmond, 1987, p. 751).

Barker chose to focus on available historical information on infant feeding practices, the health and physique of young mothers, housing, and working conditions and sanitation, as well as on features of the physical environment, such as dampness. When we think about features of the local social and physical environment that might influence health, we could probably generate a list that includes the following:

- employment opportunities
- educational provision
- transportation
- housing
- retail provision
- recreation facilities
- the prevalence of "incivilities" such as graffiti, litter, vandalism, drug dealing, crime
- policing

- land use
- health services
- environmental hazards (air pollution, noise, hazardous waste, industrial effluents)
- social networks and social cohesion
- cultural norms and values
- geology
- climate (Macintyre, 1999).

We say "probably" because there has been very little systematic research examining which aspects of an area of residence influence which facets of health, in which population groups, or over what time period. Despite the many recent attempts to partition predictors of health into compositional and contextual boxes, there has been very little empirical research directly examining the influence of local contexts on health. (Exceptions include Diez-Roux et al., 1997; O'Campo et al., 1997; Collins and Williams, 1999; Yen and Kaplan, 1999.) There has been even less research systematically evaluating the effects on health of interventions at an area level.

Much epidemiology and medical geography in Britain has tended to focus on features of the physical environment such as climate, softness or hardness of the water supply, air pollution, and exposure to toxic substances such as radon or the activities of the petrochemical or nuclear power industries (Gardner, 1973; Fox et al., 1984; Britton, 1990). More recently, attention in North America and Britain has tended to shift to features of the social environment such as psychosocial stress in the workplace or social capital and social cohesion in neighborhoods (Egolf et al., 1992; Amick et al., 1995; Wilkinson, 1996; Marmot and Wilkinson, 1999).

One issue that sometimes arises among those wishing to examine contextual influences on health is the relative importance of the physical as compared to the social environment. We believe that this distinction, like the one between composition and context, can sometimes be a false one. The reason for including climate and geology in the list above is that the physical geography of neighborhoods may provide the basic infrastructure needed for certain types of industrial or agricultural development, which in turn influence the density and type of resident population and the residents' social relations. For example, the staple industry of Nelson, Colne, and Burnley was cotton weaving, and these towns developed where and when they did because of available water power. Shipbuilding developed in Glasgow because of the navigability of the River Clyde and the proximity to iron, steel, and coal supplies. Both the cotton weaving and shipbuilding industries then developed their own typical forms of social relations and social hierarchy (including sex distribution, with women working in cotton factories at the turn of the twentieth century, while only men worked in the shipbuilding industry even up to the 1970s).

Conversely, physical features of local environments may be located there for social reasons. For example, it is more likely that toxic waste dumps, new freeways, and nuclear power stations will be built in areas whose residents are relatively politically and socially powerless (what has been termed environmental racism in the USA [Mohai and Bryant, 1992; Bullard and Wright, 1993]); big businesses may wish to put up factories in areas where they know there to be a highly educated workforce; and wealthy families or communities may surround themselves with high-security systems in order to shut out the threat of burglary or violence (e.g., the growth of "gated" communities in the United States). High-prestige housing developments are often explicitly located where they are least likely to be polluted—either physically or socially—by the dirty, the poor, or the dangerous.

In a report of studies of eight neighborhoods across Britain undergoing urban regeneration initiatives, the authors noted that local physical amenities and resources were closely associated with social relationships and symbolic meanings (Forrest and Kearns, 1999). When small shops closed, the neighborhood might lose not only access to retail outlets but also to the shopkeepers, who were key stakeholders in the local communities. When local public services such as banks or post offices closed, residents suffered not only from poorer-quality services and greater practical inconvenience, but could also feel that the removal of these services indicated lack of interest in or support for the neighborhood from service providers. Schools were important not only as locations for community activities, but also as perceived barometers of the state of the locality. Social factors such as crime and violence could hasten or trigger the closure of shops, banks, and post offices. The prevalence of delinquency and vandalism was related to physical features of the environment such as empty properties, street lighting, and organized facilities for children, as well as to social factors such as levels of policing. Finally, environmental design and layout were shown to influence patterns of social interaction. Thus, the provision of physical amenities—street lighting, street cleaning, school premises, shops, and banks—may facilitate the generation of social interaction and a "feel-good" sense about a place. Equally, a deterioration of social relations as manifested in increasing rates of crime, vandalism, and drug dealing may lead to the removal of amenities and facilities. This study of urban regeneration elegantly shows a dynamic picture of interactions over time between the physical and social infrastructures of neighborhoods (Forrest and Kearns, 1999).

Others have shown that the presence of natural elements such as trees and flowers in outdoor spaces in urban public housing developments encourages greater use of outdoor space and promotes social interactions among residents (Coley and Kuo, 1997). This might have a twofold influence on well-being through increasing exercise levels as well as the health benefits that might accrue from social interaction with others. In our work we have noted the association in the United Kingdom between greenery (trees and gardens) and better-off areas and have speculated that a simple and powerful predictor of mortality rates might be the number of trees per hectare.

In research that we have been conducting since 1987 in Glasgow, Scotland, we have used these general ideas about the importance of the physical and social environment and have been working within a framework that suggests that the following aspects of neighborhoods might be health promoting or health damaging:

1. Physical features of the environment shared by all residents in a locality (for example, air and water quality)
2. Availability of healthy environments at home, work, and play (for example, decent housing, secure and nonhazardous employment, safe play areas for children)
3. Services provided to support people in their daily lives (for example, education, transportation, street cleaning and lighting, and policing)
4. The sociocultural features of a locality (for example, the political, economic, ethnic, and religious history and the degree of community integration)
5. The reputation of an area (for example, how the area is perceived by residents, service or amenity planners, and investors) (Macintyre et al., 1993).

We have applied this framework to a study of four socially contrasting neighbourhoods in Glasgow (Ellaway et al., 1997; Ellaway and Macintyre, 1996, 1998, 2000; Forsyth et al., 1994; Macintyre and Ellaway, 1998, 1999, 1993; Sooman and Macintyre, 1995) and are now extending it to study communities throughout Scotland and neighborhoods in England and Scotland whose residents were earlier studied in two national epidemiologic clustered health surveys, the Health Survey for England and the Scottish Health Survey (Macintyre et al., 2002). In the latter study we are developing a framework with which to examine integral (i.e., not aggregated up from individual) measures of material and social capital at a neighborhood level.

In our work to date, we have observed a deprivation amplification effect, or inverse care law, that tends to apply, across the whole range of

TABLE 2–3. Area Reputation: Percentage in Each Locality Reporting, in the Last
Three Years

	Richer Neighborhood (%)	Poorer Neighborhood (%)
Refused taxi because of address	2.1	3.8
Refused ambulance because of address	1.7	4.3
Refused police because of address	2.2	7.0
Refused credit because of address	2.3	7.1

Source: Macintyre, 1997b.

potential environmental influences on health, to neighborhoods in which
more socially disadvantaged people are concentrated. In places where
there are high rates of obesity and poorer dietary habits, there are fewer
facilities for healthy physical recreation and for the purchase of healthy
foods. Areas where there are high rates of unemployment may be stig-
matized and suffer from "address discrimination" such that local residents may be less likely to obtain employment, bank loans, or other forms
of credit. Neighborhoods where there are higher rates of domestic or street
violence may find pleas for assistance from police or medical services less
likely to be answered. (See Table 2–3 below, which illustrates this from
two socially contrasting localities in Glasgow.) It could be the case that
as well as leading to a lack of services, such stigmatizing processes might
be internalized and lead to lowered self-esteem and self-efficacy.

Hence, residents in poor neighborhoods experience a "double jeop-
ardy" whereby not only are they personally poor, but they are also likely
to live in the sorts of neighborhoods that lack the infrastructure to lead a
healthy life. Conversely, a crucial thing that income, wealth, education
and, high social class help people to buy is a residence in areas with pleas-
ant environments, good schools and other services, and low crime rates.
(It is not for nothing that real estate agents say that the three most important things about a property are "location, location, location.")

THEORETICAL AND METHODOLOGICAL ISSUES

One of the main problems in the study of neighborhoods and health is
the lack of development of theories about plausible social, psychological,
and biological links between specific features of the neighborhoods and
specific health outcomes (Curtis and Rees Jones, 1998). There has been a
tendency to seek to measure features of neighborhoods by using easily

available indicators, usually census-based data on individuals aggregated up to some area level (Macintyre et al., 1993). This tends to imply a theoretical model in which the collective characteristics of one's neighbours influence health (for example, that having a lot of unemployed people in the vicinity somehow enhances one's probability of smoking). This represents the "social miasma" theory referred to in the quotation from Sloggett and Joshi above. When challenged, probably few people working in the field of neighborhood influences on health would agree that this is their underlying model, but their use of the data tends to imply it.

This raises the question of what would be appropriate and testable models of the mechanisms linking neighborhoods and health. We need to think about chains of causation: for example, from the price and availability of healthy food or local social norms and traditions about appropriate diet, through dietary patterns, to levels of obesity, and then ultimately morbidity or mortality from diseases for which obesity is a contributory factor. This then raises further questions about the reasons for the distribution and pricing of foodstuffs in different neighborhoods, the physiological processes that link dietary intake to obesity and then to manifest disease, and the contribution of other, possibly neighborhood patterned, activities such as physical exercise levels that might influence obesity.

The generation of more closely specified causal models would also help clarify the distinction between confounding and intervening variables. (For example, several authors examine area effects on health controlling for smoking, as if smoking were a possible confounder of the relationship between area and health [Yen and Kaplan, 1999; Subramanian et al., 2001]. However, it might be argued that smoking may itself be influenced by place and therefore be an intervening variable in relationships between area and health [Diehr et al., 1993; Duncan et al., 1996; Ecob and Macintyre, 2000; Ellaway and Macintyre, 1996]).

If the study of neighborhoods and health is to move forward and contribute both to etiological understanding and policy formation, it is crucial that we have better models and theories about how neighborhoods may influence health and that we use them to determine the appropriate area scale and type of area influence we wish to measure. Otherwise, we will be left with a legitimate "so what?" response to repeated demonstrations that there are neighborhood variations in a number of health indicators.

Models of neighborhood influences on health need to take into account both a temporal and spatial dimension. It is important to consider the likely time lag between neighborhood influences and their expression in health, as illustrated in the approach of David Barker, described above, who decided to explore differences between the three towns at the turn of the twentieth century as an explanation for their adult death rates in the second half of the century. If we want to understand the current health of people in neighborhoods in Glasgow, should we be looking at contemporary information about neighborhoods or at data from 10, 20, 30, or 150 years ago?

The spatial dimension relates to the size of the area over which we hypothesize influences to operate. Some influences may operate at an extremely local level (for example, exposure to noise or fumes from a local factory or the presence of a particularly good or bad primary school), while others may operate at a regional, state, or provincial level (for example, the regulation of tobacco smoking in public places or the overall level of investment in education). These spatial scales may or may not coincide with administrative or census-defined geographies or with what local residents think of as their neighborhoods.

There is no a priori reason to suppose that neighborhood influences on health (or their temporal or spatial range) will be similar for all population groups and all health outcomes. Fear of crime or violence may affect women and elderly people more than men or younger people and affect mental, but not physical, health. Children may be more affected by dampness and mold in the environment than are adults, and this may affect rates of respiratory disease but not of cancer. People with more educational and financial resources may range over wider territories for a number of activities (recreational, employment, educational, retail) than do people with a more local orientation or less money. Neighborhood stress may influence smoking levels in young mothers almost immediately but only affect levels of depression among employed men after long periods of cumulative exposure (Ellaway and Macintyre, 2001).

Many studies of neighborhoods and health are cross-sectional, that is, they relate current levels of morbidity or mortality to current features of the environment. There are several potential problems with this approach. The first is that such designs cannot deal with problems of selective, health-related, migration or stability. Of all those born in a particular neighborhood, for example, it may be that only a small percentage are still resident there by the time they are twenty years old and that this group contains the least healthy and well educated, those who are most healthy and dynamic having moved on to other areas. If we examine only those still resident we may be looking only at "unhealthy survivors" of childhood neighborhood exposures and may make incorrect inferences about the impact of the neighborhood on the health of all the children who grew up there. Second, and related, we may be focusing on current exposures (for example in housing or employment) when the real impact of the neighborhood occurred at an earlier period in childhood, although it might not be expressed in health until the late teens.

Some effects of neighborhoods on health may be direct. (For example, mold spores may directly influence young people's respiratory health without there being any cognitive or emotional mediation.) However, other effects of neighborhoods on health may be mediated through cognitive and emotional processes, which may cause methodological problems if descriptions of both neighborhood and of health are obtained from the same people. If adults report that their houses are damp and moldy and that they have frequent respiratory symptoms, this could be because of a lay belief that damp housing causes respiratory disease or because they hold a very negative view of the world that affects their perceptions of both their housing conditions and their health. These reporting biases could be just as convincing explanations of an apparent link between damp housing and respiratory symptoms as a direct physical link between damp housing and respiratory disease. It may thus be important to obtain independent measures of features of the neighborhood and of health outcomes. However, if adults report that they find local teenagers' behavior threatening and also report that they are anxious and depressed, what may be important here is their perception of threatening behavior, not the directly observable or recorded rates of those behaviors.

Some of our data from Scotland suggest that reported perceptions may reduce rather than exaggerate apparent neighborhood differences. We found marked differences in public transportation provision between our study localities when we measured this directly (by looking up local bus and train timetables), but there was less difference between the localities in the percentages of local residents reporting poor public transportation provision. When interviewed in 1992, 11% of our respondents reported household densities that would be defined as overcrowded according to the census definition (as measured by numbers of rooms and numbers of household members). However, of these, fewer than half said that they were in overcrowded accommodation. This raises the measurement issue of whether to describe features of places in insiders' or outsiders' terms. Our data consistently show bigger differences in outsiders' terms (Macintyre et al., 1993; Macintyre, 1997b). The same issue may apply to self-reported health; people in more deprived neighborhoods may have lower expectations of health compared to those in better-off neighborhoods, thereby reducing apparent neighborhood differences in rates of self-reported health.

In trying to find ways of describing neighborhoods, there is still a tendency to think of individual behaviors rather than structural or systems properties (for example, crime rates or educational achievement, rather than policing strategies or investment in education). As Mechanic noted in relation to health-related behaviors: "there is little appreciation of the extent to which life imperatives and social opportunities and constraints either enhance or inhibit harmful personal behaviours. Relative to personal behaviour change, such alternatives as the improvement of living conditions, the development of new technologies, regulatory incentives and environmental modifications receive little emphasis" (Mechanic, 1993).

If we want to look upstream at structural and environmental influences on health, it is important that we try to be more imaginative in tapping into the properties of neighborhoods and the determinants of those properties. Often, investigators from within a particular society may be blind to some of these system determinants (such as urban political structures, redistributive policies, or housing allocation systems) because they are so much taken for granted, and it may take a "stranger" to notice their importance (Ross et al., 2000). Not only must we look at the immediate neighborhood context, we must also look at the regional and national contexts if we are to understand neighborhood differences in health. For example, donating blood might have entirely different meanings in societies such as Britain, where blood donation is a voluntary and altruistic act, and societies in which donors are paid for their blood; using donation rates as an indicator of social capital might be appropriate in the former setting but highly inappropriate in the latter setting.

CONCLUSION

Interest in the effects of the local environment on human health is not new. It has been manifest for some 2,500 years and reached its peak during the public health movements of the mid to late nineteenth century in Europe and America. Interest waned with improvements in basic living conditions (the provision of clean water and air, better housing, sanitation, etc.) and the epidemiologic transition that rendered infectious diseases apparently less important than chronic diseases. Since World War II much of the focus of public health has been on individual behaviors such as smoking, drinking, diet, and exercise. More recently we have seen a resurgence of interest in the effects on health of the social and physical environment within epidemiology, geography, psychology, and sociology. It is important that this renewed interest not ignore the lessons of the past or lessons from other disciplines such as architecture, urban planning, political science, and economics.

In many industrialized societies an increasing percentage of medical research funding is being directed to human genetics. It is therefore particularly timely, in the face of the ambitious claims being made for the potential of individual-based genetic medicine, to reinstate research into the influence on human health of the environment (Macintyre, 1997a).

There is increasing acceptance of evidence that people's area of residence may influence their health either in addition to or in interaction with their individual characteristics. The advent of multilevel statistical modeling techniques and the increased availability of data about individuals and their health have provided the opportunity for numerous studies that try to unpack the relative importance of composition and context, although concerns have been raised that the application of multilevel statistical methods may have surged ahead of a theoretical framework in which to conduct meaningful and robust analyses (Blakely and Woodward, 2000). What we most lack, however, is a coherent conceptual framework for theorizing about the precise ways that particular aspects of neighborhoods may influence which aspects of health in which population groups over what time periods.

ACKNOWLEDGMENTS
Both authors are employed by the U.K. Medical Research Council. We are grateful for comments on an earlier, spoken version of this chapter from participants at the Neighbourhoods and Health Workshop in Boston in June 2000 and to Steven Cummins and Ichiro Kawachi for comments on an earlier writtten draft.

References

Amick B, Levine S, Tarlov A, and Chapman Walsh D, eds. (1995). *Society and Health*. Oxford: Oxford University Press.

Barker D, and Osmond C (1987). Inequalities in health in Britain: Specific explanations in three Lancashire towns. *BMJ* 294: 749–752.

Blakely T, and Woodward A (2000). Ecological effects in multi-level studies. *J Epidemiol Community Health* 54: 367–374.

Britton M (1990). *Mortality and Geography* (Series DS 9 ed.). London: OPCS, HMSO.

Bullard R, and Wright B (1993). Environmental justice for all: community perspectives on health and research needs. *Toxicol Ind Health* 9: 821–841.

Chadwick E (1842). *Report of an Enquiry into the Sanitary Conditions of the Labouring Population of Great Britain*. London: Poor Law Commission.

Coley R, and Kuo F (1997). Where does community grow? The social context created by nature in urban public housing. *Environment and Behavior* 29(4): 468–494.

Collins C, and Williams D (1999). Segregation and mortality: The deadly effects of racism. *Sociological Forum* 14(3): 497–523.

Curtis S, and Rees Jones I (1998). Is there a place for geography in the analysis of health inequality? *Sociology of Health & Illness* 20(5): 645–672.

Davey Smith G, Shipley M, Hole D, Hart C, Watt G, Gillis C, Marmot MG, and Hawthorne V. (1995). Explaining male mortality differentials between the west of Scotland and the south of England (abstract). *J Epidemiol Community Health* 49: 541.

Diehr P, Koepsell T, Cheadle A, Psaty B, Wagner E, and Curry S (1993). Do communities differ in health behaviours? *J Clin Epidemiol* 46: 1141–1149.

Diez-Roux AV, Nieto FJ, Muntaner C, Tyroler HA, Comstock GW, Shahar E, Cooper LS, Watson RL, and Szklo M (1997). Neighborhood environments and coronary heart disease: A multilevel analysis. *Am J Epidemiol* 146(1): 48–63.

Duncan C, Jones K, and Moon G (1996). Health related behaviour in context—a multi level modelling approach. *Soc Sci Med* 42(6): 817–830.

Ecob R, and Macintyre S (2000). Small area variations in health related behaviours: do these depend on the behaviour itself, its measurement, or on personal characteristics? *Health and Place* 6: 261–274.

Egolf B, Lasker J, Wolf S, and Potvin L (1992). The Roseto effect: A 50 year comparison of mortality rates. *Am J Public Health* 82(8): 1089–1092.

Ellaway A, and Macintyre S (1996). Does where you live predict health related behaviours? A case study in Glasgow. *Health Bull* 54(6): 443–446.

Ellaway A, Anderson A, and Macintyre S (1997). Does area of residence affect body size and shape? *Int J Obesity* 21(4): 304–308.

Ellaway A, and Macintyre S (1998). Does housing tenure predict health in the UK because it exposes people to different levels of housing related hazards in the home or its surroundings? *Health and Place* 4(2): 141–150.

Ellaway A, and Macintyre S (2000). Social capital and self rated health: Support for a contextual mechanism. *Am J Public Health* 90: 988.

Ellaway A, and Macintyre S (2001). Women in their place: Gender and perceptions of neighbourhoods and health in the West of Scotland. In Dyck I, Lewis N, and McLafferty S, eds.: *Geographies of Women's Health*, pp. 265–281.

Farr W (1975). *Vital Statistics: A Memorial Volume of Selections from the Reports and Writings of William Farr*. Metuchen, N.J.: Scarecrow Press.

Fee E, and Porter D (1992). Public health, preventive medicine and professionalization: England and America in the nineteenth century. In Wear A., ed.: *Medicine in Society. Historical essays*. Cambridge: Cambridge University Press, pp. 249–275.

Flinn MW (1965). *Report on the Sanitary Conditions of the Labouring Population of Great Britain by Edwin Chadwick*. Edinburgh: Edinburgh University Press.

Forrest R, and Kearns A (1999). *Joined-Up Places? Social Cohesion and neighbourhood regeneration*. York: Joseph Rowntree Foundation.

Fox AJ, Jones DR, and Goldblatt PO (1984). Approaches to studying the effect of socioeconomic circumstances on geographic differences in mortality in England and Wales. *Br Med Bull* 40(4): 309–314.

Gardner M (1973). Using the environment to explain and predict mortality. *Journal of the Royal Statistical Society*, Part 3: 421–440.

Halpern D (1995). *More than Bricks and Mortar? Mental Health and the Built Environment*. London: Taylor & Francis.

Hannaway C (1993). Environment and Miasmata. In Bynum W and Porter R, eds.: *The Companion Encyclopedia of the History of Medicine*. London: Routledge, vol. 1, pp. 292–308.

Jones K, and Moon G (1993). Medical geography; taking space seriously. *Progress in Human Geography* 17(4): 515–524.

Krieger N, Rowley DL, Herman AA, Avery B, and Phillips MT (1993). Racism, sexism and social class: Implications for studies of health, disease and well being. *Am J Prev Med* 9(suppl): 82–122.

Macintyre S (1997a). Social and psychological issues associated with the new genetics. *Philos Trans R Soc Lond B Biol Sci* 352: 1095–1101.

Macintyre S (1997b). What are spatial effects and how can we measure them? In Dale A, ed.: *Exploiting National Survey Data: The Role of Locality and Spatial Effects.* Manchester: Faculty of Economic and Social Studies, University of Manchester, pp. 1–17.

Macintyre S (1999). Inequalities in health—Geographical inequalities in mortality, morbidity and health-related behaviour in England. In Gordon D, Shaw M, Dorling D, and Davey Smith G, eds.: *Inequalities in Health: The Evidence Presented to the Independent Inquiry into Inequalities in Health.* Bristol: Policy Press, pp. 148–154.

Macintyre S, Ellaway A, and Cummins S (2002). Place effects on health: How can we conceptualize and measure them? *Soc Sci Med* 55:125–139.

Macintyre S, and Ellaway A (1999). Local opportunity structures, social capital and social inequalities in health: What can central and local government do? *Health Promotion Journal of Australia* 9(3): 165–170.

Macintyre S, and Ellaway A (2000). Ecological approaches: Rediscovering the role of the physical and social environment. In Berkman L and Kawachi I, eds.: *Social Epidemiology.* Oxford: Oxford University Press, pp. 332–348.

Macintyre S, Maciver S, and Sooman A (1993). Area, class and health; Should we be focusing on places or people? *Journal of Social Policy* 22: 213–234.

Marmot M, and Wilkinson R, eds. (1999). *Social Determinants of Health.* Oxford: Oxford University Press.

Mechanic D (1993). Social research in health and the American sociopolitical context: The changing fortunes of medical sociology. *Soc Sci Med* 36(2): 95–102.

Mohai P, and Bryant B (1992). Environmental Racism: Reviewing the evidence. In Bryant B and Mohai P, eds. *Race and Incidence of Environmental Hazards.* Boulder, Colo: Westview Press, pp. 163–176.

O'Campo P, Xue X, Wang M-C, and Caughy MB (1997). Neighborhood risk factors for low birthweight in Baltimore: A multilevel analysis. *Am J Public Health* 87(7): 1113–1118.

Portes A, and Landolt P (1996). The downside of social capital. *The American Prospect* (26): 18–21.

Riley M (1963). *Sociological Research 1: A Case Approach.* New York: Harcourt, Brace & World.

Robinson W (1950). Ecological correlations and the behaviour of individuals. *American Sociological Review* 15: 351–357.

Ross NA, Wolfson MC, Dunn JR, Berthelot JM, Kaplan GA, Lynch JM (2000). Relation between income inequality and mortality in Canada and in the United States: cross sectional assessment using census data and vital statistics. *BMJ* 320:898–902.

Schwartz S (1994). The fallacy of the ecological fallacy—the potential misuse of a concept and the consequences. *Am J Public Health* 84(5): 819–824.

Sloggett A, and Joshi H (1994). Higher mortality in deprived areas: Community or personal disadvantage? *BMJ* 309: 1470–1474.

Sooman A, and Macintyre S (1995). Health and perceptions of the local environment in socially contrasting neighbourhoods in Glasgow. *Health and Place* 1(1): 15–26.

Subramanian S, Kawachi I, and Kennedy B (2001). Does the state you live in make a difference? Multilevel analysis of self-rated health in the US. *Soc Sci Med.* 53(1): 9–19.

Szreter S (1984). The genesis of the Registrar General's social classification of occupations. *British Journal of Sociology* 35(4): 522–546.

Wear A (1992). Making sense of health and the environment in early modern England. Meanings of health and illness. In Wear A, ed. *Medicine in Society. Historical Essays.* Cambridge: Cambridge University Press, pp. 119–147.

Wilkinson RG (1996). *Unhealthy Societies: The Afflictions of Inequality.* London: Routledge.

Wohl AS (1983). *Endangered Lives; Public Health in Victorian Britain.* London: J. M. Dent.

Yen I, and Kaplan G. (1999). Neighborhood social environment and risk of death: multilevel evidence from the Alameda County Study. *Am J Epidemiol* 149: 898–907.

I

METHODOLOGICAL AND CONCEPTUAL APPROACHES TO STUDYING NEIGHBORHOOD EFFECTS ON HEALTH

3

The Examination of Neighborhood Effects on Health: Conceptual and Methodological Issues Related to the Presence of Multiple Levels of Organization

ANA V. DIEZ ROUX

Over the past few years there has been a resurgence of interest in the social determinants of health (Krieger, 1994; Kaplan and Lynch, 1997). At the same time there has been a move toward rethinking the uses of ecological studies and ecological variables in health research (Schwartz, 1994; Susser, 1994a; Diez Roux, 1998). And there has also been a growing sense that to better understand the causes of ill health, epidemiology needs to grapple with the presence of multiple levels of organization and their implications for both models of disease causation and empirical research (Schwartz et al., 1999). All three interrelated trends have been expressed in the study of neighborhoods and health.

The investigation of neighborhood effects on health raises a series of conceptual and methodological issues related to the presence of observations at a lower level (e.g., individuals) nested within observations at a higher level (e.g., neighborhoods). Many of these issues are generalizable to a broad set of common situations in epidemiology involving nested data structures (for example, patients nested within providers, measurements over time nested within individuals, hospitals nested within a health system, districts nested within countries). The presence of multiple levels of organization (or nested sources of variability) has two important implications (Diez Roux et al., in press). First, the units of analysis (or units for which dependent and independent variables are measured) can be defined at different levels. The units of analysis will determine the level at which variability in the outcome is examined and consequently the level about which inferences can best be made. Second, the constructs relevant to explaining variability in the outcome may also correspond to different levels of organization. Moreover, constructs defined at a higher level may be important in explaining variability at a lower level, and constructs defined at a lower level may be important in explaining variability at a higher level.

From a conceptual viewpoint, the presence of multiple levels requires the development of theories about how factors defined at different levels are related to health outcomes. This implies specifying what the relevant constructs are and the levels at which they should be defined and measured. For example, situations involving individuals nested within groups may require differentiating individual-level from group-level constructs. From a methodological viewpoint, it requires identifying the most appropriate research design for the question being investigated based on the level about which inferences are to be made and the level (or levels) at which the constructs relevant to the outcome are defined and measured. This chapter reviews the use of group-level variables in epidemiology; summarizes the characteristics of ecological studies, studies of individuals, and multilevel studies; and discusses some of the conceptual and methodological challenges that multilevel analysis faces, using the example of the investigation of neighborhood effects on health. Although the discussion focuses on the case of individuals nested within groups (e.g., neighborhoods), it is generalizable to many other situations involving observations at a lower level nested within units at a higher level.

GROUP-LEVEL VARIABLES AND GROUP-LEVEL CONSTRUCTS

One common use of group-level variables in epidemiology is as proxies for unavailable individual-level data. For example, median schooling in the geographic area where a person lives may be used as a proxy for individual-level education in the absence of individual-level information. Group-level variables are also used as proxies for individual-level data in cases in which individual-level measures are subject to much measurement error, or in which intraindividual variability makes a single measure a poor marker for the person's exposure. In these situations the ecologic measure is sometimes believed to be a better indicator of the "true" individual-level exposure than the individual-level measure itself. A distinct use of group-level variables that has been relatively uncommon in epidemiology is as measures of group-level constructs themselves. The rationale for the inclusion of these variables is that certain disease determinants may be conceptualized at the group level rather than at the individual level. Here the group-level measures are used not as proxies for individual-level data but because the group-level constructs themselves are hypothesized to be related to the outcome. For example, the construct of neighborhood unemployment is distinct from individual-level unemployment, and both may be important to health. Similarly, inequality in the distribution of income within a group measures a different construct than individual-level income.

Variables that reflect the characteristics of groups have been classified into two basic types: derived variables and integral variables (Valkonen, 1969; Lazarsfeld and Menzel, 1971; Blalock, 1984; Von Korff et al., 1992; Morgenstern, 1995). Derived variables (also termed analytical or aggregate variables) summarize the characteristics of individuals in the group (means proportions, or measures of dispersion; for example, percentage of persons with incomplete high school education, median household income, standard deviation of the income distribution). Sometimes derived group-level variables have an analogue at the individual-level (e.g., mean neighborhood income and individual-level income), but both variables may be tapping into different constructs. The group-level variable may provide information that is not captured by its individual-level analogue. For example, mean neighborhood income may be a marker for neighborhood-level factors potentially related to health (such as recreational facilities, school quality, road conditions, environmental conditions, the types of foods that are available, etc.), and these factors may affect everyone in the community regardless of their individual-level income. Similarly, community unemployment levels may affect all individuals living within a community, regardless of whether they are unemployed or not. A special type of derived variable is the average of the dependent variable within the group. The prevalence of infection in a group, for example, may affect an individual's risk of acquiring infection (Halloran and Struchner, 1991; Koopman et al., 1991a; Koopman and Longini, 1994). Similarly, an individual's likelihood of adopting a certain behavior may depend in part on the prevalence of the behavior in the community.

Integral variables (also termed primary or global variables) describe characteristics of the group that are not derived from characteristics of its members (for example, the existence of certain types of regulations, availability of health care, political systems). A special type of integral variable refers to patterns and networks of contacts or interactions among individuals within groups, which may be important in understanding the distribution of health outcomes (Koopman et al., 1991b; Koopman and Longini, 1994; Koopman and Lynch, 1999). Although these patterns are derived from how individuals are connected to one another, they are more than aggregates of individual characteristics. They can be summarized in the form of group-level attributes such as network size or structure (Lazarsfeld and Menzel, 1971; van den Eeden and Huttner, 1982). Although derived and integral variables are sometimes presented as conceptually distinct, they are closely interrelated. Derived variables operate by shaping certain integral properties of the group. For example, the composition of a group may influence the predominant types of interpersonal contacts, values, and norms or may shape organizations or regulations within the group that affect all members (Valkonen, 1969).

In considering the use of group-level variables in epidemiology as well as in interpreting the results of studies that use ecological, or group-level variables, it is crucial to differentiate group-level and individual-level constructs and specify the types of constructs the variables included in the analyses are purported to be measuring. In some cases this distinction may be complex. On one hand, individual-level variables can be used to categorize people into groups, such as age groups. However, age itself remains an individual-level attribute. Of course, it is possible that age groups themselves may have emergent group-level properties (related, for example, to the types and patterns of interactions between individuals), which may be related to the outcome being studied. Another issue is that many variables measured at the individual-level (such as individual social class or race–ethnicity) may be meaningfully understood only in the context of how individuals are related to one another in groups or societies. Although they derive their meaning (and implications for health) from how individuals are related to one another in society (or groups), they remain individual-level constructs (although they are not individually determined). Thus, there is no direct correspondence between "group-level" variables and "social" variables on the one hand, and "individual-level" variables and "biological" variables on the other hand.

STUDIES WITH GROUPS AS THE UNITS OF ANALYSIS: ECOLOGICAL STUDIES

Ecological studies are studies in which groups are the units of analysis. Both independent and dependent variables are measured for groups, and variability in outcomes across groups is examined as a function of group-level variables. Ecological studies have often been used to investigate the relation between area characteristics and morbidity and mortality rates. The sizes of the areas investigated have ranged from relatively large (e.g.,

Wing et al., 1992; Tyroler et al., 1993; Raleigh and Kiri, 1997) to small (e.g., Briggs and Leonard, 1977; Paul-Shaheen et al., 1987; Townsend, 1988; Eames et al., 1993). The group-level variables most commonly investigated have been derived variables constructed by aggregating the socioeconomic characteristics of individuals living within areas.

Ecological studies are most appropriate when investigators are interested in explaining variation among groups (i.e., drawing inferences regarding the causes of intergroup variability in the outcome), and the constructs of interest can be conceptualized as group-level properties. Because of the unavailability of information on the cross-classification of individual-level exposures and outcomes within groups, ecological studies are limited in their ability to examine the role of individual-level constructs as confounders, mediators, or effect modifiers of the relation between group-level variables and the outcomes. For example, ecological studies documenting a relation between area deprivation and mortality are unable to determine whether this is confounded by individual-level characteristics of the persons living in different areas, how it is mediated by individual variables, or whether the effect of area deprivation varies by individual characteristics. The absence of individual-level data also makes it impossible to differentiate the contextual from the compositional effects of derived variables (a variant of the more general problem of absence of information on individual-level confounders) (Duncan et al., 1998). Both the contextual and the individual-level effects are confounded in the ecological association. For example, a study documenting associations between measures of area deprivation and mortality cannot determine whether the association is due to the contextual effect of living in a deprived area or to the fact that many deprived individuals live in deprived areas. Of course, from a public health perspective, the ecological association may itself be of interest, regardless of whether it is confounded by individual-level variables or whether it results from contextual or compositional effects.

The methodological problem inherent in drawing inferences regarding individual-level associations based on group-level data (the ecological fallacy) is well known and often discussed in epidemiology (Piantadosi et al., 1988; Greenland and Robins, 1994; Morgenstern, 1995). The absence of information on individual-level confounders or effect modifiers (which may vary from group to group) is one of the sources of the ecological fallacy. Another source (which is less often highlighted in discussions of the ecological fallacy because of the implicit assumption that all disease determinants are individual-level constructs) is the presence of contextual effects of derived variables (an effect of the aggregate measure over and above the effects of its individual-level namesake). Even in

the absence of individual-level confounders or effect modifiers that differ from group to group, associations at the group and individual level
may differ because the group variable (e.g., area deprivation) and the individual level variable (e.g., individual-level deprivation) are tapping into
different constructs.

In considering the inferences that can be drawn from ecological studies, it is important to bear in mind that characteristics of individuals may
be important even in drawing inferences regarding variability in the outcomes across groups (i.e., variables defined at a lower level may be important in explaining variability at a higher level). Ignoring the role of
individual-level variables in explaining group-level associations may lead
to what some have called the sociologistic fallacy (Riley, 1963). For example, suppose a researcher finds that communities with higher rates of
transient population have higher rates of schizophrenia and then concludes
that higher rates of transient population lead to social disorganization,
breakdown of social networks, and increased risk of schizophrenia among
all community inhabitants. However, suppose that schizophrenia rates
are only elevated for transient residents (because transient residents tend
to have fewer social ties, and individuals with few social ties are at greater
risk of developing schizophrenia). That is, rates of schizophrenia are high
for transient residents and low for nontransient residents, regardless of
whether they live in communities with a high or a low percentage of transient residents. If this is the case, the researcher would be committing the
sociologistic fallacy in attributing the higher schizophrenia rates to social
disorganization affecting all community members rather than to differences across communities in the percentage of transient residents.

Studies with Individuals as the Units of Analysis: Individual-Level Studies

In individual-level studies both dependent and independent variables are
measured for individuals, and the causes of interindividual variation are
examined. These studies are most appropriate when investigators are interested in explaining variation among individuals (i.e., drawing inferences regarding the causes of interindividual variability). When studies
with individuals as the units of analysis are limited to individuals from
a single "group," they cannot examine the role of group-level constructs
in causing individual-level outcomes (or as effect modifiers of individual-
level predictors), because group-level characteristics are obviously invariant within groups (Schwartz and Carpenter, 1999). Although studies

of individuals sometimes pool individuals across potentially meaningful "groups," they often lack information on the groups to which individuals belong. Thus, they cannot examine the role of group-level constructs as antecedents of individual-level variables, as independent predictors of outcomes, or as confounders of individual-level associations. They cannot determine whether the effect of a given individual-level variable is present only in certain group contexts or varies from group to group as a function of group characteristics.

Just as ecological studies are limited in their ability to draw inferences regarding variability across individuals in the outcomes (individual-level inference), studies of individuals are limited in their ability to draw inferences regarding group to group variability in the outcomes. The methodological problem inherent in drawing inferences regarding intergroup variability based on individual-level data has sometimes been called the atomistic fallacy (the counterpart of the ecological fallacy). It arises because individual-level measures do not necessarily measure the same construct as their group-level analogues and because information on potentially important group-level confounders or effect modifiers is often unavailable (or cannot be examined) in studies of individuals, either because individuals are drawn from a single group or because information on group-level variables is not collected.

In addition, just as individual-level variables may be important in explaining variability across groups, group-level variables may be important in explaining variability in the outcomes across individuals. The failure to consider important group-level factors in drawing individual-level inference has been termed the psychologistic (or individualistic) fallacy (Riley, 1963; Valkonen, 1969). (The term *psychologistic fallacy* is not the most appropriate because the individual-level factors used to explain the outcome are not always exclusively psychological. Other authors have used the term *individualistic fallacy*, [Valkonen, 1969], but this term has also been used as a synonym of the *atomistic fallacy* described above [Alker, 1969; Scheuch, 1969]). For example, a study based on individuals might find that immigrants are more likely to develop depression than are natives. However, suppose this is true only for immigrants living in communities where they are a small minority. A researcher ignoring the contextual effect of community composition might attribute the higher overall rate in immigrants to the psychological effects of immigration per se or even to genetic factors, ignoring the importance of community-level factors and thus committing the psychologistic fallacy (Riley, 1963; Valkonen, 1969). The potential fallacies in ecological and individual-level studies are summarized in Table 3–1.

TABLE 3–1. Types of Fallacies

Unit of Analysis	Level of Inference	Type of Fallacy
Group	Individuals	Ecologic
Group (relevant individual-level variables excluded)	Groups	Sociologistic
Individual	Groups	Atomistic*
Individual (relevant group-level variables excluded)	Individuals	Psychologistic*

*Also called individualistic by some authors.
Source: Diez-Roux (1998).

CONTEXTUAL ANALYSIS

When studies of individuals include individuals from several meaningful groups, characteristics of the groups to which individuals belong can be examined in individual-level analyses by appending the group characteristic to each observation. For example, group-level variables can be included in regression equations with individuals as the units of analysis. These types of analyses have been called contextual analyses (Blalock, 1984; Iversen, 1991). Contextual effects models can include multiple group-level and individual-level variables as well as their interactions. Special methods may be necessary to account for residual correlation between outcomes within groups that may persist after accounting for individual-level and group-level variables included in the analyses. The residual correlation violates the assumption of independence of observations and may lead to incorrect standard errors and inefficient estimates (Diggle et al., 1994). With the exception of recent work on neighborhood effects, contextual analysis is still uncommon in epidemiology, perhaps because the prevalent assumption is that all relevant disease determinants are reducible to individual-level constructs and can be measured at the individual level.

Several studies have investigated the contextual effects of neighborhood environments by including neighborhood characteristics (usually derived variables) in individual-level equations and examining associations between neighborhood characteristics and the outcomes before and after controlling for individual-level variables (Anderson et al., 1997; Robert, 1998; Waitzman and Smith, 1998; LeClere et al., 1998; Slogget and Joshi, 1998; Yen et al., 1998; Davey Smith et al., 1998: Elreedy et al., 1999; Diez-Roux et al., 2001). Because it allows the investigation of neighborhood effects after controlling for individual-level variables, contextual analysis can be used to separate out the effects of group context and composition. It can also be used to examine interactions between group-level and individual-level variables. However, the unit of analysis remains the individual, and only interindividual variation is examined. In contrast to modern multilevel analysis methods (see below), contextual analysis does not allow examination of group-to-group variability per se or of the factors associated with it.

MULTILEVEL ANALYSIS

Recently, multilevel analysis has emerged as a new analytic strategy in several fields, including education, sociology, and public health (see Chapter 4, as well as Mason et al., 1983; Hermalin, 1986; Bryk and Raudenbush, 1992; Von Korff et al., 1992; DiPrete and Forristal, 1994; Paterson and Goldstein, 1995; Wu, 1995; Rice and Leyland, 1996; Duncan et al., 1998; Kreft and de Leeuw, 1998). Although the terms contextual analysis and multilevel analysis often have been used synonymously (Van den Eeden and Hutner, 1982; Hermalin, 1986), today's multilevel models are more general than were early contextual models in that they allow examination of intergroup as well as interindividual variability. Multilevel analysis simultaneously examines groups (or samples of groups) and individuals within them (or samples of individuals within them). Variability at both the group level and the individual level can be examined, and the role of group-level and individual-level constructs in explaining variation among individuals and among groups can be investigated. For example, a study may have information on a sample of neighborhoods and on the individual-level characteristics of a sample of individuals within each neighborhood. Researchers may be interested in investigating how neighborhood-level and individual-level factors are related to health outcomes, as well as the extent to which between-neighborhood and between-individual variability in the outcomes are explained by variables defined at both levels. Multilevel analysis methods allow the simultaneous investigation of both types of research questions. Thus, multilevel analysis allows researchers to deal with the microlevel of individuals and the macrolevel of groups or contexts simultaneously (Duncan et al., 1998). Multilevel models can be used to draw inferences regarding the causes of interindividual variation and the extent to which it is explained by individual-level or group-level variables, but inferences can also be made regarding intergroup variation, whether it exists in the data, and to what extent it is accounted for by group- and individual-level characteristics. The statistical details as well as advantages and limitations of multilevel models are discussed in Chapter 4 and in other published papers (Bryk and Raudenbush, 1992; DiPrete and Forristal, 1994; Goldstein, 1995; Duncan et al., 1998; Kreft and de Leeuw, 1998; Snijders and Bosker, 1999; Diez-Roux, 2000).

In the investigation of neighborhood effects on health, multilevel analysis has been used with the two purposes outlined above. On one hand, multilevel analysis has been used to examine between-neighborhood and within-neighborhood variability in outcomes and the degree to which between-neighborhood variability is accounted for by neighborhood-level and individual-level variables (Humphreys and Carr-Hill, 1991; Duncan et al., 1993; Jones and Duncan, 1995; Ecob, 1996; Gould and Jones, 1996; Shouls et al., 1996; Hart et al., 1997; Boyle and Willms, 1999; Duncan et al., 1999). Another related objective of the use of multilevel analysis in the investigation of neighborhood effects has been to estimate associations of neighborhood characteristics with individual-level outcomes after adjustment for individual-level confounders, usually individual-level measures. Thus, for example, neighborhood characteristics such as deprivation or other indicators of socioeconomic context have been found to be associated with adverse health outcomes after accounting for individual-level indicators of social class (Humphreys and Carr-Hill, 1991; Kleinschmidt et al., 1995; Ecob, 1996; Shouls et al., 1996; O'Campo et al., 1997; Diez-Roux et al., 1997; Matteson et al., 1998; Duncan et al., 1999; Yen and Kaplan, 1999). In deriving these estimates, multilevel models are used chiefly as a way to account for residual correlation between outcomes within neighborhoods, an objective that can also be achieved using contextual analysis and accounting for residual intraneighborhood correlation in other ways, as noted above. The types of study designs based on unit of analysis, level at which variability is examined, and constructs most appropriately investigated are summarized in Table 3–2.

THEORETICAL AND METHODOLOGICAL CHALLENGES IN MULTILEVEL ANALYSIS

In allowing the simultaneous examination of between-group and within-group variability and the contribution of individual-level and group-level factors to both sources of variability, multilevel analysis provides a link between ecological and individual-level studies and resolves many of the limitations of these study designs. However, although the last few years have witnessed an explosion of the statistical methods of multilevel analysis, the use of multilevel analysis (and contextual analysis generally)

TABLE 3–2. Types of Study Designs Based on Unit of Analysis, Level at Which Variability Is Examined, and Constructs Most Appropriately Investigated

Type of Study	Unit of Analysis	Level at Which Variability Is Examined	Constructs Investigated as Potential "Causes" of Variability	
			Group Level	Individual Level
Ecologic	Groups	Groups (utility for interindividual variability limited)	Yes	Only group-level proxies
Individual level	Individuals	Individuals (utility for intergroup variability limited)	No (Yes in contextual)	Yes
Multilevel	Groups and individuals	Groups and individuals	Yes	Yes

Source: Diez Roux et al. (2002).

raises a series of important conceptual and methodological challenges. Many of these challenges are closely linked to the need to develop theoretical models of the ways in which constructs defined at different levels influence individual-level outcomes. In the absence of this theoretical development, multilevel analysis runs the risk of being reduced to the investigation of meaningless groups or of finding associations and patterns that are difficult to interpret or understand. Although common to multilevel analysis generally, many of these challenges can be illustrated with the example of the investigation of neighborhood effects of health.

DEFINING RELEVANT "GROUPS" AND GROUP-LEVEL VARIABLES

A key issue in multilevel analysis is defining the relevant "groups" to be included in the analysis. The definition of *groups* is closely linked to the theoretical model underlying the research and the research question being investigated. In the investigation of neighborhood effects, defining the relevant "groups" implies deciding how *neighborhoods* (or other geographic areas relevant to the outcome) should be defined. The definition of *neighborhoods* is no simple task. Many different criteria can be used to define *neighborhoods*, including historical criteria, geographical criteria, residents' perceptions, and administrative boundaries. Definitions based on these different criteria will not necessarily overlap. Moreover, the size and definition of the relevant geographic area may differ based on the outcome being studied and the processes presumed to operate (Furstenberg and Hughes, 1997; Gephart, 1997). In some cases these areas may not be thought of as neighborhoods in the traditional sense at all. The definition and operationalization of relevant areas (or neighborhoods) based on the underlying processes presumed to operate is a key challenge in the investigation of neighborhood effects on health (Diez-Roux, 2001).

A related issue is identifying the group-level variables to be investigated. As in the case of the definition of the relevant "group," the group-level variables selected should be based on the theoretical model and the specific hypothesis being tested. The key issue becomes specifying the relevant group-level constructs and developing operational definitions and measures of them. Here it is crucial to distinguish measures of true group-level constructs from group-level proxies of unavailable individual-level data. Failure to distinguish conceptually group-level properties from individual-level properties leads to confusion regarding the interpretation of any group effects observed. The specification of relevant constructs and the levels at which they are defined and measured is a key challenge to multilevel analysis. Most existing quantitative research on neighborhood effects has examined the effects of neighborhood socioeconomic context (constructed by aggregating the characteristics of individuals within neighborhoods) on individual-level outcomes after controlling for the socioeconomic position of individuals (Robert, 1999). Neighborhood socioeconomic context may serve as a proxy for a variety of neighborhood characteristics that vary across neighborhoods. However, there has been little examination of the specific attributes of neighborhoods that are relevant or of the processes involved (MacIntyre et al., 1993; see also discussion in Chapters 2 and 15). Specifying the relevant neighborhood properties and processes as well as developing operational measures that can be examined in quantitative studies is an important need in this field. The examination of specific neighborhood factors also raises additional methodological issues derived from the fact that many neighborhood properties are interrelated and may influence one another, making the isolation of their effects difficult.

Specifying the Role of Individual-Level Constructs

Another important challenge to multilevel analysis is specifying the role of individual-level constructs both in the theoretical model and in the specific hypotheses being tested. This will, in turn, determine how individual-level variables will be incorporated into the empirical analyses. Because disease is expressed in individuals, group-level effects ultimately will be mediated through individual-level processes (just as the effects of individual-level variables ultimately will be mediated through cellular and molecular processes). Strictly speaking, therefore, group-level attributes cannot affect individuals "independently" of all individual-level attributes, but this does not imply that group-level constructs are reducible to individual-level constructs. The extent to which an individual-level variable is conceptualized as a confounder or a mediator depends on the particular research question and its underlying theoretical model. A large part of quantitative research on neighborhood effects has examined the effects of neighborhood socioeconomic characteristics after controlling for the socioeconomic position of individuals in an attempt to separate out context from composition (Duncan et al., 1998). Although analytically useful, this approach is also artificial because neighborhood context may influence the socioeconomic trajectories of individuals, and living in disadvantaged neighborhoods may be one of the mechanisms leading to adverse health outcomes in persons of low socioeconomic position. Group-level and individual-level constructs may also interact. For example, the effects of neighborhood environments may differ by individual-level attributes such as age or socioeconomic position. Although a few studies have investigated interactions between neighborhood socioeconomic context and individual-level indicators of social position, results have not been entirely consistent regarding the types of interactions that occur (Robert, 1999). The investigation of interactions is promising in terms of elucidating the processes through which neighborhoods may affect health but is also challenging from a methodological point of view, as it requires sufficient sample size as well as variability in individual-level indicators within neighborhoods.

In addition, multilevel models generally do not allow examination of the full range of complex and reciprocal interrelationships among group-level and individual-level variables (Blalock, 1984). For example, multilevel models do not model the possibility that individual-level properties (or individual-level relations among variables) may influence group characteristics (Mason, 1991; DiPrete and Forristal, 1994), and, vice versa, that group characteristics may shape individual-level independent variables. This is pertinent to the investigation of neighborhood effects on health because many neighborhood and individual characteristics are likely to be interrelated. Individuals may shape the neighborhoods in which they live, and neighborhoods may, in turn, affect individuals within them. A simple example can be found in the examination of dietary patterns. The dietary habits of individuals may influence food availability in their neighborhoods, and neighborhood food availability may, in turn, influence the dietary preferences of individuals. Although modifications to multilevel models to allow the examination of some of these types of reciprocal relations have been proposed (Entwisle, 1991; Mason, 1991), they may be better addressed using other methodological approaches.

SOURCES OF DATA AND STUDY DESIGN

To date, most empirical applications of multilevel analysis have relied on existing data sources. For example, in the examination of neighborhood effects, studies have generally linked data on individuals to census data for the census-defined areas in which they live. An important strength of this approach is the availability of standardized data for a wide range of areas. Disadvantages include possible limitations of the census areas used to proxy "neighborhoods" as well as limited information on measures of neighborhood attributes that may be more directly relevant to understanding the processes underlying neighborhood effects. A better understanding of whether and how neighborhoods are important to health may require new data collection on specific neighborhood attributes and studies specially designed to test hypotheses regarding the processes through which neighborhood effects could be mediated. Although ideal, the collection of new data on theoretically defined areas is complex and may be impractical over a broad range of areas. Strategies that combine the use of existing standardized data on a broad range of areas with new data collection on a subset of areas (as in the West of Scotland Twenty-07 Study) (MacIntyre et al., 1989) are a promising alternative. In addition, more qualitative approaches may also be useful in understanding some of the processes linking neighborhood environments to health. Qualitative research may contribute to the development of hypotheses that can be tested in large, quantitative datasets and may be of help in understanding the results of quantitative studies. The integration of quantitative and qualitative approaches would constitute a major innovation in epidemiology generally.

An additional dimension that has yet to be fully incorporated into investigations of neighborhood effects on health is the longitudinal dimension. Although several longitudinal studies have related neighborhood characteristics to mortality or incidence over time (Haan et al., 1987; Anderson et al., 1997; Waitzman and Smith, 1998; Davey Smith et al., 1998; Yen and Kaplan, 1999), neighborhood characteristics have generally been assessed at one point in time. The investigation of the effects of neighborhood environments over the lifecourse as well as the impact of moving from one neighborhood to another or changes over time in neighborhoods themselves will require study designs that follow both neighborhoods and individuals over time. The analysis of this type of longitudinal data also implies increasing methodological complexity. A final caveat is that observational studies are inherently limited in their ability to conclusively identify causal neighborhood effects on health. The use of experimental designs (Katz et al., 2001) and the evaluation of neighborhood-level interventions may help strengthen inferences regarding the presence neighborhood effects.

CONCLUSION

The recognition in public health and epidemiology that factors defined at multiple levels may be important in understanding the causes of ill health has stimulated thinking on the implications this has for study design and empirical research. Multilevel analysis has emerged as an analytical technique that allows the examination of both intergroup and interindividual variability in the outcomes as well as how group-level and individual-level constructs are related to variability at both levels. Research on neighborhood effects on health is one substantive area in which this analytical approach has been applied. Despite the advent of sophisticated statistical models, important challenges remain. Many of these stem from the need to articulate theories that specify the processes through which group-level (i.e., neighborhood-level) and individual-level factors jointly influence health outcomes, theories that can be operationalized and tested. Like other statistical methods, multilevel analysis will help describe, summarize, and quantify patterns present in the data, but it will not explain these patterns; explanation will emerge from reciprocal interplay between theory formulation and empirical testing.

In considering alternative study designs it is important to emphasize that multilevel analysis is not necessarily the "ideal" analytical technique for all research questions. The selection of the appropriate study design should be based on the specific research question to be investigated, including the level of organization for which inferences are to be drawn, as well as the levels of organization of the constructs of interest. For many research questions studies with groups or individuals as the units of analysis may be perfectly appropriate. In addition, when examining the effects of group-level variables on individual-level variables, traditional contextual effects models with appropriate adjustment for residual correlation may be a simpler and adequate alternative to the more complex multilevel models, if estimating between-group variability is not of specific interest.

Finally, in investigating neighborhood effects (or the effects of any given "group" or context), it is important to remember that the continuum of levels of organization does not end with neighborhoods (or with the group being examined). For example, neighborhoods themselves exist within the broader social, economic, and policy "contexts" of states, regions, countries, and social systems. Factors defined at these levels generate differences among neighborhood environments and may also contribute to enhancing or buffering the impact of these neighborhood differences on health. In addition, neighborhoods are only one of the many "groups" or "contexts" to which individuals belong. For some people, and for some outcomes, other contexts (such as, for example, the work context) that may or may not be geographically defined may be more relevant to health than "neighborhood" or area of residence. Broadening discussion, theorizing, and empirical research on the causes of ill health to incorporate these multiple levels and multiple contexts is likely to enhance our understanding of the causes of ill health generally and will help generate more effective actions to reduce health disparities.

ACKNOWLEDGMENTS
This work was supported in part by R29 HL59386-1 (National Heart, Lung and Blood Institute of the National Institutes of Health).

References

Alker HR (1969). A typology of ecological fallacies. In Dogan M and Rokkam S, eds.: *Social Ecology*. Boston: MIT Press, pp. 69–83.

Anderson R (1997). Mortality effects of community socioeconomic status. *Epidemiology* 8: 42–47.

Blalock HM (1984). Contextual-effects models: Theoretical and methodological issues *Annual Review of Sociology* 10: 353–372.

Boyle MH and Willms JD (1999). Place effects for areas defined by administrative boundaries *Am J Epidemiol* 149: 577–585.

Briggs R and Leonard W (1977). Mortality and ecological structure: A canonical approach *Soc Sci Med* 11: 757–762.

Bryk AS and Raudenbush SW (1992). *Hierarchichal Linear Models: Applications and Data Analysis Methods*. Newbury Park, Calif.: Sage.

Davey Smith G, Hart C, Watt G, Hole D, Hawthorne V (1998). Individual social class, area-based deprivation, cardiovascular disease risk factors, and mortality: The Renfrew and Paisley study *J Epidemiol Comm Health* 52: 399–405.

Diez-Roux A, Nieto F, Muntaner C, Tyroler HA, Comstock GW, et al. (1997). Neighborhood environments and coronary heart disease: A multilevel analysis. *Am J Epidemiol* 146: 48–63.

Diez-Roux AV (1998). Bringing context back into epidemiology: Variables and fallacies in multilevel analysis *Am J Public Health* 88: 216–222.

Diez-Roux AV (2000). Multilevel analysis in public health research *Ann Rev Public Health* 21: 193–221.

Diez Roux AV, Stein Merkin S, Arnett D, Chambless L, Massing M, Nieto FJ, Sorlie P, Szklo M, Tytoler HA, Watson RL (2001). Neighborhood residence and incidence of coronary heart disease. *New Engl J Med* 345: 99–106.

Diez-Roux AV (2001). Investigating area and neighborhood effects on health. *Am J Public Health* 91: 1783–1789.

Diez Roux AV, Schwartz S, Susser E. (2002). Ecological variables and ecological studies in public health research. In Detels R, McEwen J, Beaglehole R, Tanaka H, eds. *The Oxford Textbook of Public Health*. Fourth Edition, London: Oxford University Press, pp. 493–508.

Diggle PJ, Liang KY, Zeger SL (1994). *Analysis of Longitudinal Data*. New York: Oxford University Press.

DiPrete TA and Forristal JD (1994). Multilevel models: Methods and substance *Annual Review of Sociology* 20: 331–357.

Duncan C, Jones K, Moon G (1993). Do places matter? A multi-level analysis of regional variation in health-related behavior in Britain *Soc Sci Med* 37: 725–733.

Duncan C, Jones K, Moon G (1998). Context, composition, and heterogeneity: Using multilevel models in health research *Soc Sci Med* 46: 97–117.

Duncan C, Jones K, Moon G (1999). Smoking and deprivation: Are there neighbourhood effects? *Soc Sci Med* 48: 497–505.

Eames M, Ben-Shlomom Y, Marmot MG (1993). Social deprivation and premature mortality: Reional comparison across England *BMJ* 307: 1097–1102.

Ecob R (1996). A multilevel modelling approach to examining the effects of area of residence on health *J R Statist Soc* A 159: 61–75.

Elreedy S, Krieger N, Ryan PB, Sparrow D, Weiss ST, Hu H (1999). Relations between individual and neighborhood-based measures of socioeconomic position and bone lead concentrations among community exposed men *Am J Epidemiol* 150: 129–141.

Entwisle B (1991). Micro-macro theoretical linkages in social demography: A commentary. In Huber J, ed.: *Macro-Micro Linkages in Sociology.* Newbury Park, Calif.: Sage, pp. 280–286.

Furstenberg FF, Hughes ME (1997). The influence of neighborhoods on children's development: A theoretical perspective and a research agenda. In Brooks-Gunn J, Duncan GJ, Aber JL, eds.: *Neighborhood Poverty: Vol II: Policy Implications in Studying Neighborhoods.* New York: Russell Sage, pp.

Gephart MA (1997). Neighborhoods and communities as contexts for development. In Brooks-Gunn J, Duncan GJ, Aber JL, eds.: *Neighborhood Poverty: Vol I: Context and Consequences for Children.* New York: Russell Sage, 1997, pp. 1–33.

Goldstein H (1995). *Multilevel Statistical Models.* New York: Halsted Press.

Gould M, Jones K (1996). Analyzing perceived limiting long-term illness using U. K. Census microdata *Soc Sci Med* 42: 857–869.

Greenland S, Robins J (1994). Ecologic studies, biases, misconceptions, and counter-examples *Am J Epidemiol* 139: 747–760.

Haan M, Kaplan G, and Camacho T (1987). Poverty and health: Prospective evidence from the Alameda County Study *Am J Epidemiol* 125: 989–998.

Halloran ME, Struchiner CJ (1991). Study design for dependent happenings. *Epidemiology* 2: 331–338.

Hart C, Ecob R, Davey Smith G (1997). People, places, and coronary heart disease risk factors: a multilevel analysis of the Scottish Heart Health Study archive *Soc Sci Med* 45: 893–902.

Hermalin A (1986). The multilevel approach: Theory and concepts. The methodology for measuring the impact of family planning programs on fertility. In *Population Studies, Addendum Manual IX, 66.* New York: United Nations, pp. 15–31.

Humphreys K, Carr-Hill R (1991). Area variations in health outcomes: Artefact or ecology *Int J Epidemiol* 20: 251–258.

Iversen G (1991). *Contextual Analysis.* Newbury Park, Calif.: Sage.

Jones K, Duncan C (1995). Individuals and their ecologies: Analysing the geography of chronic illness within a multilevel modelling framework *Health Place* 1: 27–40.

Kaplan GA, Lynch JW (1997). Whither studies on the socioeconomic foundations of population health? *Am J Public health* 87: 1409–1411.

Katz LF, King, J, and Liebman JB (2001). Moving to opportunity in Boston: early results of a randomized mobility experiment. *QJ Econ* 116:607–654.

Kleinschmidt I, Hills M, Elliott P (1995). Smoking behavior can be predicted by neighborhood deprivation mesures *J Epidemiol Comm Health* 49: S72–S77.

Koopman JS, Lynch J (1999). Individual causal models and population system models in epidemiology *Am J Public Health* 89: 1170–1174.

Koopman JS, Longini IM, Jacquez JA, Simon CP, Ostrow DG, Martin WR, Woodcock DM (1991b). Assessing risk factors for transmisson of infection *Am J Epidemiol* 133: 1199–1209.

Koopman JS, Longini IM (1994). The ecological effects of individual exposures and nonlinear disease dynamics in populations *Am J Public Health* 84: 836–842.

Koopman JS, Prevots DR, Vaca Marin MA, Dantes HG, Zarate Aquino ML, Longini IM, Sepulveda J (1991a). Determinants and predictors of dengue infection in Mexico *Am J Epidemiol* 133: 1168–1178.

Kreft I, deLeeuw J (1998). *Introducing Multilevel Modeling.* London: Sage.

Krieger N (1994). Epidemiology and the web of causation. Has anyone seen the spider? *Soc Sci Med* 39: 887–903.

Lazarsfeld PF, Menzel H (1971). On the relation between individual and collective properties. In Etzioni A, ed.: *A Sociological Reader on Complex Organizations.* New York: Holt, Rinehart & Winston, pp. 499–516.

Leclere F, Rogers R, Peters K (1998). Neighborhood social context and racial differences in women's heart disease mortality *J Health Soc Behav* 39: 91–107.

MacIntyre S, Annamdale E, Ecob R, Ford G, Hunt K, Jamieson B, Maciver S, West P, Wyke S (1989). The West of Scotland Twenty-07 Study: Health in the community. In Martin C and MacQueen D, eds.: *Readings for a New Public Health.* Edinburgh: Edinburgh University Press, pp. 56–74.

Macintyre S, Maciver S, Sooman A (1993). Area, class, and health: Should we be focusing on places or people? *J Soc Policy* 22: 213–234.

Mason W, Wong G, Entwisle B (1983). Contextual analysis through the multilevel linear model. In Leinhardt S, ed.: *Sociological Methodology 1983–1984.* San Francisco: Josey Bass, pp. 72–103.

Mason W (1991). Problems in quantitative comparative analysis: Ugly ducklings are to swans as ugly scatter plots are to . . . ? In Huber J, ed.: *Macro-Micro Linkages in Sociology.* Newbury Park, Calif.: Sage, pp. 231–243.

Matteson D, Burr J, Marshall J (1998). Infant mortality: A multi-level analysis of individual and community risk factors *Soc Sci Med* 47: 1841–1854.

Morgenstern H (1995). Ecologic studies in epidemiology: Concepts, principles, and methods *Annu Rev Public Health* 16: 61–81.

O'Campo P, Xue X, Wang M, M OB (1997). Neighborhood risk factors for low birthweight in Baltimore: A multilevel analysis *Am J Public Health* 87: 1113–1118.

Paterson L, Goldstein H (1991). New statistical methods for analysing social structures: An introduction to multilevel models *British Education Research Journal* 17: 387–393.

Paul-Shaheen P, Deane J, Williams D (1987). Small area analysis: A review and analysis of the North American literature *J Health Polit Policy Law* 12: 741–809.

Raleigh VS, Kiri VA (1997). Life expectancy in England: Variations and trends by gender, health authority and level of deprivation *J Epidemiol Comm Health* 51: 649–658.

Rice N, Leyland A (1996). Multilevel models: Applications to health data *Journal of Health Services Research and Policy* 1: 154–164.

Riley MW (1963). Special problems of sociological analysis. In *Sociological Research I: A Case Approach*, New York: Harcourt, Brace, and World, pp. 700–725.

Robert S (1998). Community-level socioeconomic status effects on adult health *J Health Soc Behav* 39: 18–37.

Robert S (1999). Socioeconomic position and health: the independent contribution of community socioeconomic context *Annu Rev Sociology* 25: 489–516.

Scheuch EK (1969). Social context and individual behavior. In Dogan M and Rokkam S, eds.: *Social Ecology.* Boston: MIT Press, pp. 133–155.

Schwartz S, Carpenter K (1999). The right answer for the wrong question: Consequences of type III error for public health research *Am J Public Health* 89: 1175–1180.

Schwartz S (1994). The fallacy of the ecological fallacy: The potential misuse of a concept and its consequences *Am J Public Health* 84: 819–824.

Schwartz S, Susser E, Susser M (1999). A future for epidemiology? *Annu Rev Public Health* 20: 15–33.

Shouls S, Congdon P, Curtis S (1996). Modelling inequality in reported long term illness in the UK: Combining individual and area characteristics *J Epidemiol Comm Health* 50: 366–376.

Sloggett A, Joshi H (1998). Deprivation indicators as predictors of life events 1981–1992 based on the UK ONS Longitudinal Study. *J Epidemiol Commun Health* 52: 228–233.

Snijders T, Bosker R (1999). *Multilevel Analysis: An Introduction to Basic and Advanced Multilevel Modeling.* London: Sage.

Susser M (1994a). The logic in ecological: I. The logic of analysis *Am J Public Health* 84: 825–829.

Susser M (1994b). The logic in ecological: II. The logic of design *Am J Public Health* 84: 830–835.

Townsend P, Phillimore P, Beattie A (1988). *Health and Deprivation. Inequality and the North.* London: Routledge.

Tyroler HA, Wing S, Knowles MG (1993). Increasing inequality in coronary heart disease mortality in relation to educational achievement: Profile of places of residence. United States, 1962–87 *Ann Epidemiol* 3(suppl): S51–S54.

Valkonen T (1969). Individual and structural effects in ecological research. In Dogan M and Rokkam S, eds.: *Social Ecology.* Boston: MIT Press, pp. 53–68.

van den Eeden P, Huttner HJ (1982). Multi-level research *Currents in Sociology* 30: 1–178.

Von Korff M, Koepsell T, Curry S, Diehr P (1992). Multi-level research in epidemiologic research on health behaviors and outcomes *Am J Epidemiol* 135, 1077–1082.

Waitzman N, Smith K (1998). Phantom of the area: Poverty-area residence and mortality in the United States *Am J Public Health* 88: 973–976.

Wing S, Barnett E, Casper M, Tyroler HA (1992). Geographic and socioeconomic variation in the onset of decline of coronary heart disease mortality in white women *Am J Public Health* 82: 204–209.

Wu Y-W (1995). Hierarchical linear models: A multilevel data analysis technique *Nursing Res* 44: 123–126.

Yen I, Kaplan G (1998). Poverty are residence and changes in physical activity level *Am J Public Health* 88: 1709–1712.

Yen I, Kaplan G (1999). Neighborhood social enviornment and risk of death: Multilevel evidence from the Alameda County study *Am J Epidemiol* 149: 898–907.

4

Multilevel Methods for Public Health Research

S. V. SUBRAMANIAN
KELVYN JONES
CRAIG DUNCAN

Where you live makes a difference to your health over and above who you are (Jones and Moon, 1993; Roberts, 1999; Berkman and Kawachi, 2000; Macintyre, 2000). People's lives are lived in different settings, including residential neighborhoods, workplaces, and schools as well as more macrolevel contexts such as metropolitan areas, regions, and states. Over and above individual influences on health, researchers are increasingly emphasizing the role that contexts and environments play in shaping health and health inequalities in the population.

Such a conceptual perspective is intrinsically *multilevel*, that is, factors that affect health are viewed as simultaneously operating at the *level of individuals* and at the *level of contexts*. The term *multilevel* has also been used to advocate a multidisciplinary perspective on public health (Anderson, 1999). Our use of the term, however, is from an analytical perspective, that is, in relation to the *levels of analysis* in public health research. We begin by outlining the conceptual motivation behind multilevel analyses and by identifying a core set of research questions that this approach addresses. We then introduce the idea of multilevel structures and discuss simple and complex multilevel models. We emphasize that the key strength of multilevel models lies in modeling heterogeneity at different levels. After introducing the basic structure of a multilevel model, using the example of individuals nested within neighborhoods, we show how this framework can be extended to additional contextual levels (e.g., neighborhoods nested within regions). The estimation procedures underlying such models are then discussed. Our aim is to show how a multilevel framework can provide a general, unified approach to data analysis and how this can be achieved by extensions to the basic hierarchical structure of individuals nested within contexts. We conclude with a discussion of issues that researchers should be aware of when applying multilevel methods.

WHY MULTILEVEL METHODS AND ANALYSES?

The problem of the "ecological fallacy" (Robinson, 1950; Selvin, 1958) is well known in epidemiology (Susser, 1994). It refers to the invalid transfer of results obtained at the ecological level to the individual level. A symmetrical fallacy, known as the "individualistic fallacy", occurs by failing to take into account the ecology, or context, within which individual relationships happen (Alker, Jr., 1969). The issue common to both types of fallacy is, therefore, the failure to recognize the existence of unique relationships observable at multiple levels, each being important in its own right. Specifically, we can think of an *individual relationship* (e.g., poor individuals are more likely to have poor health); an *ecological–contextual relationship* (e.g., places with a high percentage of poor individuals are more likely to have higher rates of poor health); and an *individual–contextual relationship* (e.g., the greatest likelihood of being in poor health is found for poor individuals in places with a high percentage of poor people).

From a statistical standpoint, if individual data are aggregated to a contextual level, then information is lost and statistical analysis loses power. If data are disaggregated to the individual level, but are not independent of one another, then the result is fewer independent data values. Ordinary statistical tests demand that data values for individual observations be independent. Failing to recognize the dependent nature of the data values, along with the source of the dependency, can lead to finding significant relationships where none exist. A multilevel methodological and statistical perspective provides one comprehensive framework to address the above concerns.

CONCEPTUAL CONSIDERATIONS IN MULTILEVEL PUBLIC HEALTH RESEARCH

Some core concepts are intrinsic to adopting a multilevel perspective, which we outline here.

Contextual and Compositional Sources of Variation

Evidence for variations in poor health between different settings, or contexts, can arise from factors that are intrinsic to, and measured at, the contextual level. In other words, the variation is due to what can be described as *contextual*, *area*, or *ecological* effects. Alternatively, variations between places may be *compositional*, that is, certain types of people who are more likely to be in poor health due to their individual characteristics happen to live in certain places. The question, therefore, is not whether variations exist between different settings (they always do), but what is their source, that is, are the variations across settings compositional or contextual? The notions of contextual and compositional sources of variation have general relevance and are applicable whether the context is administrative (e.g., political boundaries), temporal (e.g., different time periods), or institutional (e.g., schools or hospitals). *The research question underlying this concern is: are there significant contextual differences in individual health between settings (such as neighborhoods), after taking into account the individual compositional characteristics of the neighborhood?*

Contextual Heterogeneity

Beyond disentangling the contextual and compositional sources of variation, contextual differences may be *complex* such that they may not be the same for all types of people. For example, while neighborhood contexts may matter for the health outcomes of one population group (e.g., low social class), they may not have any influence on the health status of other groups (e.g., high social class). *The research question in this case is: are the contextual neighborhood differences in poor health different for different types of population groups, after taking into account the individual composition of the neighborhood?*

Individual Heterogeneity

Within particular contexts one group's health experience may be more or less variable than another's over and above the average differences. For example, people of low social class, in addition to being contextually heterogeneous in terms of health outcomes, may experience more variability compared to other groups. *The related question is: are individual differences in poor health different for different types of population groups, after taking into account neighborhood context and the average effects of individual demographic and socioeconomic factors?*

Individual–Contextual Interaction

Contextual differences, in addition to people's characteristics, may also be influenced by the different characteristics of neighborhoods. Stated differently, individual differences may interact with contexts. For example, poor people (individual characteristic) may experience different levels of health depending on the poverty level (place characteristic) of the area in which they live. *The research question of interest is: what is the average relationship between individual poor health and neighborhood-level socioeconomic characteristics, and does the effect of neighborhood-level socioeconomic characteristics on individual health differ for different types of individuals based on their demographic and socioeconomic characteristics, after taking into account the complex effects of individual demographic and socioeconomic factors, as well as the neighborhoods in which individuals reside?*

Multiple Hierarchical Contexts

Contextual settings themselves can be conceptualized and measured at multiple levels such that individual health experiences are not simply influenced by people's proximate environment (e.g., neighborhoods) but also their macroecologic settings (e.g., states). Moreover, neighborhoods rarely exist in a vacuum, and considering their broader contextual settings can be vital given the functional interconnectedness between geographic levels. An analysis of health variations should consider both the immediate contextual setting of people (e.g., neighborhoods) and also the macrocontextual settings to which both people and neighborhoods belong (e.g., states). *A related question of interest is: what additional contextual levels are relevant for the health outcome under consideration, and what is the relative importance of different contexual levels?*

Changing People, Changing Places

Contexts change over time, as do the circumstances and health of people. Simultaneously incorporating time and space dimensions involves asking the following research question: *while the prevalence of poor health may have declined over time, have neighborhood contextual disparities declined, and, if so, for which type of population groups?*

Interrelated Outcomes

Health outcomes themselves are often interrelated. For instance, people often engage simultaneously in high-risk behaviors, such as smoking and excess drinking. Each of these behaviors typically have a qualitative (yes or no) and a quantitative (how much) aspect. For instance, whether a person smokes may reveal nothing about the number of cigarettes smoked. There may be neighborhoods where few people smoke, but those who do, smoke heavily; an average figure would be very misleading. An ideal modeling approach should allow consideration of multiple responses and allow us to ask: *are neighborhoods with a high percentage of smokers also high in the number of cigarettes smoked, and/or are neighborhoods that are high on smoking also high on drinking, after taking into account individual, compositional differences?*

Overlapping "Cross-Classified" Contexts

Not only are contexts hierarchically multiple, they may also overlap. For instance, health behaviors such as smoking may be influenced not only by the neighborhoods in which people live but also by their work environment. Clearly, workplaces and residential neighborhoods need not be nested neatly one within the other. Thus, the relevant question is: *what is the relative contribution of different contextual settings that may not be nested within one another, but overlap (e.g., neighborhoods and workplaces)?* A related situation is one in which individual health behaviors are influenced not only by the characteristics of the neighborhood in which they occur but also by characteristics of adjoining areas.

As can be seen, the focus of the conceptual approach outlined above is on ascertaining heterogeneity in health either through multiple contexts, multiple times, or multiple outcomes. Standard statistical approaches, however, cannot deal with these requirements because (1) they operate at a single level, and (2) the emphasis is on modeling average relationships and not on the underlying heterogeneity per se. Multilevel statistical methods provide a unified and powerful approach to address these issues (de Leeuw and Kreft, 1986; Bryk and Raudenbush, 1992; Longford, 1993; Goldstein, 1995).

Multilevel methods are pertinent when the research problem under investigation has a multilevel structure and/or when a process is thought to operate at more than one level. It is important to note that multilevel models are not simply about modeling average relationships, but their unique strength lies in modeling the different sources of variability that underlie such relationships that are observable at different levels of analysis.

MULTILEVEL STRUCTURES: AN OVERVIEW

It is well known that once groupings are created (consisting of individuals), even if their origins are essentially "random", individuals end up being influenced by their group membership. Such groupings can be spatial (e.g., areas) or nonspatial (e.g., ethnicities), and in this chapter our focus is on the former. Hierarchies are one way of representing the dependent, or correlated, nature of the relationship between individuals and their groups. Thus, for instance, we can conceptualize a two-level structure of *many* level-1 units (e.g., individuals) nested within *fewer* level-2 groups (e.g., neighborhoods or

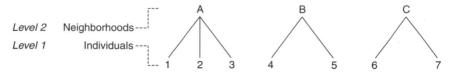

FIGURE 4–1. A two-level hierarchical structure of individuals in neighborhoods.

places) as illustrated in Figure 4–1. For instance, in Figure 4–1, individuals 1, 2, and 3 are shown to be clustered and more alike, given their grouping to the neighborhood context A, while individuals 6 and 7 are more alike given their grouping to the neighborhood context C. Because individual outcomes are anticipated to be dependent on the neighborhoods in which they occur, responses within a neighborhood are more alike than different. When dependency is anticipated in the "population", or "universe", they represent population-based, or naturally occurring, hierarchies.

Multilevel structures, however, may also arise as a consequence of study design. For reasons of cost and efficiency, many large-scale surveys adopt a multistage design. For example, a survey of health status might involve a three-stage design, with regions sampled first, then neighborhoods, and then individuals. A design of this kind generates a three-level hierarchical structure of individuals at level 1, nested within neighborhoods at level 2, which in turn are nested in regions at level 3. Individuals living in the same neighborhood can be expected to be more alike (i.e., they are autocorrelated, or clustered) than they would be if the sample were truly random. Similar autocorrelation can be expected for neighborhoods within a region. As a consequence, such a clustered sample does not contain as much information as simple random samples of similar size, and ignoring this autocorrelation can result in an increased risk of finding a relationship where none exists (Skinner et al., 1989).

While the conventional approach to such correlated data structures is to treat the clustering as a nuisance that needs to be minimized and/or adjusted/corrected, multilevel models view such hierarchical structures as a feature of the population that is of substantive interest. Indeed, "once you know that hierarchies exist, you see them everywhere" (Kreft and de Leeuw, 1998). Individuals, neighborhoods, and regions are seen as distinct structures of the population that should be measured and modeled.

INTRODUCING MULTILEVEL CONCEPTS: VARYING RELATIONSHIPS

One of the main attractions of multilevel models for public health research is their ability to allow relationships to vary across different contextual set-

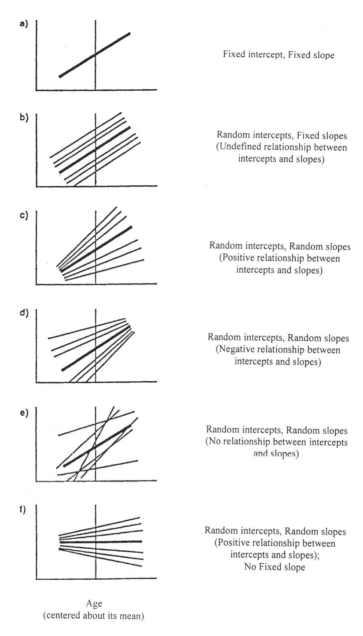

a) Fixed intercept, Fixed slope

b) Random intercepts, Fixed slopes
(Undefined relationship between
intercepts and slopes)

c) Random intercepts, Random slopes
(Positive relationship between
intercepts and slopes)

d) Random intercepts, Random slopes
(Negative relationship between
intercepts and slopes)

e) Random intercepts, Random slopes
(No relationship between intercepts
and slopes)

f) Random intercepts, Random slopes
(Positive relationship between
intercepts and slopes);
No Fixed slope

Age
(centered about its mean)

FIGURE 4–2. Varying relationships: a graphical typology.

tings. We illustrate this with a two-level structure consisting of individuals at level 1 nested within neighborhoods at level 2 with a single continuous outcome (e.g., a score measuring individual illness symptoms) and a single continuous individual (compositional) predictor (e.g., age) centered about its mean. Figure 4–2 illustrates a range of hypothetical graphic models for representing this data structure. In Figure 4–2(a), the poor health–age relationship is shown as a straight line with a positive slope: older people generally have worse health. This model conceptualizes health status only in terms of an individual's age, and the neighborhood context is ignored. This is remedied in Figure 4–2(b), in which the relationships in each of the neighborhoods (six here, but typically more) are represented by a separate line at a varying distance from the underlying average relationship shown by the thicker line. The parallel lines imply that while the poor health–age relationship in each neighborhood is the same, some neighborhoods have uniformly higher rates of poor health than do others.

In Figure 4-2(c)–(f) the contextual variations in poor health–age are allowed to become more complex. In Figure 4–2(c), the pattern is such that neighborhoods make very little difference for the young, but there is a greater degree of neighborhood variation in poor health among the old. Conversely, Figure 4–2(d) shows relatively large neighborhood differentials in poor health for the young. Figure 4–2(e) shows some neighborhoods where the young are in poor health, and others where it is the old. The final graph, Figure 4–2(f), shows that there is no overall, or average, relationship between poor health–age (the single thicker line is horizontal), but specific neighborhoods have distinctive relationships.

The different patterns in Figure 4–2 are achieved by allowing the average (fixed) "intercept" and the average (fixed) "slope" to vary (be random) across neighborhoods. Multilevel models specify the different intercepts and slopes for each context as coming from a distribution at a higher level. The different forms of relationships represented in Figure 4–2(c)–(f) are a result of how the intercepts and slopes are associated. Graphical models represented in Figures 4–2(c)–(f) are also called "random-slopes" or "random coefficients" models because the patterns are achieved by allowing the fixed slope to vary across neighborhoods. Figure 4–2(b), meanwhile, is the simplest form of multilevel model and is referred to as a "random-intercepts" or "variance components" model, as only intercepts are allowed to vary across neighborhoods.

For instance, in Figure 4–2(c) the relationship between poor health and age is strongest in neighborhoods (a steeper slope) where poor health rates are quite high for average age groups (a high intercept). Stated differently, there is a positive association between the intercepts and the slopes. In Figure 4–2(d) high intercepts are shown to be associated with shallower slopes, that is, a negative association between the slopes and the intercepts. The complex criss-crossing in Figure 4–2(e) results from a lack of pattern between the intercepts and the slopes, such that the health achievement rates of a neighborhood at average age tell us nothing about the direction and magnitude of the poor health–age relationship. The distinctive feature of Figure 4–2(f) results from the slopes varying around zero. In other words, while typically there is no poor health–age relationship, in some neighborhoods the slope is positive, in others negative. In this case, a single-level model would reveal no relationship whatsoever between poor health and age, and as such the "average" relationship would not occur anywhere.

FROM GRAPHS TO EQUATIONS

All statistical regression equations have the same underlying function, which can be expressed algebraically as:

Response = Fixed/Average Parameters
$$+ \text{(Random/Variance Parameters)}$$

We begin with a single individual level regression model:

$$y_i = \beta_0 x_{0i} + \beta_1 x_{1i} + (e_{0i} x_{0i}) \tag{1}$$

where y_i is the response, a continuous poor health score for individual i; x_0 is a set of ones to represent the constant; and x_1 is the continuous predictor, age. In this model, if age, x_1, is centered about its mean, β_0, the intercept gives the average health status for an individual of average age. The slope, β_1, gives the average change in poor health for a unit change in age. The intercept and the slope parameter represent the fixed part of the regression model and provide estimates of the average poor health–age relationship. The random part represents the individual differences from the fixed regression line and is given by e_{0i}. Making the usual assumptions of independent and identical distributions (IID), these residuals are usually summarized in a single variance term, σ_{e0}^2.

The antithesis of this individual model (in which health depends only on individual characteristics, such as age) is one in which health depends *only* on the neighborhood in which a person lives. This is achieved by specifying a micro model, with the response, intercept, and the individual random term now indexed to distinguish between j neighborhoods:

$$y_{ij} = \beta_{0j} x_{0ij} + e_{0ij} x_{0ij} \tag{2}$$

and further specifying a macro model at the neighborhood level in which the intercept is allowed to vary:

$$\beta_{0j} = \beta_0 + u_{0j} \tag{3}$$

The poor health rate in each of the j neighborhoods now depends on the fixed average, β_0, plus a random difference allowed to vary for each neighborhood (u_{0j}). Because the neighborhood differences are allowed to vary according to a higher level distribution (and making the usual IID assumptions), this distribution can be summarized by its overall mean, β_0, and its variance, σ^2_{u0}. This model presumes, as does much of census-based mapping of health outcomes, that a description of poor health can be summarized by a single rate for each place.

Both models considered so far are potentially deficient. In equation (1), a single individual model is fitted to all neighborhoods, thereby suppressing important contextual differences that may underlie average relationships. For instance, if the graphical model in Figure 4–2(f) is true, with no average relationship between poor health and age but each neighborhood showing positive or negative relationships, the individual model would be extremely misleading.

In relation to equations (2) and (3), meanwhile, the apparent neighborhood differences might be artifacts of the differential composition of neighborhood populations. Consequently, the model may be overemphasizing or underestimating the "true" contextual differences between neighborhoods. For example, an apparently high neighborhood specific rate could be merely the result of that neighborhood having a larger number of older people, a group who, in general, are more likely to be in poor health (composition-based neighborhood difference).

The converse is also possible, whereby genuinely large contextual effects are masked by failing to control for a neighborhood's composition. Such a result can occur, for instance, when a neighborhood with a genuinely high rate of poor health has relatively high numbers of young people, who, despite enjoying a lower rate of poor health on average, are nonetheless more likely to be ill compared to the old in other neighborhoods.

In a model that fails to adequately specify individual characteristics, the context (the difference a place makes) is confounded with the compositional (what is in a place). This can be remedied by combining the individual-only model specified in equation (1) with the context-only model specified in equations (2) and (3).

Central to developing a multilevel model is the specification of models at each desired level and their combination into an overall model. Equation (1) can be rewritten as a revised micro model with the response, intercept, and the individual random term now suitably indexed with the subscript j to distinguish neighborhoods:

$$y_{ij} = \beta_{0j}x_{0ij} + \beta_1 x_{1ij} + e_{0ij}x_{0ij} \tag{4}$$

and with the between neighborhood macro model outlined in equation (3)

$$\beta_{0j} = \beta_0 + u_{0j} \tag{5}$$

Substituting the macro model into the micro model gives us:

$$y_{ij} = (\beta_0 + u_{0j})x_{0ij} + \beta_1 x_{1ij} + e_{0ij}x_{0ij} \tag{6}$$

Multiplying variables by terms inside the parentheses and grouping the fixed and random parts together yields a full multilevel model of random intercepts:

$$y_{ij} = \beta_0 x_{0ij} + \beta_1 x_{1ij} + (u_{0j}x_{0ij} + e_{0ij}x_{0ij}) \tag{7}$$

In this model, the poor health of individuals depends on their age and a differential effect for the neighborhood in which they reside. The neighborhood-specific level 2 random term (u_{0j}) now represents neighborhood differences after allowing for age composition and individual variation (the level 1 random term e_{0ij}, the individual differences after allowing for age and between-neighborhood differences).

Such a model assumes that neighborhoods are uniformly high or low in terms of poor health rates and is equivalent to Figure 4–2(b). Such an assumption may be overly simplistic, for the age effect may vary across neighborhoods. Incorporating this complexity requires that all of the β parameters are indexed in the micro model, such that:

$$y_{ij} = \beta_{0j}x_{0ij} + \beta_{1j}x_{1ij} + e_{0ij}x_{0ij} \tag{8}$$

and are allowed to vary in a set of macro models:

$$\beta_{0j} = \beta_0 + u_{0j} \tag{9}$$

$$\beta_{1j} = \beta_1 + u_{1j} \tag{10}$$

As before, substituting the macro models into the micro model gives us:

$$y_{ij} = (\beta_0 + u_{0j})x_{0ij} + (\beta_1 + u_{1j})x_{1ij} + e_{0ij}x_{0ij} \tag{11}$$

and following the similar procedure of multiplying variables by terms inside the brackets and grouping the fixed and random parts together gives us a full multilevel model of random intercepts and random slopes:

$$y_{ij} = \beta_0 x_{0ij} + \beta_1 x_{1ij} + (u_{0j}x_{0ij} + u_{1j}x_{1ij} + e_{0ij}x_{0ij}) \tag{12}$$

The key change is that the age effect in neighborhood j in equation (10) consists of a fixed average age effect across all neighborhoods, β_1, and a differential age effect that is specific to each neighborhood, u_{1j}. The novel features of a multilevel model are, therefore, the level-2 random terms (u_{0j}, u_{1j}) at the neighborhood level.

The model in equation (12) does not, however, allow for heterogeneity between individuals within neighborhoods. Indeed, the standard assumption of ordinary least squares regression models is that residuals at level 1 have a constant variance (the assumption of homoskedasticity). As the variability about the fitted average line is presumed to be constant, it is summarized in a single variance term σ_{e0}^2. Such homoskedastic assumptions may be quite unrealistic; people of different ages may be differentially variable in terms of health status. While older people may have similar health status, young people may be much more variable.

Anticipating and modeling heteroskedasticity, or heterogeneity, at the individual level is particularly important in multilevel analysis, as there may be confounding across levels: what may appear to be contextual heterogeneity (level 2) could be due to a failure to take account of the between-individual (within context) heterogeneity (level 1). In addition, heterogeneity at level 1 also has implications for the fixed part predictions and inferences. Heterogeneity at level 1 can be incorporated by allowing the fixed parameter, β_1, associated with age, x_{1ij}, to vary at the individual level, giving us the following multilevel model:

$$y_{ij} = \beta_0 x_{0ij} + \beta_1 x_{1ij} + (u_{0j} x_{0ij} + u_{1j} x_{1ij} + e_{0ij} x_{0ij} + e_{1ij} x_{1ij}) \qquad (13)$$

The model now estimates two sets of residuals at level 1: e_{0ij}, which is associated with x_{0ij}, the constant; and e_{1ij}, which is associated with x_{1ij}, individual age. Using the model specified in equation (13), we now discuss the key characteristics of a multilevel statistical model.

MODELING INDIVIDUAL AND CONTEXTUAL HETEROGENEITY

Multilevel models are essentially concerned with modeling both the average and the variation around the average. To accomplish this, they consist of two sets of parameters: those summarizing the average relationship(s) and those summarizing the variation around the average at both the level of individuals and neighborhoods. Thus, in equation (13) the parameters β_0 and β_1 are fixed and give the average poor health–age relationship. The remaining subscripted parameters in the brackets are random (allowed to vary) and represent the differences in poor health between neighborhoods and between individuals within neighborhoods.

Representing the between-neighborhood differences in equation (13) are two terms, u_{0j}, and u_{1j}, associated with x_{0ij} and x_{1ij}, respectively. However, it is not the neighborhood-specific values that are estimated by multilevel models. Rather, they estimate the variance and the covariance based on the underlying distribution of the neighborhood specific differences. Making the usual IID assumptions, the neighborhood differences at level 2 can be summarized through a variance–covariance parameter matrix consisting of the intercept variance (σ_{u0}^2), slope variance (σ_{u1}^2), and covariance (σ_{u0u1}). Following a well-known result (Weisberg, 1980), the combined variability for two random variables at level 2 can be written as:

$$Var(u_{0j}x_{0ij} + u_{1j}x_{1ij}) = \sigma_{u0}^2 x_{0ij}^2 + 2\sigma_{u0u1}x_{0ij}x_{1ij} + \sigma_{u1}^2 x_{1ij}^2 \qquad (14)$$

In terms of differences between individuals at level-1, there are also two terms in equation (13). Making the same assumptions and following a similar procedure, we obtain:

$$Var(e_{0ij}x_{0ij} + e_{1ij}x_{1ij}) = \sigma_{e0}^2 x_{0ij}^2 + 2\sigma_{e0e1}x_{0ij}x_{1ij} + \sigma_{e1}^2 x_{1ij}^2 \qquad (15)$$

Thus, the between-neighborhood variation *and* between-individual (within neighborhood) variation is estimated in relation to age based on the variance parameters for the constant and the predictor variable and their covariance at each level. Thus, the fixed parameters give the average poor health–age relationship, while the random parameters combine to form quadratic functions representing differences between neighborhoods and between individuals (within neighborhoods).

Heterogeneity as a Quadratic Function

More generally, the size and the magnitude of the three random parameters at each level reflect the structure and form of the heterogeneity in the poor health–age relationships. Figure 4–3 presents one set of illustrative results. Figure 4–3(a) shows the shape of the between-neighborhood variation in relation to age; Figure 4–3(b) shows the shape of the between-individual variation in relation to age. Figure 4–3(c) and 4–3(d), meanwhile, plots the average poor health–age relationship (solid line) and the corresponding 95% predictive intervals for the neighborhood-level population heterogeneity (dashed lines) and individual level heterogeneity (dashed lines). These are approximated as the predicted regression line based on the fixed part ± 1.96 times the square root of the estimated

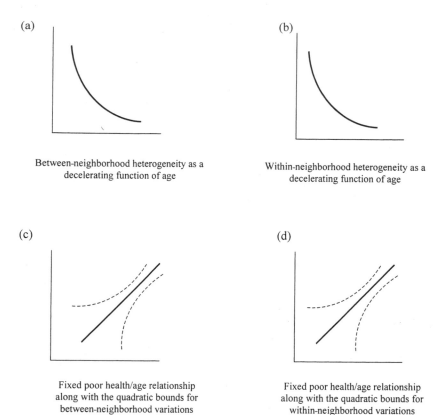

(a)

Between-neighborhood heterogeneity as a
decelerating function of age

(b)

Within-neighborhood heterogeneity as a
decelerating function of age

(c)

Fixed poor health/age relationship
along with the quadratic bounds for
between-neighborhood variations

(d)

Fixed poor health/age relationship
along with the quadratic bounds for
within-neighborhood variations

FIGURE 4–3. Plotting within and between neighborhood heterogeneity as a quadratic function of an individual predictor variable.

between-neighborhood and between individual variance. From the graphs we see that both between-neighborhood variation, Figure 4–3(a), and between-individual (within-neighborhood) variation, Figure 4–3(b), are a *decelerating* function of age. Such a situation would occur when all the variances are nonzero and both the covariances are negative. As is evident, the sign of the covariance term(s) is of key interpretative significance. As shown here, if it is negative, variation decreases as the predictor variable increases, and if it is positive, variation increases as the predictor variable increases. As Figure 4–3(c) shows, the neighborhood differences occur around the average relationship in which older people are more likely to be in poor health (a positive fixed intercept and a positive fixed slope). This graph also confirms that in the population the greatest differences between neighborhoods are for the young, Figure 4–3(c), and the variability for young people in the population is also larger than that for the older people, Figure 4–3(d). While in this illustration we consider only one predictor variable, it is possible to allow additional predictor variables to be random at the neighborhood and individual level.

Heterogeneity as a Linear Function

Specifying a quadratic variation between individuals and between neighborhoods may not be appropriate, and instead of differences increasing or decreasing at an accelerating or decelerating rate, they may change at a linear rate. We can, therefore, specify the heterogeneity at each level as a linear function of age. While we would still write the model in equation (13), we would only estimate one variance and one covariance at each level rather than the full set of variances and covariances. Thus, we would specify:

$$Var(u_{0j}x_{0ij} + u_{1j}x_{1ij}) = \sigma_{u0}^2 x_{0ij}^2 + 2\sigma_{u0u1}x_{0ij}x_{1ij} \tag{16}$$

$$Var(e_{0ij}x_{0ij} + e_{1ij}x_{1ij}) = \sigma_{e0}^2 x_{0ij}^2 + 2\sigma_{e0e1}x_{0ij}x_{1ij} \tag{17}$$

Although estimating a covariance when there is only one variance might seem contradictory, such a specification is entirely feasible (Goldstein, 1995; Rasbash et al., 2000). Put differently, if all three random parameters in equations (14) and (15) are significant, then the differences will be seen as a complex quadratic function of individual predictor age. On the other hand, if the size of the variances $\sigma_{u1}^2 x_{1ij}^2$ and $\sigma_{e1}^2 x_{1ij}^2$—which contribute to the quadratic functional form—are not substantial and/or are zero *but* the size of the covariances $\sigma_{u0u1}x_{0ij}x_{1ij}$ and $\sigma_{e0e1}x_{0ij}x_{1ij}$ are significant and substantial, then the between-neighborhood and between individual variation will be seen as a linear function of age. In light of this, and especially when we have several predictor variables that are allowed to vary at both the levels, it is important to view all the parameters jointly, and it is the functional form of the heterogeneity that should be interpreted.

Figure 4–4 illustrates one set of possible results for a model based on linear variance functions. For both between-neighborhood variation, Figure 4–4(a), and between-individual (within-neighborhood) variation, Figure 4–4(b), these are negative. As before, they would be based on nonzero variances and negative "covariances," although now there would be only two of the former, one at each level. The neighborhood differences again occur around the average relationship in which older people are less healthy, with smaller between-neighborhood, Figure 4–4(c), and smaller between-individual (within-neighborhood) differences, Figure 4–4(d).

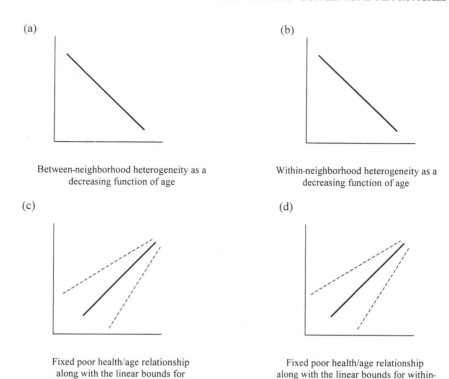

(a)

(b)

Between-neighborhood heterogeneity as a
decreasing function of age

Within-neighborhood heterogeneity as a
decreasing function of age

(c)

(d)

Fixed poor health/age relationship
along with the linear bounds for
between-neighborhood variations

Fixed poor health/age relationship
along with the linear bounds for within-
neighborhood variations

FIGURE 4–4. Plotting within and between neighborhood heterogeneity as a linear function of an individual predictor variable.

Variance as a Constant Function

Rather than specify quadratic or linear functions, it may, of course, be appropriate to specify a constant function, such that between-neighborhood and between-individual within-neighborhood variation is unchanging with age, thus specifying:

$$Var(u_{0j}x_{0ij}) = \sigma_{u0}^2 x_{0ij} \tag{18}$$

$$Var(e_{0ij}x_{0ij}) = \sigma_{e0}^2 x_{0ij} \tag{19}$$

and the underlying multilevel model would be as specified in equation (7). In this simplest case, therefore, the variance function at each level consists of only one parameter associated with x_{0ij}, because the differences are unchanging with age. Regarding equation (18), while there are still neighborhood differences, these are held to be the same at all ages. Equation (19), meanwhile, corresponds to the usual assumption of ho-

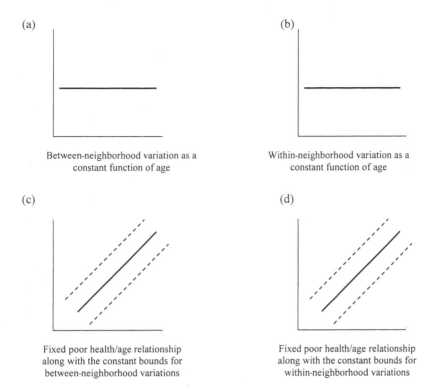

(a)

Between-neighborhood variation as a
constant function of age

(b)

Within-neighborhood variation as a
constant function of age

(c)

Fixed poor health/age relationship
along with the constant bounds for
between-neighborhood variations

(d)

Fixed poor health/age relationship
along with the constant bounds for
within-neighborhood variations

FIGURE 4–5. Plotting within and between neighborhood heterogeneity as a constant function of an individual predictor variable.

moskedasticity of the level 1 residual terms. As before, one set of possible results for this model can be graphed, and this is done in Figure 4–5. This confirms that while there are differences between neighborhoods, Figure 4–5(a), and between individuals, Figure 4–5(b), these do not change with age. Accordingly, the 95% predictive interval lines for neighborhood-level heterogeneity, Figure 4–5(c), and the individual heterogeneity (within-neighborhoods) in the population are parallel, Figure 4–5(d).

Because the variance functions are based on random parameters, they relate to the broader population of neighborhoods rather than simply the specific sampled neighborhoods. This way of handling neighborhood heterogeneity is in direct contrast to techniques such as analysis of variance/analysis of covariance (ANOVA/ANCOVA) or the specification of indicator neighborhood dummies in the fixed part. These approaches are neither efficient nor parsimonious (Jones and Bullen, 1994). Because they use traditional OLS estimation procedures, they are unable to handle the between-individual heterogeneity because this violates the assumption of homoskedasticity. At the same time, inferences of between-neighborhood heterogeneity are based on only the specific neighborhoods explicitly identified and not the wider population from which they are drawn.

It should, however, be noted that at the neighborhood level, predictions of specific relationships (u_{0j}, u_{1j}) can be obtained once the overall variance functions have been estimated. Thus, a multilevel estimation procedure can be viewed as a two-stage process. In the first, the overall variance functions are estimated together with the fixed parameters. In the second, these overall fixed and random parameters are combined with neighborhood-specific intercepts and slopes. If a particular neighborhood has few observations or there is little variation in the predictor variable(s), the predictions for such a neighborhood will be down-weighted or shrunk toward the overall fixed relationship (Morris, 1983). A reliably estimated within-neighborhood relationship will, however, be largely immune to this shrinkage. In Bayesian terminology these predictions are known as the posterior residual estimates. By using shrinkage estimators, multilevel models have the potential to avoid the misestimation problems caused by small numbers and sampling fluctuations in traditional methods based on single-level regressions (Jones and Bullen, 1994).

In the preceding paragraphs, we showed how multilevel models are not just concerned with the "average" or "fixed effect," but about how people, groups, and neighborhoods vary. This is achieved through the specification of variance functions based on random parameters. Crucially, there are no built-in assumptions about the heterogeneity that exists at a particular level. Instead, it is possible to specify differential functional forms (constant, linear, or quadratic) at each level and evaluate which receives the best empirical support from the data. For instance, as shown in Figure 4–6, while the between-neighborhood variation can be a positive quadratic function of age, Figure 4–6(a), the between-individual (within neighborhood) could decrease with age according to a linear function, Figure 4–6(b). In Figure 4–6(c) the dashed lines represent 95% predictive intervals for neighborhood-level population heterogeneity, and in Figure 4–6(d) the dashed lines represent the bounds for the individual heterogeneity, after taking account of the neighborhood heterogeneity, around the average regression line. While older people are less variable, Figure 4–6(d), there are larger neighborhood differences for such people, Figure 4–6(c).

VARIANCE PARTITIONING IN MULTILEVEL MODELS

In multilevel models, residual variation in the response is partitioned into components that can be attributed to the different levels of analysis. Much interest is focused on the amount of variation attributable to the higher level

(a)

(b)

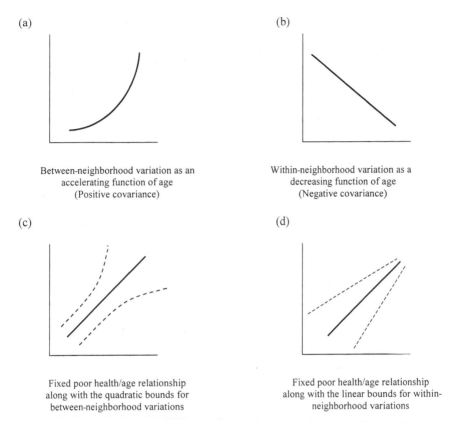

Between-neighborhood variation as an
accelerating function of age
(Positive covariance)

Within-neighborhood variation as a
decreasing function of age
(Negative covariance)

(c)

(d)

Fixed poor health/age relationship
along with the quadratic bounds for
between-neighborhood variations

Fixed poor health/age relationship
along with the linear bounds for within-
neighborhood variations

FIGURE 4–6. Plotting within neighborhood heterogeneity as a linear function of individual predictor variable and between neighborhood heterogeneity as a quadratic function of individual predictor variable.

(such as neighborhoods), because this provides a quantitative estimate of "where the action lies". Thus, for example, the variance partitioning coefficient (VPC) (Goldstein et al., 2002) for equation (7) can be defined as:

$$VPC = \sigma_{u0}^2 x_{0ij} / \sigma_{u0}^2 x_{0ij} + \sigma_{e0}^2 x_{0ij} \tag{20}$$

Equation (20) divides the level 2 variance by the total variance (level 2 + level 1 variance). This statistic is also known as the Intra-Unit Correlation (in survey literature referred to as intra-class correlation, ICC). ICC gives us the correlation between two individuals within the same level 2 unit but with different x_i values for different individuals. As a result, VPC and ICC will have the same formula in a random intercepts model, as the x_i values relate only to the constant, x_0, which is the same for each individual. However, in a complex random-slopes model, as specified in equations (12) or (13), we have a variance function at level 2 that is related to the individual predictor variable, x_1, and as such we cannot have a summary ICC statistic, because x_1 can take different values for different individuals, hence the terminology, VPC (Goldstein et al., 2002). The VPC in complex random slopes models as specified in equation (12) is given by:

$$VPC = \sigma_{u0}^2 x_{0ij}^2 + 2\sigma_{u0u1} x_{0ij} x_{1ij} + \sigma_{u1}^2 x_{1ij}^2 / \sigma_{u0}^2 x_{0ij}^2$$
$$+ 2\sigma_{u0u1} x_{0ij} x_{1ij} + \sigma_{u1}^2 x_{1ij}^2 + \sigma_{e0}^2 x_{0ij} \quad (21)$$

The VPC in equation (21) can be extended to allow for individual heterogeneity in its linear or quadratic form.

MODELING CATEGORICAL PREDICTORS

While, so far, our example was based on a continuous predictor (age), multilevel models can readily analyze categorical predictor variables. Figure 4–7 illustrates the interpretation of neighborhood heterogeneity with categorical predictors. We consider social class as a two-category individual variable, high social class and low social class, and these are shown on the horizontal x-axis, with the response being a continuous score of poor health (y-axis) in Figure 4–7.

Figure 4–7(a) presents the simplest outcome: differences between social groups but no variation between neighborhoods. With only one fixed average for each group, it shows an individual-level model in which the same relationship is fitted to all neighborhoods. Figure 4–7(b) represents a two-level model with each of six neighborhoods having its own poor health–social class relationship. The thick solid lines represent the average poor-health rates for the two groups, while the symbol lines (one for each neighborhood) represent the variation between neighborhoods around the average line. Because the individual relationship between social class and poor health is also shown in the model, the graph implies that the variation between neighborhoods is not solely due to the varying social composition of neighborhoods and is, therefore, contextual. The neighborhood differences, however, are assumed to be simple, such that neighborhoods that are high for one group are also high for the other and vice versa (similar to the random-intercepts model) as shown by the similar ordering of symbols for both social class categories in Figure 4–7(b). Thus, while there is a (contextual) geography of poor health, it can be summarized in one map.

We can, however, anticipate the neighborhood variation to be significantly different for the two groups. This difference consists of two dimensions. First, the amount (range) of neighborhood variation can be dif-

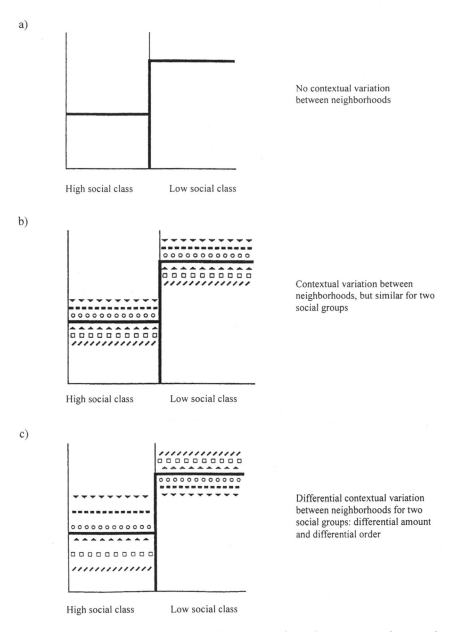

a) — No contextual variation between neighborhoods

High social class　　Low social class

b) — Contextual variation between neighborhoods, but similar for two social groups

High social class　　Low social class

c) — Differential contextual variation between neighborhoods for two social groups: differential amount and differential order

High social class　　Low social class

FIGURE 4–7. Varying relationships with categorical predictors: a graphic typology.

ferent for the two groups. In Figure 4–7(c) high social class people, on average, tend to have lower chances of being in poor health, but their neighborhood variation is relatively large compared to low social class people. For low social class people, it is the reverse: they have a higher probability of being in poor health, on average, but they have a smaller variation between neighborhoods. The second aspect of the neighborhood difference relates to the ordering. Thus, neighborhoods that are high for one group may be low for the other and vice versa, as shown in Figure 4–7(c) with the ordering of symbols being different.

When individual categorical predictors are allowed to vary at their own level (that is, at level 1), it is important to note that individuals cannot belong to, for example, both social class groups. Investigating whether the individual social class effect (compositional) varies by neighborhood, such that neighborhoods matter differently for high social class and low social class (contextual heterogeneity) and whether one group is more variable than the other (individual heterogeneity) would require the following statistical form:

$$y_{ij} = \beta_0 x_{0ij} + \beta_1 x_{1ij} + (u_{0j} x_{0ij} + u_{1j} x_{1ij} + e_{1ij} z_{1ij} + e_{2ij} z_{2ij}) \tag{22}$$

In order to implement equation (22), we have created two new separate indicator variables: z_{1ij} is an indicator variable (1 if low social class, 0 otherwise), and z_{2ij} is the indicator variable for high social class (1 if high social class, 0 otherwise). It is important to note that the new indicator variables are associated *only* with the level 1 residual terms. The fixed parameter, β_0, gives the average poor health score for high social class associated with constant, x_{0ij}, and β_1 estimates the average differential for low social class associated with the contrast coded dummy, x_{1ij}. Thus, the average poor health score for low social class would be given as $\beta_0 + \beta_1$.

Making the usual IID assumptions, the residuals at level 2 (u_{0j}, u_{1j}) and at level 1 (e_{1ij}, e_{2ij}) can be summarized through a set of variances and covariances. Thus, σ_{u0}^2 would estimate the between-neighborhood variation for high social class, while σ_{u1}^2 gives the differential variance for low social class, that is, the extent to which the variance for low social class is different from high social class. The between-neighborhood variation for low social class would be given by $\sigma_{u0}^2 x_{0ij}^2 + 2\sigma_{u0u1} x_{0ij} x_{1ij} + \sigma_{u1}^2 x_{1ij}^2$.

If the covariance term is positive ($+ \sigma_{u0u1}$), then the variation for low social class will be greater compared to that for high social class, and neighborhoods that have high rates for one group will tend to be relatively higher for the other. A negative covariance ($-\sigma_{u0u1}$), meanwhile, could imply either that low social class is less variable or that neighborhoods that are high for one group are relatively low for the other, as was shown in Figure 4–7(c). The exact interpretation would depend on the relative size of the covariance in relation to the variance, σ_{u1}^2.

At the individual level, $\sigma_{e1}^2 z_{1ij}$ gives the variability for high social class, while $\sigma_{e2}^2 z_{2ij}$ directly estimates the variability for low social class. Because individuals cannot belong to more than one category, there is not enough information to estimate the full "quadratic" function at level 1, as was specified in equation (15) in the case of the continuous predictor variable.

Allowing different specifications in different parts is an important characteristic of a multilevel model. For instance, in the above illustration, the fixed effect of social class was specified as a difference, as was the contextual heterogeneity at the neighborhood level. Put differently, the model in equation (22) ascertains the average social class gap and the extent to which the social class gap varies across neighborhoods at level 2. However, at level 1, individual heterogeneity between social class groups was specified separately and not as a difference from the other. Furthermore, the "linear" formulation that was discussed in relation to continuous predictor variables at the neighborhood level can be extended to categorical predictor variables as well (Bullen et al., 1997). This flexibility is particularly useful when we have a range of categorical predictors with each of the categorical predictors having two or more categories.

INDIVIDUAL–CONTEXTUAL INTERACTIONS

An attractive feature of multilevel models—one that is commonly used in health research—is their ability to model contextuality as a function of characteristics that relate to neighborhoods in addition to individual characteristics. At the same time, the nature and type of interactions between individual characteristics and neighborhood characteristics can also be assessed.

We illustrate the idea of such cross-level interactions by building on our running example of a two-level model (individuals at level 1 within neighborhoods at level 2), with the response being a score for poor health for each individual. We consider the categorical individual predictor, social class (with high social class as a reference and low social class specified as a contrast indicator variable) and a continuous neighborhood-level contextual predictor (e.g., socioeconomic deprivation index). Figure 4–8 portrays a range of hypothetical graphical models. In Figures 4–8(a)–(h), the y-axis represents the poor health score and the x-axis represents the neighborhood socioeconomic deprivation index. The dashed line represents low social class, and the solid line represents high social class.

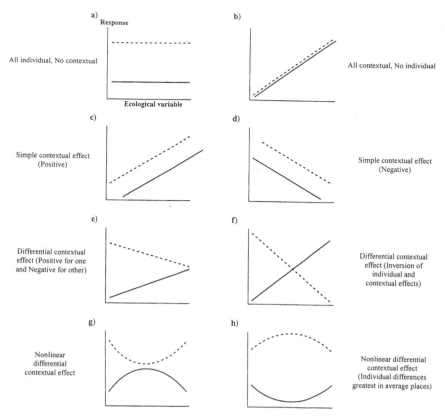

FIGURE 4–8. Individual and contextual relationships: a graphical typology.

Figure 4–8(a) shows marked differences between high social class and low social class but no contextual effect for neighborhood socioeconomic deprivation (all individual, no contextual). Figure 4–8(b) represents the converse: a small difference between the two social groups but a large contextual effect of socioeconomic deprivation (all contextual, no individual). The parallel lines in Figure 4–8(c) and 4–8(d) show both individual and contextual effects. In Figure 4–8(c) the neighborhood socioeconomic deprivation is shown to have a detrimental effect on the health of the individuals, and the reverse is shown in Figure 4–8(d). The key point is that the contextual effect of socioeconomic deprivation is seen to be the same for both high social class and low social class. Put differently, while neighborhood socioeconomic deprivation explains the prevalence of poor health, it does not account for the inequalities in health between the social class groups.

    In Figure 4–8(e) contextual effects are different for different groups. They are shown to be positive for high social class and negative for low social class, such that in neighborhoods with the highest level of socio-economic deprivation, health inequalities are minimal. Thus, neighborhood-level socioeconomic deprivation is not only related to average health achievements but also shapes social inequalities in health. Figure 4–8(f) represents the case in which contextual effects are strong enough to invert the individual effects. Figures 4–8(g) and 4–8(h) show models in which nonlinear terms are of importance, such that the smallest or largest group inequalities in health are found at "average" levels of socioeconomic deprivation and not at the extreme levels of neighborhood socioeconomic deprivation.

Relating this to equation (22), a neighborhood-level continuous predictor variable, socioeconomic deprivation, n_j, referring to the context of the neighborhood, is now introduced. Crucially, the contextual variables in the multilevel model are specified in the macromodels and then combined into the overall model. Thus, the underlying macromodels for equation (22) are now:

$$\beta_{0j} = \beta_0 + \alpha_0 n_{1j} + u_{0j} \tag{23}$$

$$\beta_{1j} = \beta_1 + \alpha_1 n_{1j} + u_{1j} \tag{24}$$

which results in the overall multilevel model:

$$y_{ij} = \beta_0 x_{0ij} + \beta_1 x_{1ij} + \alpha_0 n_{1j} x_{0ij} + \alpha_1 n_{1j} x_{1ij} \\ + (u_{0j} x_{0ij} + u_{1j} x_{1ij} + e_{1ij} z_{1ij} + e_{2ij} z_{2ij}) \tag{25}$$

The separate specification of micro and macromodels correctly recognizes that the contextual variables are predictors of between-neighborhood differences, after allowing for individual compositional variables. The α parameters represent the relationship between neighborhood differences (after controlling for the individual variable, social class) and the contextual variable, n_j. Thus, α_0 assesses the relationship between high social class (at the individual level) and the socioeconomic deprivation of the neighborhood. The parameter α_1 represents the differential contextual effect for low social class. This formulation makes clear that it is only through multilevel models that cross-level interactions between individual and contextual characteristics can be robustly specified and estimated.

MULTIPLE SPATIAL CONTEXTS

Most of the existing accounts of multilevel methods have been largely restricted to two-level structures, typically with individuals at level 1 and places at level 2. In this section we extend the model to consider the multiplicity of spatial levels in public health. For instance, in the United States, geographical units such as block groups (BGs), census tracts (CTs), counties, and states may each exert a differential influence on health in the population. Despite this, most research examining the effects of context on health has conceptualized contextual effects at only one level of geography.

Multiple hierarchical geographic levels may be needed to explain the mechanisms by which contexts at different levels affect health. The multiplicity of geographic levels raises a fundamental issue: determining the number of levels necessary to analyze a particular health outcome and the relative importance of different levels. Failure to address this issue can result in variability being attributed to the wrong contextual level. Consider, for example, a hierarchy of different geographic levels in which BGs are nested within CTs which in turn, are nested within counties within states. If poor health had a strong dependence at the BG level but the analysis only considered the CT level, incorrect inferences would be made at both the individual level *and* the CT level.

To appreciate the importance and implications of including this additional spatial level (level 3), a series of graphical typologies is useful (Subramanian, Duncan, et al., 2001). For the purposes of clarity and ease of understanding, we start with the simple case, shown in Figure 4–9, in which we assume that the differences between places at two spatial levels are the same for both the social class groups. We continue with the use of the term *neighborhoods* to represent level 2 spatial units and introduce the term *regions* to represent level 3 spatial units.

In Figure 4–9, the y-axis represents the individual score for poor health, the solid thick line represents the fixed average, the thinner solid lines represent the regions, while the dashed and the dotted lines represent neighborhoods within regions A and B, respectively. In Figure 4–9(a) it can be seen that while regions vary significantly around the average line, such that one is high (Region B) and one is low (Region A), the neighborhoods within each lie close to their respective region lines. This suggests that there is no need to include neighborhoods as a level and that a structure of individuals nested within regions is sufficient to capture the main source of geographic variation. In Figure 4–9(b) the converse is portrayed: while the differences between regions are insignificant (i.e., they are grouped close to the overall average line), those between neighborhoods are substantial. This would suggest the greater importance of the neighborhood level compared to the region level. Finally, Figure 4–9(c) anticipates a situation with significant variation at both region and neigh-

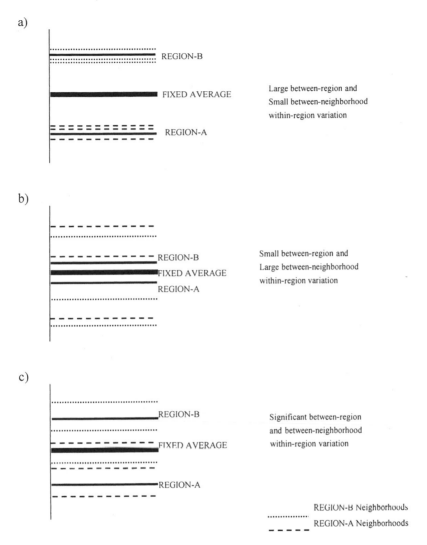

FIGURE 4–9. Partitioning variation at multiple spatial levels.

borhood levels. While the relative importance of each might vary, both levels need to be included in an empirical model.

Ascertaining the relative importance of different spatial scales, after taking into account (individual) compositional effects, can provide important clues about the level "at which the action lies." A multilevel framework is ideally and readily suited to this task. Thus, underlying Figure 4–9 is a multilevel model based on a three-level structure of individuals (level 1) nested within neighborhoods (level 2) nested within regions (level 3). The micro model can be written as:

$$y_{ijk} = \beta_{0jk}x_{0ijk} + \beta_1 x_{1ijk} + e_{0ijk}x_{0ijk} \tag{26}$$

with an additional subscript k to represent the regions. In addition, there would be a macro model at the neighborhood level (level 2):

$$\beta_{0jk} = \beta_{0k} + u_{0jk} \tag{27}$$

where β_{0k} is the poor health proportion for region k and u_{0jk} is the differential for the jth neighborhood in the kth region. There would also be a macro model at the region level (level 3):

$$\beta_{0k} = \beta_0 + v_{0k} \tag{28}$$

where β_0 is the average poor health score and v_{0k} is the differential for the kth region, to form an overall three-level random-intercepts model:

$$y_{ijk} = \beta_0 x_{0ijk} + \beta_1 x_{1ijk} + (v_{0k}x_{0ijk} + u_{0jk}x_{0ijk} + e_{0ijk}x_{0ijk}) \tag{29}$$

Depending on the relative size of the neighborhood and region level variance terms (σ_{u0}^2 and σ_{v0}^2, respectively), that summarize the place-specific differentials at each level, this model would produce one of the patterns shown in Figure 4–9.

MULTILEVEL RESIDUAL MAPPING

While it is the variances that are estimated in a multilevel model at each of the specified levels, it is possible to estimate place-specific (posterior) residuals at each of the contextual levels. Residual mapping is an extremely useful application of multilevel models, especially when interest lies in simultaneous multiple geographies and when *all* the units at each of the geographic level can be observed in the analysis (e.g., the census) (Subramanian et al., 2001). In order to appreciate this, Figure 4–10 unpacks the way in which residuals are constructed when there are two spatial levels.

The region-specific residuals (v_{0k}) at level 3 represent the difference from the fixed average line, β_0. For example, Region A will have a negative residual given its lower rate of poor health compared to the overall average; Region B, in contrast, will have a positive residual given its higher rate compared to the average. Neighborhood-specific residuals

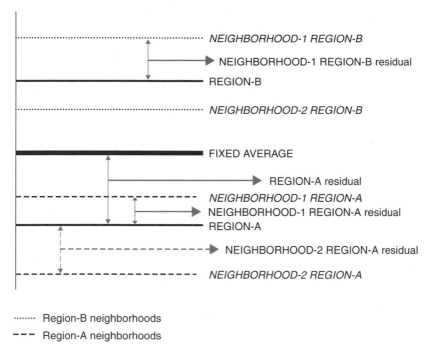

FIGURE 4–10. Residuals at multiple spatial levels.

(u_{0jk}) at level 2, meanwhile, are measured as the difference from the regions to which they belong (hence, the subscript jk) and *not* as a difference from the fixed average as shown in Figure 4–10 for Neighborhood 1 in Region A and Neighborhood 2 in Region A. Consider Neighborhood 1 in Region A in Figure 4–10. From a conventional perspective, this neighborhood would be considered a "healthy place" (given that it is below the average). From a multilevel perspective, however, this neighborhood would be considered an "unhealthy place" given the healthy context of the region (low rate) to which it belongs, and as such it would have a positive neighborhood residual.

Such ideas are extremely useful for social policy (Goldstein and Spiegelhalter, 1996). As an example, consider Neighborhood 2 in Region A, and Neighborhood 2 in Region B in Figure 4–10. Both neighborhoods are seen to be performing well, with low rates of poor health (negative neighborhood residuals). The similarity in neighborhood effects is, however, occurring in entirely different contexts and as such may be telling quite different stories. While low rates in Neighborhood 2 in Region A are being achieved within a favorable context (a low-rate region), in Neighborhood 2 in Region B they are occurring within an unfavorable context (a high-rate region).

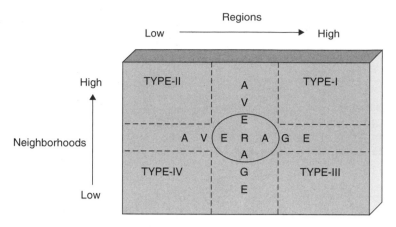

FIGURE 4–11. Illustrating multilevel geographic typologies.

As this example illustrates, we have a nuanced way of evaluating and monitoring the performance of particular places. One possibility, as shown in Figure 4–11, is to have a simple fourfold typology of neighborhood health performance: Type I—unhealthy neighborhoods in unhealthy regions; Type II—unhealthy neighborhoods in healthy regions; Type III—healthy neighborhoods in unhealthy regions; and Type IV—healthy neighborhoods in healthy regions.

The purpose of such typologies is not simply methodological, but substantive and practical. For instance, Type I neighborhoods are doubly disadvantaged ("unhealthy" neighborhoods in "unhealthy" regions), while Type IV neighborhoods suggest a virtuous reinforcement of contextual advantage ("healthy" neighborhoods in "healthy" regions). For Type II and Type III neighborhoods, meanwhile, contextual advantage at one level offsets disadvantage at the other. Determining the cut-off points for what can be considered "healthy" and "unhealthy" is critical, and care must be taken while identifying specific places, an issue to which we shall return later in this chapter. Nonetheless, our aim here is to illustrate the potential of a multilevel approach for evaluative and monitoring exercises that are usually of interest for public health departments.

PARAMETER ESTIMATION IN MULTILEVEL STATISTICAL MODELS

In this section we provide a brief overview of the estimation strategies that are used to fit multilevel models. Using observed data, a multilevel model estimates the regression coefficients (fixed parameters) and the variance components (random parameters). These parameters are usually generated using the maximum likelihood (ML) estimators that provide population values that maximize the so-called likelihood function, which gives the probability of observing the sample data given the parameter estimates. ML estimators, therefore, are parameter estimates that maximize the probability of finding the sample data we have actually found (Hox, 1995). The ML estimators are available using the Newton-Raphson Fisher scoring, iterative generalized least squares, or the expectation maximization algorithms (Longford, 1993).

Computing the ML estimators requires an iterative procedure. At the beginning starting values for the various parameter estimates (usually based on the ordinary least squares regression estimates) are generated. In the next step the computation procedure improves upon the starting values to produce better estimates via generalized least squares. This step is repeated (iterated) until the changes in the estimates between two successive iterations become very small, indicating convergence, with the parameter estimates now being ML estimators. Lack of convergence could suggest model misspecification in the fixed part, misspecification of the variance–covariance structure (either too simple or too complex), or small sample sizes at different levels.

Two different varieties of ML estimators are used in the available software for multilevel modeling. One is the full information maximum likelihood (FIML), in which both the regression coefficients and the variance components are included in the likelihood function. The other is the restricted maximum likelihood (REML), and here only the variance components are included in the likelihood function. The difference is that FIML treats the estimates for the regression coefficients as known quantities when the variance components are estimated, while REML treats them as estimates that carry some amount of uncertainty (Bryk and Raudenbush, 1992; Goldstein, 1995). While REML is more realistic and is recommended, especially when the number of groupings is small (Bryk and Raudenbush, 1992), FIML is computationally less demanding and allows for greater comparison across different model specifications.

The ML theory is based on several assumptions, and three that are critical from an applied perspective are (1) the random parameters at all levels are normally distributed; (2) the level 2 random parameters are independent of the level 1 random parameters; and (3) the sample size is large and tends to infinity. In practice, these assumptions will, at best, be met only approximately. Violations of these assumptions could lead to bias of the estimators and incorrect standard errors. In recent years, however, Bayesian estimation using Gibbs sampling (Gilks et al., 1996; Browne, 2002), quasi-likelihood estimation together with bias correction procedures (Goldstein and Rasbash, 1996) have been developed as alternatives. For inference, interval estimates are obtained directly from Gibbs sampling and via large sample deviance statistics or bootstrapping for likelihood function estimation.

We now turn to identifying some key extensions to the multilevel models outlined so far. We consider two types of extensions: the first relates to complex multilevel structures and the second relates to modeling specifications.

EXTENSIONS TO MULTILEVEL STRUCTURES

It is important to note that redesigning the data structure is a way by which some problematic issues are circumvented within multilevel frameworks.

Modeling Spatially Aggregated Data

While we have so far discussed the multilevel structure in terms of individuals at level 1 and places at level 2, we argue that a similar framework of people within places can be established using routinely available aggregate data (e.g., census and mortality data). As is well known, analyses of aggregated data confound the microscale of people and the macroscale of places. Although regrettable, this situation is usually tolerated owing to the other obvious attractions of these data sets (e.g., large, extensive coverage of places at multiple levels). A multilevel approach offers a solution to this problem (Subramanian et al., 2001).

Table 4–1 provides hypothetical data on deaths for two social groups in a format typical for spatially aggregated data. Thus, in Area 1, 9 out of 50 in the low social class category died in a particular year; in Area 2,

TABLE 4–1. Hypothetical Counts of Death and Total Population by Social Class by Areas

	Counts of Death out of Total Population	
Areas	Low Social Class	High Social Class
1	9 out of 50	2 out of 50
2	5 out of 90	5 out of 95
. . . .	. . . .	. . . .
49	10 out of 80	0 out of 50
50	20 out of 90	0 out of 0

5 out of 95 in the high social class category died, and so on. In this table individuals are grouped as "types" (low and high social class) and are represented as "cells": of a table that contains counts of death for each social group in every area. Importantly, by using the compact, aggregated form of Table 4-1, data agencies can preserve individual confidentiality.

Five points need to be made about this table. First, it is vital to note that underlying Table 4–1 is simply a set of individual records that happens to be presented in a tabular format but that can easily be changed into an individual record format. Second, just as individuals nest within areas, producing a two-level hierarchical data structure, so do the cells presented in Table 4–1. This is shown in Figure 4–12. Third, although here the data is cross-tabulated by only one individual characteristic, exactly the same principles apply when there is a greater degree of cross-tabulation. Fourth, if in an area there are no people of a particular type (e.g., missing high social class in Area 50 in Table 4–1), this poses no special problems, as multilevel data structures can be unbalanced as shown in Figure 4–12. Finally, there is good reason for invoking the notion of cells even when data is available in an individual record format because the amount of information, and therefore the associated computing time, can be reduced without any substantial loss of information.

Consequently, routinely available aggregated data can readily be adapted to a multilevel data structure with table cells at level 1 (representing the population groups) nested within places at level 2. The counts within each cell give the number of people with the outcome of interest (e.g., number of deaths) together with the "denominator" (the total population). The proportion so formed becomes the response variable, and the cell characteristics, meanwhile, are the individual predictor variables. Such a structure now lends itself to all the analytical capabilities that were discussed earlier (Subramanian et al., 2001).

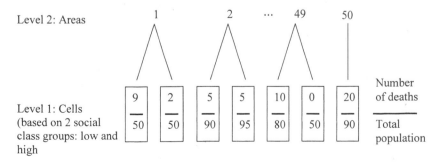

FIGURE 4–12. Two-level structure of cells at level 1 within areas at level 2.

Nonhierarchical Cross-Classified Structures

Individuals live their lives in a number of overlapping settings, such as neighborhood, workplace, home, and so on. Such contexts do not always lend themselves to a neat hierarchical structure. Instead, the different settings may overlap at the same level, producing a *crossed* structure. The importance of such structures has been long recognized and they are now technically and computationally tractable (Goldstein, 1994; Jones et al., 1998). The "quasi-hierarchical" format employed within cross-classified multilevel models enables an assessment of the relative importance of a number of different, overlapping contexts after allowing for the differential composition of each. Such models identify contexts that have a confounding influence, thus ascertaining the contexts that have the greatest significance. For example, a cross-classified model of health behavior (e.g., smoking) could be formulated with individuals at level 1 and *both* residential neighborhoods and workplaces at level 2, as shown in Figure 4–13(a). If account is not taken of this cross-classified structure, what may appear to be between-workplace variation could actually be between-neighborhood variation, and vice versa.

A related structure occurs if, for a single level 2 classification (e.g., neighborhoods), level 1 units (e.g., individuals) may belong to more than one level 2 unit. The individual can be considered to belong simultaneously to several neighborhoods, with the contributions of each neighborhood being weighted in relation to its distance (if the interest is spatial) from the individual.

Repeated Measures of People and Places

Health outcomes and behaviors as well as their causal mechanisms are rarely stable and invariant over time, producing data structures that involve repeated measures. Two possibilities arise depending on the unit that is repeatedly measured. When individuals are repeatedly measured within a panel design, the outcomes taken at different times form level 1. The same outcomes measured over different times are nested within individuals at level 2, which in turn nest within higher-level units (e.g., neighborhoods). This structure is shown in Figure 4–13(b) and allows the assessment of individual change within a contextual setting.

The other possibility is repeated cross-sectional surveys in which places are monitored at regular time intervals (repeatedly measuring places over time). The structure would then be individuals at level 1, time/years within places at level 2, and places at level 3, as shown in Figure 4–13(c). Such a structure permits an investigation of trends within geographic settings controlling for their compositional make-up. Multilevel models could be used

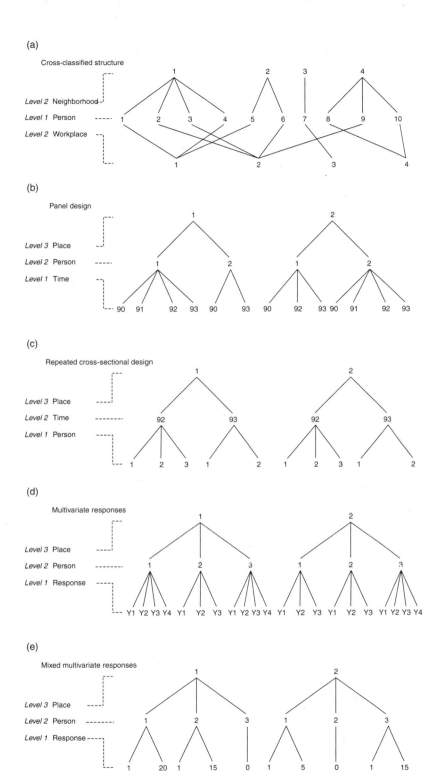

FIGURE 4–13. A range of multilevel structures.

to explore what sorts of individuals and what sorts of places have changed over time with respect to health outcomes and other characteristics.

Multiple Yet Related Outcomes

Multivariate multilevel models can handle situations in which a number of different but related response measurements are made on individuals (Duncan, 1997). The key feature is that the set of responses (outcomes) is nested within individuals. The response could be a set of outcomes that relate to, for instance, different aspects of health behavior (e.g., smoking and drinking). Crucially, such responses could be a mixture of "quality" (do you smoke/do you drink) and "quantity" (how many/how much). A multilevel structure on different aspects of health behavior could be measurements (e.g., smoking and drinking both at level 1) nested within individuals (level 2) within neighborhoods (level 3). The substantive benefit of this approach is that it is possible to assess whether different types of behavior are related to individual characteristics in the same or different ways. Moreover, the residual covariances at level 2 and level 3 measure the "correlation" of behaviors between individuals and between places. Technical benefits in terms of efficiency result if the response is correlated and if there are many missing responses, as in matrix sample designs. Figure 4–13(d) presents a structure in which the responses at level 1 capture four different aspects of health behaviors, and Figure 4–13(e) portrays the idea of "mixed" (quality and quantity) responses on a particular aspect of health behavior. Thus, for example, person 1 in place 1 is a smoker and smokes 20 cigarettes, while person 3 in place 1 is a non-smoker and as such the response related to number of cigarettes smoked does not apply.

While for the purpose of clarity and ease of understanding we have discussed each of the multilevel structures separately, readers are urged to think about these structures in an integrated manner. For instance, in a model of health behaviors, in addition to a mixed multivariate structure (e.g., smoke or not, how many; drink or not, how much), individuals could be repeatedly measured across multiple time periods, who in turn are then cross-nested across neighborhoods and workplaces. The mixed multivariate response would then be the level 1 units that are nested within time periods at level 2, within individuals at level 3, and neighborhoods and workplaces at level 4.

EXTENSIONS TO MODEL SPECIFICATIONS

We have already discussed how multilevel methods offer an extremely powerful framework to (1) disentangle compositional and contextual effects; (2) model between contextual and between individual (within context) heterogeneity; (3) model interaction effects between individual and contextual characteristics; and (4) model variation across multiple spatial scales. In this section we draw attention to additional model specifications that we consider important.

Modeling Heterogeneity at Multiple Spatial Levels

The three-level framework presented in equation (29) considered between-neighborhood variation at level 2 and between-region variation at level 3 as a constant function that was unchanging across the social class groups. This assumption can be relaxed such that between-context variation at both the spatial levels can be modeled as a function of social class. Such models are extremely useful in order to explore the relative importance of different spatial levels for different types of population groups. For instance, for individuals of low social class it may be the regions that matter more than the neighborhoods, while it might be the reverse for those of high social class. In addition, such models allow a mapping of the differential geographies for different social classes at each of the geographic level.

Allowing the Effect of Contextual Variables to Vary

Typically, contextual variables (e.g., neighborhood-level socioeconomic index) are modeled in the fixed part of the multilevel model. However, as we emphasize in this chapter, a unique advantage of multilevel models is their ability to model variability in the fixed average relationships, both at their own level (that is, the level at which they are observed and measured) and at higher levels. For instance, the effect of neighborhood-level socioeconomic deprivation may not be uniform across all regions and may vary across the regions. Furthermore, highly deprived neighborhoods may also be characterized by a greater degree of heterogeneity. Considering both these formulations is vital to develop a rich empirical description of the role of neighborhood socioeconomic deprivation on poor health and to condition the inferences and predictions that are derived based on fixed average relationships.

Interaction between Contextual Levels

The notion of cross-level interaction that we discussed earlier using Figure 4–8 can be usefully extended to contextual variables at different geographic levels (e.g., one relating to neighborhood characteristics and the other representing region characteristics). Such interactions explore the influence of a contextual variable at the region level for different types of neighborhoods. This idea is particularly significant given the direct interest in characterizing and measuring places. Furthermore, this extension is also intrinsic to earlier arguments in which we emphasized the importance of interpreting neighborhood patterning in relation to regions, given their functional interconnectedness. For example, a neighborhood characteristic (e.g., low and high socioeconomic deprivation index) and region characteristic (e.g., per capita expenditure on health) may interact in ways such that region health expenditure levels may manifest in different ways, depending on the type of neighborhood such that the same level of expenditure may produce better results in low-deprivation neighborhoods compared to high-deprivation neighborhoods.

Nonlinear Multilevel Models

So far we have illustrated the methodological concepts by considering a continuous response variable that has a normal distribution. However, a large number of outcomes of interest in public health research are not continuous and do not have Gaussian (normal) distributive properties. While not discussed in detail here, multilevel models are capable of handling a wide range of responses, and "generalized multilevel models" exist to deal with binary outcomes, proportions (such as logit, log–log, and probit models), multiple categories (such as multinomial and ordered multinomial models), and counts (such as Poisson and negative binomial distribution models) (Leyland and Goldstein, 2001). Indeed, all these outcomes can be modeled using any of the hierarchical and nonhierarchical structures discussed previously (Rasbash et al., 2000).

These models work, in effect, by assuming a specific, non-normal distribution for the random part at level 1, while maintaining the normality assumptions for random parts at higher levels. Consequently, much of the discussion presented in this chapter focusing at the neighborhood and region level (higher contextual levels) would continue to hold regardless of the nature of the response variable. It may, however, be noted that the computation of VPC, which we discussed earlier, in complex nonlinear models is not as straightforward as it is in normal models and is an issue of applied methodological research (Goldstein et al., 2002; Browne, Subramanian et al., 2002). Research developments are currently underway in which multilevel perspectives have been extended to survival and event history models, metaanalysis, structural equation modeling, instrumental variable analysis, and factor analysis (Goldstein, 1998).

MULTILEVEL METHODS: A CRITICAL PERSPECTIVE

There has been an enthusiastic rush to use multilevel modeling techniques in recent years (for an excellent review of multilevel applications in health research see Diez Roux, 2001, 2002, in press). In their enthusiasm researchers have often overlooked certain fundamental methodological issues that may have critical conceptual and empirical implications. Having discussed the nature and scope of multilevel methods, we now turn to some of these key issues.

Operationalizing Context

The validity of multilevel models relies entirely on the researchers' conceptualization and operationalization of the analytical levels. Practical convenience often has guided the selection and identification of contexts. For instance, in the United States, block groups and/or census tracts (spatial administrative units) are commonly used to define the neighborhood setting. Whether such administrative units accurately delimit the boundaries of what constitutes a "neighborhood" is debatable. Related to this issue are problems of missing levels and outcome-contingent hierarchies.

Recent studies have shown that the variance apportioned to different levels may be over or underestimated depending on the ignored nature and number of levels. While there are technical reasons to expect the apportioned variance to change between a two-level and a three-level model (Hutchison and Healy, 2001; Tranmer and Steel, 2001), there are implications for making neighborhood-level inferences and also for the fixed part estimates. While we do not advocate abandoning the use of administrative units to define contexts, there is a need to be conceptually clear about the selection (or omission) of levels in the analysis.

Second, the conceptual and operational multilevel structure may differ depending on the outcome that is being analyzed. Often, regardless of the health outcome, the same set of hierarchical levels is used. Future applications, therefore, need to not only justify the analysis in terms of the choice of levels but also in terms of the extent to which the choice depends on the outcome under investigation.

Closely related to this issue is the level-contingent nature of different contextual predictor variables. For instance, certain contextual variables (e.g., the extent of income inequality in an area) may be more meaningful at the higher level of aggregation (e.g., region) than at lower levels of aggregation (e.g., neighborhoods), while others such as cognitive perceptions of social capital may be more meaningul at lower levels of aggregation. In summary, multilevel models are only as good (or as bad) as the underlying theories used to justify the levels and choice of covariates at each of the identified levels.

Endogeneity of Contextual Effects

Because individuals do, to some extent, choose where to live, "unobserved" individual or family factors can be mistaken for neighborhood effects. Similar unobserved factors may also characterize neighborhoods and other spatial levels of analysis. This problem of endogeneity, whereby an unobserved variable is related to a set of predictors *and* the response, is only beginning to be addressed in the context of multilevel methods. The issue of endogeneity is even more complex in multilevel analysis because the unmeasured influences of omitted variables in the fixed part gets incorporated in the random part of the model, thereby violating the assumption of the independence of regressors and model disturbances (Rice et al., 1998). Three ways of dealing with this issue have been suggested in the multilevel literature. The first is to include data that actually "measure the crucial omitted variable" (Duncan and Raudenbush, 1999). The second is to apply specially developed multilevel instrumental variable estimation techniques (Spencer, 1998; Spencer and Fielding, 2000), which is the standard solution to endogeneity problems in single-level regression now extended to multilevel regression models. The third is to use a repeated measures, cross-classified structure, longitudinal fixed-effects model based on the nesting of panel observations for those who change neighborhoods within a cross-classified structure with time-varying covariates at each level of the analysis (Rasbash and Goldstein, 1994). This strategy, of course, is extremely data intensive and involves intensive computational demands. It is recommended that future applications be sensitive to the causal implications that the issue of endogeneity poses for multilevel research.

Limits to Context-Specific Predictions

Multilevel models, through the estimation of the posterior residuals at the higher level, provide an extremely useful way of measuring and monitoring performances of higher-level units (e.g., neighborhoods, hospitals) (Goldstein and Spiegelhalter, 1996). While this is extremely useful, it is important to realize that the primary function of multilevel models is to model population heterogeneity at different levels (e.g., individuals, neighborhoods) and *not* to generate context-specific predictions. Because multilevel models treat the neighborhoods as a sample realized from a population of neighborhoods, the main focus is on the variability between neighborhoods rather than the specific effect of each neighborhood. Therefore, while predictions for specific neighborhoods are possible, these are not simply point estimates; degrees of uncertainty are associated with them as well as any ranking that derives from them (Goldstein and Spiegelhalter, 1996). Specifically, neighborhood-specific estimates depend on the sample size in specific neighborhoods. Neighborhoods with small sample sizes will have large confidence intervals; they will also contribute little to the estimation of the population parameters given the precision weighting used (Jones and Bullen, 1994). These considerations are extremely important before "naming" (and "shaming") specific places and institutions.

Power and Sample Size Considerations

As we have emphasized, multilevel models are not about modeling each neighborhood separately, but, rather, the sample of neighborhoods is seen as one realization from a population of neighborhoods. When designing a powerful multilevel study it is important, therefore, to consider two things: the determination of sample sizes at the various levels of analysis, and ensuring the property of exchangeability. We first discuss the issue of sampling in multilevel analysis.

It is vital that the study design have "adequate" numbers of units at *all* the levels of analysis. In general, by increasing sample sizes at all levels, estimates and their standard errors become more accurate to some extent. The analysis of binomial data in particular requires larger samples than the analysis of normally distributed data (Hox, 1998). Determination of sample sizes at level 1 and level 2 units for efficiency, unbiasedness, and consistency of parameter estimates is not entirely straightforward, and this is especially the case if we are interested in the random slopes component. In a two-level random intercepts model, the sample design question is analogous to computing the effective sample size in two-stage cluster sampling as given by Kish, 1965. Effective sample size of a two-stage cluster sampling design, n_{eff}, is computed by:

$$n_{eff} = n/[1 + (n_{clus} - 1)\rho] \tag{30}$$

where n is the total number of individuals in the study, that is, the actual sample size; n_{clus} is the number of individuals per neighborhood; and ρ is the intraclass correlation. However, the analogy is not straightforward for random slopes models, because the ICC for these models is a function of the independent variable, as was shown in equation (21). Neither are such calculations straightforward in three-level models.

Consensus has yet to be developed on the precise power of calculations within multilevel models. Some argue for a sample of at least 30 groups with at least 30 individuals in each group (Kreft, 1996). This advice is considered sound provided interest is largely in the fixed parameters. Modification to this "rule" is advised if interest is in estimating cross-level interactions and/or variance and covariance components (Hox, 1998). For the former a 50/20 rule is generally recommended (about 50 neighborhoods with at least 20 individuals per neighborhood), and for a variance–covariance components model about 100 neighborhoods with about 10 individuals per neighborhood is suggested. Indeed, if this is the case, then one has to be cautious about making neighborhood-specific predictions. These "rules" take into account that there are costs attached to data collection, such that if the number of neighborhoods is increased, the number of individuals per neighborhood decreases (Snijders and Bosker, 1993; Snijders, 2001).

Exchangeability of the Sample

Multilevel models treat the higer-level units as a sample drawn from a common population and inferences are made about this population. However, just because multilevel models operate in this way does not guarantee that they are appropriate in any particular instance. Crucial exchangeability judgments exist that are often neglected (Morris, 1995). Specifically, researchers need to ensure that the sample of neighborhoods does come from, can be exchanged with, and is similar to the population that they wish to make inferences about, with this being true for each specific neighborhood for which they have data. If there are reasons to believe that certain neighborhoods are truly independent or that they come from different populations, they should not be regarded as exchangeable with the remaining random sample of neighborhoods and, as such, should be treated as fixed effects. While one option is to perform diagnostics after the model is fitted and/or conduct multilevel analysis with those neighborhoods that are believed to share exchangeable properties and without those neighborhoods that are believed to violate the exchangeability assumption, a conceptually sound approach is to carefully plan the selection of neighborhoods at the design stage, analogous to the sampling of individuals in a survey (Draper, 1995).

CONCLUDING REMARKS

Multilevel models, in conclusion, have several features that make them attractive for public health research. In this chapter we sought to explain and emphasize how these methods offer an extremely flexible yet unified framework for conceptualizing and investigating substantive ideas related to contextuality and heterogeneity. Specifically, variability and the correlated nature of data structures are seen as the norm, not an aberration, and consequently multilevel methods neither ignore nor adjust for them, but rather anticipate and model them. In doing so, we showed that these methods encourage and foster refinement in our thinking about different levels of causation.

At the same time, the full potential of multilevel methodologies is yet to be realized. Reviewing applications of multilevel methods in public health research to date reveals three methodological motivations: (1) the need to obtain more accurate estimates and standard errors of the individual correlates that influence health (that is, the need to adjust for any autocorrelation in the response); (2) to establish the average fixed contribution of compositional and contextual factors; and (3) to establish fixed cross-level interaction effects between individual and contextual factors. While not discounting the relevance of these motivations, the methodological focus has been, and continues to be, on the fixed part of the multilevel model, with very little focus on the random part. Furthermore, research applications have also not moved beyond the simple two-level structure of individuals at a lower level nested within a spatial setting at a higher level.

Multilevel methods, we have argued, provide a theoretical and technical framework that can help reconceptualize much of public health research. Specifically, they compel the researcher to reflect on the multilevel nature of causal processes and raise questions that are not simply about fixed averages but rather about the variability and heterogeneity of populations. Indeed, multilevel methods are changing the way we think about "individual effects" and "contextual effects." From an initial view of interpreting these effects in terms of "who you are in relation to where you are," multilevel methods encourage us to think along the lines of "who you are *depends* on where you are." While the methodological capability of multilevel models to disentangle compositional (individual) and contextual effects related to spatial variations has been well demonstrated, the multilevel framework has also redefined the construct of individual compositional explanations. Indeed, as Macintyre and Ellaway (2000) point out, "your SES and income are partly a product of your place of upbringing, rather than being intrinsically personal attributes."

While being attractive both conceptually and technically, multilevel methods are also undoubtedly complex and should not be approached in simplistic terms. Indeed, simplistic use of complex methodological tools can lead to interpretive confusion and a potential overstatement of what may validly be concluded from a given piece of research (Draper, 1995). These comments are not meant to discourage the use of multilevel methods. Rather, as we have emphasized, multilevel models can raise new research agendas and provide important insights into existing knowledge. At the same time, as one of the pioneers in this field reminds us, multilevel methods, like all statistical methods, should be used "with care and understanding" (Goldstein, 1995).

REFERENCES

Alker, HA, Jr. (1969). A typology of ecological fallacies. In Dogan M and Rokkan S, eds.: *Quantitative Ecological Analysis*. Cambridge, Mass: Massachusetts Institute of Technology Press, pp. 69–86.

Anderson NB (1999). Solving the puzzles of socioeconomic status and health: The need for integrated, multilevel, interdisciplinary research. *Ann NY Acad Sci* 896: 302–312.

Berkman LF and Kawachi I, eds. (2000). *Social Epidemiology*. New York: Oxford University Press.

Browne WJ (2002). MCMC Estimation in MLWIN, Version 1.0. London: Centre for Multilevel Modelling, University of London.

Browne WJ, Subramanian SV, et al. (2002). *Variance Partitioning in Multilevel Logistic Models that Exhibit Over-dispersion*. London: Center for Multilevel Modelling.

Bryk AS and Raudenbush SW (1992). *Hierarchical Linear Models: Applications and Data Analysis Methods*. Newbury Park, Engl: Sage Publications.

Bullen N, Jones K, et al. (1997). Modelling complexity: Analysing between-individual and between-place variation—a multilevel tutorial. *Environment and Planning A* 29(4): 585–609.

de Leeuw J and Kreft KGG (1986). Random coefficients models for multilevel analysis. *Journal of Educational Statistics* 11: 57–85.

Diez Roux AV (2001). Investigating neighborhood and area effects on health. *Am J Public Health* 91(11): 1783–1789.

Diez Roux AV (2002). Invited commentary: Places, people, and health. *Am J Epidemiol* 155(6): 516–519.

Diez Roux AV (2003). The examination of neighborhood effects on health: Conceptual and methodological issues related to the presence of multiple levels of organization. In Kawachi I and Berkman LF, eds.: *Neighborhoods and Health*. New York: Oxford University Press, pp. 43–64.

Draper D (1995). Inference and hierarchical modeling in the social sciences. *Journal of Educational and Behavioral Statistics* 20: 115–147.

Duncan C (1997). Applying mixed multivariate multilevel models in geographical research. In Westert GP and Verhoeff RN, eds.: *Place and People: Multilevel Modelling in Geographical Research*. Utrecht: Royal Dutch Geographical Society and Faculty of Geographical Sciences, Utrecht University, pp. 100–115.

Duncan G and Raudenbush S (1999). Assessing the effects of context in studies of child and youth development. *Educational Psychologist* 34: 29–41.

Gilks W, Richardson S, et al. (1996). *Markov Chain Monte Carlo in Practice*. London: Chapman & Hill.

Goldstein H (1994). Multilevel cross-classified models. *Sociological Methods and Research* 22: 364–375.

Goldstein H (1995). *Multilevel Statistical Models*. London: Arnold.

Goldstein H (1998). Multilevel models. In Armitage P and Colton T, eds.: *Encyclopaedia of Biostatistics*. Vol. 4. Chicester: Wiley. pp. 2725–2731.

Goldstein H, Browne W, et al. (2002). *Partitioning Variation in Multilevel Models*. London: Institute of Education, University of London.

Goldstein H and Rasbash J (1996). Improved approximations for multilevel models with binary responses. *J R Stat Soc A* 159: 505–513.

Goldstein H and Spiegelhalter D (1996). League tables and their limitations: Statistical issues in comparisons of institutional performance (with discussion). *J R Stat Soc A* 159: 385–443.

Hox J (1998). Multilevel modeling: When and why. In Balderjahn I, Mather R, and Schader M, eds.: *Classification, data analysis, and data highways*. New York: Springer Verlag, pp. 147–154.

Hox J (1995). *Applied Multilevel Analysis*. Amsterdam: TT-Publikaties.

Hutchison D and Healy M (2001). The effect of variance component estimates of ignoring a level in a multilevel model. *Multilevel Modelling Newsletter* 13(2): 4–5.

Jones K and Bullen N (1994). Contextual models of urban house prices: A comparison of fixed- and random-coefficient models developed by expansion. *Economic Geography* 70: 252–272.

Jones K, Gould MI, et al. (1998). Multiple contexts as cross-classified models: The labor vote in the British general elections of 1992. *Geographical Analysis* 30: 65–93.

Jones K and Moon G (1993). Medical geography: Taking space seriously. *Progress in Human Geography* 17(4): 515–524.

Kish L (1965). *Survey Sampling*. New York: Wiley.

Kreft I and de Leeuw J (1998). *Introducing Multilevel Models*. London: Sage.

Kreft IGG (1996). *Are Multilevel Techniques Necessary? An Overview Including Simulation Studies*. Los Angeles: Calfornia State University Press.

Leyland AH and Goldstein H, eds. (2001). *Multilevel Modelling of Health Statistics*. Wiley Series in Probability and Statistics. Chichester, England: Wiley.

Longford N (1993). *Random Coefficient Models*. Oxford: Clarendon Press.

Macintyre S (2000). The social patterning of health: Bringing the social context back in. *Medical Sociology Newsletter* 26: 14–19.

Macintyre S and Ellaway A (2000). Ecological approaches: Rediscovering the role of physical and social environment. In Berkman LF and Kawachi I, eds.: *Social Epidemiology*. New York: Oxford University Press., pp. 332–348.

Morris C (1983). Parametric empirical Bayes. *Journal of the American Statistical Association* 78: 47–65.

Morris C (1995). Hierarchical models for educational data: An overview. *Journal of Educational and Behavioral Statistics* 20: 190–199.

Rasbash J, Browne W, et al. (2000). *A User's Guide to MLwiN, Version 2.1*. London: Multilevel Models Project, Institute of Education, University of London.

Rasbash J and Goldstein H (1994). Efficient analysis of mixed hierarchical and cross-classified random structures using a multilevel model. *Journal of Educational and Behavioural Statistics* 19(4): 337–350.

Rice N, Jones A, et al. (1998). Multilevel models where the random effects are correlated with the fixed predictors: A conditioned iterative generalised least squares estimator (CIGLS). *Multilevel Modelling Newsletter* 10(1): 10–14.

Roberts S (1999). Socioeconomic composition and health: The independent contribution of community socioeconomic context. *Annual Review of Sociology* 25: 489–516.

Robinson S (1950). Ecological correlations and the behaviour of individuals. *American Sociological Review* 15: 351–357.

Selvin HC (1958). Durkheim's suicide and problems of empirical research. *American Journal of Sociology* 63: 607–619.

Skinner C, Holt D, et al., eds. (1989). *The Analysis of Complex Surveys*. New York: Wiley.

Snijders TAB (2001). Sampling. In Leyland AH and Goldstein H, eds.: *Multilevel Modelling of Health Statistics*. Chichester, Engl: Wiley, pp. 159–174.

Snijders TAB and Bosker RJ (1993). Standard errors and sample sizes for two-level research. *Journal of Educational Statistics* 18: 237–259.

Spencer N (1998). Consistent parameter estimation for lagged multilevel models. Statistics Technical Report Paper 1. Hertfordshire, University of Hertfordshire Business School, Report No. UHBS: 19.

Spencer N and Fielding A (2000). An instrumental variable consistent estimation procedure to overcome the problem of endogenous variables in multilevel models. *Multilevel Modelling Newsletter* 12(1): 4–7.

Subramanian SV, Duncan C, et al. (2001). Multilevel perspectives on modeling census data. *Environment and Planning A* 33(3): 399–417.

Susser M (1994). The logic in the ecological. *Am J Public Health* 84: 825–835.

Tranmer M and Steel DG (2001). Ignoring a level in a multilevel model: Evidence from UK census data. *Environment and Planning A* 33: 941–948.

Weisberg S (1980). *Applied Linear Regression*. New York: Wiley.

SELECTED READINGS

For fundamental ideas underlying multilevel models, see:
Raudenbush SW and Bryk AS (2002). *Hierarchical Linear Models: Applications and Data Analysis Methods*. 2nd edition. Thousand Oaks, California: Sage Publications.

Goldstein H (1995). *Multilevel Statistical Models*. 2nd edition, London: Arnold. (An electronic version of this book can be downloaded free from the following website http://www.arnoldpublishers.com/support/goldstein.htm, accessed September 9, 2002.)

Longford N (1993). *Random Coefficient Models*. Oxford: Clarendon Press.

For an applied perspective on multilevel models, see:
Bullen N, Jones K and Duncan C (1997). *Modelling Complexity: Analysing Between-Individual and Between-Place Variation—A Multilevel Tutorial*. Environment and Planning A 29(4): 585–609.

Hox J (2002). *Multilevel Analysis: Techniques and Applications*. Mahwah, NJ: Lawrence Erlbaum Associates.

Leyland AH and Goldstein H, eds. (2001). *Multilevel Modelling of Health Statistics*. Wiley Series in Probability and Statistics. John Wiley & Sons Ltd.: Chichester.

Snijders T and Bosker R (1999). *Multilevel Analysis: An Introduction to Basic and Advanced Multilevel Modeling*. London: Sage Publications.

For hands-on practical tutorial based learning, see:

http://multilevel.ioe.ac.uk and http://tramss.data-archive.ac.uk/Software/ MLwiN.asp, (accessed September 9, 2002.)

Rasbash J et al., *A user's guide to MLwiN, Version 2.1.* 2000, London: Multilevel Models Project, Institute of Education, University of London. (An electronic version of this book can be downloaded free from http://multilevel.ioe.ac.uk/ download/manuals.html; accessed September 9, 2002.)

Browne WJ (2002). MCMC Estimation in MLwiN, Version 1.0. London: Centre for Multilevel Modelling, University of London. (An electronic version of this book can be downloaded free from http://multilevel.ioe.ac.uk/dev/develop.html; accessed September 9, 2002.)

5

The Quantitative Assessment of
Neighborhood Social Environments

STEPHEN W. RAUDENBUSH

Researchers in social science and public health have become increasingly interested in the social and physical environments of urban neighborhoods. These densely populated residential areas create or constrain opportunities for social interaction and physical exercise. They supply role models and peers, positive or negative, for developing youths. Neighbors may assist parents in child care, but they may also instill fear of crime. Local social networks may aid in job seeking, or they may steer youths away from productive employment. Elderly people may find the local neighborhood a familiar and congenial landscape with gathering places of old friends, but they may find neighborhoods forbidding and alien territories to be avoided whenever possible.

NEIGHBORHOODS AND HEALTH

Scholarly interest in urban neighborhoods coincides with increasing collaboration among social science disciplines and public health. This coincidence in time is not accidental. Jencks and Mayer (1990), Massey and Denton (1993), and Wilson (1987) supply theories and evidence connecting the social organization of neighborhoods with children's cognitive growth, with youths' antisocial behavior, and with adult employment and economic well-being. However, such cognitive, social, and economic outcomes are reliably correlated with mental and physical well-being (Adler et al., 1993; House and Williams, 1996). Understanding the processes that link these outcomes is a major puzzle for research and policy in social welfare and public health.

While neighborhoods may affect health indirectly by influencing human developmental outcomes predictive of health, their effects may be more direct. Predatory crime in neighborhoods poses a clear risk of injury and death. Ambient violence also promotes fear and may increase stress and reduce opportunities for physical activity, with implications for later outcomes such as hypertension and heart disease. Social cohesion may supply social networks that generate social support and useful health-related information (Berkman and Syme, 1979; House et al., 1988; Kaplan et al., 1994). Such networks may also promote transmission of venereal disease, alcoholism, and drug addiction. Pro-social institutions, parks, and churches may both reflect and activate the positive potential of neighborhoods, while a density of liquor stores, bars, adult entertainment stores, and alcohol and tobacco advertisements may reflect a lack of local political power and also promote health-reducing behaviors. Urban neighborhoods will vary in exposures to toxic chemicals such as lead in water, paint, and air; industrial pollutants; and emissions from trucks, buses, and cars.

The Measurement of Neighborhood Characteristics

The preceding paragraphs suggest that neighborhood effects on human development and health occur as a result of differences in neighborhood social organization and certain physical characteristics of neighborhoods. To measure these neighborhood properties requires a variety of active research strategies. Neighborhood social cohesion, norms of social support, perceptions of violence and fear, and active engagement in local institutions are intersubjective phenomena that require perspectives of local residents themselves. Interviewing is a sensible mode of data collection for these processes. In contrast, assessing the presence of bars, public drinking, adult entertainment businesses, tobacco advertising, and toxic chemicals require direct observation. Aspects of social disorder such as abandoned cars and buildings, defaced property, broken glass, garbage, litter, presence of drug paraphernalia, condoms on the street, and public displays of prostitution also require direct observation. Such indicators of disorder directly indicate public health problems (garbage, broken glass, drug paraphernalia), or they may cue criminals that local residents are unwilling or incapable of protecting social order (Wilson and Kelling, 1982) while simultaneously suggesting to local residents that walking in the area is unsafe and unpleasant and therefore to be avoided.

While interviewing and direct observation are the logical modes of data collection for tapping neighborhood processes directly linked to human development and public health, most large-scale quantitative studies of neighborhood effects have, until recently, relied entirely on administrative data sources such as the U.S. decennial census, vital health statistics, and police records. Such administrative data are relatively inexpensive to collect, and they contain scientifically valuable information. They enable broadly replicable studies of the social composition of neighborhoods and the social and spatial distribution of key outcomes including educational attainment, employment, income, and public health outcomes such as birthweight, infant mortality, homicide and suicide rates, disease rates, and mortality. Neighborhood-level data on social composition can be combined with individual data to support multilevel studies of the demographic and spatial distribution of social and health outcomes. Such studies are essential to epidemiology and generate a wealth of empirical associations that cry out for explanation. However, to test such explanations requires specification of relevant neighborhood (as well as person-level) processes. To tap these processes requires data collection beyond administrative records to include interviewing and direct observation.

The Problem of "Ecometrics"

A strategy for neighborhood assessment requires, then, the construction of interview protocols and observation schemes. These will consist of variables such as social cohesion, perceived violence, and social disorder as well as items selected as indicators of those variables. Data from these items must be combined in some way to construct observable measures of the variables of interest. One must assume that the measures will be fallible: they will correspond imperfectly with the variable they are intended to measure. A comprehensive methodology is also required for evaluating the validity and reliability of such imperfect measures of neighborhood properties. This strategy corresponds to the well-developed methodology of psychometrics, the science of assessing the quality of measures of mental functioning. When applied to the assessment of social environments to evaluate ecological rather than psychological measures, we shall refer to this methodology as ecometrics rather than psychometrics (Raudenbush and Sampson, 1999).

Ecometrics can employ statistical methods commonly associated with psychometrics, but the application of these methods requires additional complexity. For example, when we interview or test a participant in a psychological study, we aggregate data across related items to produce measures of that person's skills and attitudes. Item consistency along with the number of items in a scale contribute to reliability. When we use interview data to characterize a neighborhood, we first aggregate across items within a scale to construct a measure of each resident's perceptions. However, our goal is to assess the neighborhood using residents as informants. We therefore aggregate across informants who share residence in the physical space designated as "the neighborhood" in order to characterize that neighborhood. Reliability will depend not only on item consistency and the number of items (which contribute to our understanding of each informant's perceptions), but also on the degree of intersubjective agreement among informants and the number of informants sampled (which contribute to our characterization of the neighborhood these informants share). Suppose, for example, that we could "know" with perfection the perceptions of each resident. Our "psychometric" reliability would be perfect. However, if the residents informing us about their neighborhood had a low level of agreement, such that considerable random variation existed among the responses of residents within the neighborhood, the "ecometric" reliability would tend to be low. We might, however, overcome a comparatively low level of informant agreement by sampling a large number of residents, averaging over the random variation to discern the "signal" of interest, the property of the neighborhood on which residents do agree. The ecometrics of observational data have a similar structure. We might observe certain items on one side of a street (a face-block) of an area designated as "a neighborhood." However, to discern what is shared across the face-blocks of a neighborhood requires aggregation across such local data. The reliability of the assessment will depend on the number of items per measure and their consistency, but also on the consistency of results across face-blocks.

The notion of intersubjective agreement in an interview, or of inter-face-block agreement in an observational study, provides one basis for testing the notion of "neighborhood" that motivates the study. If residents sampled within a spatial area designated a priori as a neighborhood agree no more than what might be expected from any random sample of persons, we have evidence either that the measure at hand is badly flawed or that the concept of neighborhood is an a priori construction with no validity. Similarly, if the face-blocks observed within such an area bear little resemblance to one another, one has a basis for challenging the notion that the aggregation of such face-blocks constitutes a neighborhood. We shall develop other methods for evaluating the construct validity of variables defined on neighborhoods in the material that follows.

Ecometric assessment entails sources of bias not found in psychometric assessment. As we interview adults within each neighborhood, we may find that neighborhoods vary in the types of informants in our sample. It may be, for example, that some neighborhoods yield a large number of elderly informants, while other neighborhoods produce mostly younger informants. We might tend to find that older informants report lower levels of ambient violence in neighborhoods than do younger adult informants—even though all such informants share residence in the same physical area. Presumably, this reporting difference would result from the fact the younger adults spend more time out of the house on the streets and at later hours of the night. This difference in routine activities would produce a difference in perceptions that would masquerade as neighborhood differences unless this tendency of older residents to report less violence were adjusted for statistically. Moreover, it is essential that the adjustment be based on the "within-neighborhood" association (the extent to which age is related to perception within the neighborhood) rather than the "total association" (which includes both the within-neighborhood association and the real difference between neighborhoods that is associated with the fact that some neighborhoods are composed of residents of older age, on average, than other neighborhoods).[1]

Similar biases arise in observational data. Observers will tend to see more adults publicly drinking in the late afternoon than in the early afternoon. If certain neighborhoods are observed later in the afternoon than are others, these "time-of-day" effects will masquerade as neighborhood differences. Such biases should be controlled by design to the extent possible. However, it will generally not be possible to ensure that each neighborhood is observed at exactly the same time of day. Thus, some statistical adjustment is required to control the time-of-day effects not eliminated by design. Other possible sources of bias are day-of-week effects, seasonal effects, and observer effects.

Statistical Analysis

Ecometric assessment is intrinsically multilevel. When neighborhoods are the objects of measurement and interviews supply the data, the lowest level of variation involves items within persons. The sample size at that level is the number of items. The next level of variation involves persons within neighborhoods. The sample size at that level is the number of persons per neighborhood area. The third and highest level of variation is the neighborhood. That sample size is the number of neighborhoods.

When observations of face-blocks are aggregated to construct neighborhoods, three levels of variation also arise. The lowest level of variation involves items within face-blocks. The sample size at that level is the number of items. The next level of variation involves face-blocks within neighborhoods. The sample size at that level is the number of face-blocks sampled within a given neighborhood area. The third and highest level of variation is again the neighborhood.

The statistical model used to assess the reliability and validity of ecometric measures must also be multilevel. We illustrate the modeling

> **Level 1**
>
> * Variation between item responses within each scale for each person
> * Adjusts for missing data and varying item "difficulty"
>
> **Level 2**
>
> * Variation between respondents within neighborhood clusters
> * Adjusts for possible bias arising from: sex, marital status, home ownership, ethnicity, age, years in household, and socioeconomic status of respondent
>
> **Level 3**
>
> * Variation between neighborhood clusters
>
> **Yield**
>
> * Informant agreement as indicated by the intracluster correlation
> * Reliability for discriminating between neighborhood clusters
> * Construct validity in associations with census data, official crime data, and observational data

FIGURE 5–1. Models for uncertainty in assessing neighborhoods: community survey.

framework first with respect to interview data and second with respect to observational data.

ASSESSMENT OF MEASURES BASED ON INTERVIEW DATA

Figure 5–1 shows the structure of the three-level model used in the Project on Human Development in Chicago Neighborhoods (PHDCN) to assess the quality of neighborhood measures based on interviewing.[2] At the first level of analysis, the item response within a person is the outcome. It depends on the person's "true perception" plus a random effect attributable to item inconsistency. Such item inconsistency creates random measurement error within persons. At the second level of analysis, the person's true perceptions vary across persons as a function of the "true neighborhood score" on the variable, plus effects attributable to measured demographic variables, plus random error. The effects of measured demographic variables create potential biases because neighborhoods are likely to vary systematically in the demographic compositions of their samples of informants. The random effects at this second level represent random person-specific inconsistency that increases measurement error at the neighborhood level. Finally, the third and highest level of variation lies between neighborhoods, the units of key interest.

Ecometric Properties

Estimation of the three-level model yields a wealth of useful data about the properties of measures. For each measure we can assess the degree of item inconsistency (the level 1 variance) and the degree of intersubjective disagreement (level 2 variance) as well as the degree of variation of interest, that is, variation between neighborhoods (level 3 variance). Based on these variance components estimates, we can construct a measure of intersubjective agreement, that is, the percentage of variation in peoples' true perceptions that lie between neighborhoods. This is known as the "intracluster correlation," or ICC. Similarly, we can estimate the reliability of measurement of the neighborhood-level measure. This reliability may be computed as

Reliability

$$= \frac{neighborhood\ variance}{neighborhood\ variance + \dfrac{person\ variance}{no.\ of\ persons} + \dfrac{item\ inconsistency}{(no.\ of\ items)^*(no.\ of\ persons)}} \quad (1)$$

This reliability analysis can be extremely useful in the design of new research. If a pilot study shows a large component of variation between persons (that is, low intersubjective agreement), one would tend to plan the main study to include a large sample of informants. On the other hand, a large item inconsistency would suggest increasing the number of items. Based on an estimate of the cost of adding an item relative to the cost of adding a new informant, one might optimize the design, minimizing the denominator of Equation 1 with respect to the number of items, then setting the number of persons per neighborhood large enough to achieve a desired level of reliability.

The multilevel model also enables us to estimate the extent to which survey-based measures are biased by within-neighborhood effects of demographic variables on responses (coefficients associated with level 2 explanatory variables). We may also estimate "item severities" and use these estimates as a check on construct validity, but we defer discussion on this to the section on observational measures.

Some Results for PHDCN's Interview Study

Sampson, Raudenbush, and Earls (1997) used a multilevel research design to construct and evaluate measures of neighborhood social organization. Within each of 343 Chicago neighborhoods, between 20 and 50 households were selected according to a multistage probability sample. The total sample size was 8,782, with a response rate of 75%. Within each household a randomly chosen adult was interviewed concerning conditions and social relationships in the local neighborhood.

Extending this analysis, Table 5–1 displays five scales that tap theoretically relevant aspects of the physical and social properties of neighborhoods as perceived by Chicago residents. Included in Table 5–1 are the items composing each scale, the inter-rater agreement (ICC), and the scale reliability at the neighborhood level.

Table 5–1 reveals that the ICCs are modest, ranging from .13 for informal social control to .36 for social disorder. Because these correlations are variance ratios, it is clear that in no case does most of the variation in ratings lie between neighborhoods. The relatively modest ICCs are similar to those found in other studies that looked at contexts such as schools and even families.

Although the inter-rater agreement appears modest, only a moderate sample size of raters per neighborhood cluster is required to achieve reasonably high inter-rater reliabilities at the neighborhood level. This association between sample size of raters and reliability is graphed in Figure 5–2, for informal social control (which has the lowest inter-rater agreement) and social disorder (which has the highest inter-rater agreement). The curves for the other three measures lie between the two curves in Figure 5–2 because their inter-rater agreements are neither as low as that for informal social control nor as high as that for social disorder. It is clear that sampling 20 raters per neighborhood produces inter-rater reliabilities ranging from .70 to .90, while 40 raters yields reliabilities ranging from .83 to .95. The curves make vividly clear the diminishing returns to investments in raters beyond a given number to yield acceptable reliability.

Further analysis revealed some redundancy among the scales. For example, the correlation between social control and social cohesion, disattenuated for measurement error, was $r = .88$. This result was conceptually sensible. Informal social control taps the extent to which neighbors can be relied upon to intervene to protect the public order. Without some degree of social cohesion, which involves neighbors knowing and trusting one another and having shared values, informal social control would appear impossible. In addition, the exertion of such informal control would likely enhance social cohesion: people get to know each other by working together for common goals. The two sets of items appeared closely linked the larger the notion of collective efficacy (Sampson et al., 1997). Thus, the two measures were combined to create a more parsimonious, reliable, and readily interpretable measure of an ecological construct with strong theoretical connections to crime reduction.

TABLE 5–1. Selected Variables from the PHDCN Community Survey
(8782 respondents; 343 NCs)

Scale	ICC	Reliability
Social Disorder	.36	.89
Litter		
Graffiti		
Vacant or deserted houses		
Drinking in public		
Selling or using drugs		
Teenagers/adults causing trouble		
Perceived Violence	.25	.82
Fights in which a weapon was used		
Violent arguments between neighbors		
Gang fights		
Sexual assaults		
Robbery		
Social Cohesion	.24	.80
Close-knit neighborhood		
Helpful people		
People get along with one another		
People share the same values		
People can be trusted		
Social Control		
Neighbors are willing to:	.13	.74
Do something about children skipping school		
Do something about children painting graffiti		
Do something about children showing disrespect to adults		
Do something about someone being beaten or threatened		
Do something to keep the fire station open		
Neighborhood Decline	.18	.75
Personal safety gotten worse		
Neighborhood looks worse		
People in neighborhood less helpful		
Level of police protection worse		

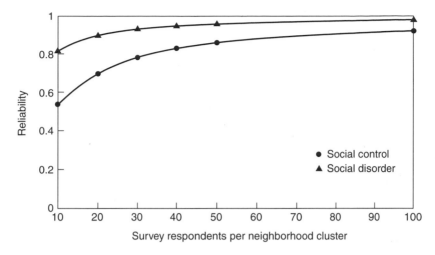

Figure 5–2. Reliabilities of community survey measures of social disorder and social control.

Assessments of Measures Based on Observational Data

We illustrate the logic of direct observation of urban neighborhoods using data designed to measure two variables: physical disorder (10 items) and social disorder (7 items).[3] The first is a scale intended to capture the level of physical disorder, consisting of items indicating the presence or absence of empty beer bottles in the street, sidewalk, or gutter; cigarettes or cigars; drug paraphernalia; condoms; garbage; abandoned cars; and graffiti. Although some of the items were measured initially on an ordinal scale, the data behaved essentially as dichotomous items, coded for analysis as 1 = presence and 0 = absence of the indicator of disorder.

The second scale is intended to capture direct evidence of social disorder. All items were coded from video tape. They include presence of prostitutes, drug sales, adults fighting, drunken adults, public drinking, peer gangs, and adults loitering. In general, indicators of social disorder were present far less frequently than were indicators of physical disorder.

Figure 5–3 shows the structure of the three-level model used in the PHDCN to assess the quality of neighborhood measures based on systematic social observation.[4] At the first level of analysis, the item responses within each face-block person are the outcome. The probability that a given aspect of disorder will arise within that face-block is viewed as depending on the level of disorder (either physical or social) on that face-block at that time plus a random effect attributable to item inconsis-

Level 1

    * Variation between item scores within each scale for each
      face-block
    * Creates an interval scale from binary responses

Level 2

    * Variation between face blocks within neighborhood clusters
    * Adjusts for possible bias arising from time of day

Level 3

    * Variation between neighborhood clusters

Yield

    * Face-block consistency as indicated by the intracluster correlation
    * Reliability for discriminating between neighborhood clusters
    * Construct validity in associations with census data, official
      crime data, and community survey data

FIGURE 5–3. Models for uncertainty in assessing neighborhoods: systematic social observation.

tency. The item inconsistency creates random measurement error within face-blocks. At the second level of analysis, the face-block's level of disorder varies across face-blocks as a function of the "true neighborhood score" on the variable, plus the effect of the time of day of the observation. The effect of time of day creates a potential bias if neighborhoods are observed at different times of day. The random effects at this second level represent random face-block–specific inconsistency that increases measurement error at the neighborhood level. Finally, the third and highest level of variation lies between neighborhoods, the units of key interest.

Ecometric Properties

Estimation of the three-level model yields considerable data about the properties of measures. For each measure we can assess the degree of consistency across face-blocks within a neighborhood (the ICC). Similarly, we can estimate the reliability of measurement of the neighborhood-level measure. This reliability may be computed as

$$\text{Reliability} = \frac{\textit{neighborhood variance}}{\textit{neighborhood variance} + \dfrac{\textit{face}-\textit{block variance}}{\textit{n of face}-\textit{blocks}} + \dfrac{\textit{item inconsistency}}{\textit{(no. of items)}^*\textit{(no. of face}-\textit{blocks)}}} \tag{2}$$

As in the case of interview data, this reliability analysis can be useful in the design of new research. If a pilot study shows a large component of variation between face-blocks, one would be inclined to plan the main study to include a large sample of face-blocks. On the other hand, a large item inconsistency would suggest increasing the number of items. Based on cost estimates, one might optimize the design to minimize the denominator of equation 2 with respect to the number of items, then set the face-blocks per neighborhood large enough to a achieve a desired level of reliability.

Two other summaries of evidence are useful. The item-response model at level 1 identifies "item severities." These are the log-odds of observing a given indicator of disorder, holding constant the true level of disorder of the face-block. One can examine these severities to see whether indicators viewed theoretically as severe (e.g., observing needles and syringes) do, in fact, have higher severities than items viewed theoretically as less severe (e.g., seeing garbage on the street).

Finally, the example below is multivariate: two kinds of disorder (physical and social) are of interest. One would want to know how strongly correlated these are, after taking into account measurement error. If the correlation is sufficiently high, one might view the two variables as reflecting a single underlying dimension.

Some Results for PHDCN's Observational Study

Item severity

In Table 5–2, items with negative coefficients have low probabilities of occurrence and thus are rarer and, presumably, more "difficult," or "severe," than are items with positive coefficients. Thus, in the physical disorder scale, the presence of cigarettes or cigars and garbage on the street or sidewalk, along with the presence of empty beer bottles, are comparatively less severe than the presence of gang graffiti, abandoned cars, condoms, or drug paraphernalia (needles and syringes). Thus, item severity conforms to intuitive expectations. The exception is political graffiti, which is exceptionally rare yet not generally regarded as especially severe. A nice feature of the physical disorder scale is that the item severities vary substantially, a feature of a "well-behaved" scale.

In contrast, all of the severities in the social disorder scale are clumped at the severe end except for the item indicating adults loitering or congregating. Although the item severities are not well separated, their ordering does correspond to theoretical expectation, with adults loitering and drinking alcohol being less severe than adults fighting, prostitution, or drug sales.

TABLE 5–2. Model Fitting Results: Item Severity at Face-Block Level

Item	Coefficient	SE
Physical Disorder		
Intercept	−2.215	0.225
Cigarettes, cigars on street or gutter	3.456	0.032
Garbage or litter on street or sidewalk	2.431	0.031
Empty beer bottles visible in street	1.126	0.032
Tagging graffiti	0.338	0.036
Graffiti painted over	(0)	(reference item)
Gang graffiti	−0.667	0.043
Abandoned cars	−1.297	0.046
Condoms on sidewalk	−2.569	0.071
Needles/syringes on sidewalk	−2.893	0.082
Political message graffiti	−5.028	0.269
Social Disorder		
Intercept	−7.017	(0.153)
Adults loitering or congregating	3.884	(0.227)
People drinking alcohol	0.590	(0.280)
Peer group, gang indicators present	(0)	(reference item)
People intoxicated	−0.106	(0.325)
Adults fighting or hostilely arguing	−0.512	(0.366)
Prostitutes on street	−0.599	(0.376)
People selling drugs	−0.696	(0.388)

Time of day

Table 5–3 provides estimates of the effects of time of day. One would expect social interactions in public view to occur with relatively little frequency early in the morning and more frequently later on. This would presumably be true of those social interactions indicative of disorder as well, and that is what the results show. Note that there is a near linear positive trend in time for social disorder with coefficients of −0.766, −0.715, −0.363, −0.057, −0.134, and 0.000 as the day progresses. No such trend is apparent in the case of physical disorder. All other model estimates are adjusted for any time-of-day effects.

TABLE 5–3. Model Fitting Results: Time of Day Effects at NC Level (N = 80)

Item	Coefficient	SE
Physical Disorder		
7:00–8:59	0.213	0.043
9:00–10:59	0.036	0.031
11:00–12:59	0.057	0.036
1:00–2:59	0.073	0.040
3:00–4:59	0.020	0.033
5:00–6:59	(0)	(reference time)
Social Disorder		
7:00–8:59	−0.766	0.180
9:00–10:59	−0.715	0.115
11:00–12:59	−0.363	0.137
1:00–2:59	−0.057	0.129
3:00–4:59	−0.134	0.107
5:00–6:59	(0)	(reference time)

Variance–covariance components and related quantities:
physical disorder
Estimation of the variance–covariance components provides the necessary data to compute useful indicators of data quality. For physical disorder the estimated variance between face-blocks is 0.734, while the estimated variance between NC's is 0.475. Thus, the estimated ICC for physical disorder is 0.475/(0.475 + 0.734) = 0.39. Thus, about 39% of the variation in the physical disorder of face-blocks is estimated to be between NC's. This fact, when combined with the typical frequency of "yes" responses and the large number of face-blocks per NC, yields a high average reliability of 0.98 at the NC level. Thus, the data enable us too distinguish among NC's with high reliability. The reliability for distinguishing among face-blocks within NC's is estimated to be much lower, at 0.36. This reflects the dependance of the reliability at the face-block level on the number of items. More items would be required to increase this reliability.

Variance–covariance components and related quantities:
social disorder
The social disorder scale behaves quite differently. The point estimate of
the variance within NC's for social disorder is zero. This result does not
imply that face-blocks within NC's are homogeneous. Rather, the result
appears to reflect the extreme rarity of "yes" responses to most social disorder items. The data are simply too sparse at the face-block level to facilitate stable estimation of variance between face-blocks within NC's, yet
the variation between NCs is quite substantial, leading to a respectable
NC-level reliability estimate of 0.84. Although the frequency of indicators
of social disorder is rare at the face-block level, when we aggregate over
the many face-blocks within an NC, we are able to achieve a respectable
between-NC reliability.

Implications for research design
Applying the logic of generalizability analysis, we can use our data to inform the design of new research. Figure 5–4 plots the expected NC-level
reliability of the two scales as a function of the number of face-blocks sampled. For physical disorder there appears to be little point in sampling
more than 80 to 100 face-blocks per NC if the sole aim is to obtain reasonable NC reliability. The same is not true for social disorder. More face-
blocks are required for adequate reliability in measuring social disorder
(as compared to physical disorder).

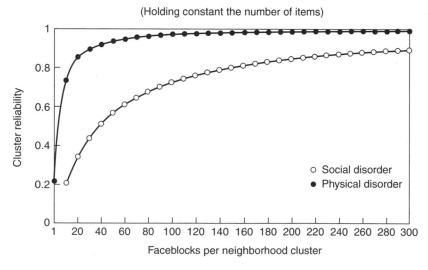

FIGURE 5–4. NC reliability as a function of face-blocks sampled.

Physical disorder results provide good news for the next analyses of the PHDCN data. It is clear that physical disorder can be reliably measured at much lower levels of aggregation than the NC. Thus, it is feasible to construct physical disorder measures at the level of the block group or census tract,[5] creating a measure that is more proximal geographically to the longitudinal cohort subjects of PHDCN than is the NC. Our results are less encouraging about the measurement of social disorder at lower levels of aggregation because of the low frequency of "yes" responses on most social disorder items.

Dimensionality
The correlation between physical disorder and social disorder is estimated to be .58. This is the estimated correlation of the two latent variables and is therefore automatically adjusted for measurement error in each. The implication is that physical and social disorder as conceived here are quite strongly related, although not so strongly as to be viewed as a single dimension. There is reason to pursue sound measures of each construct separately.

Convergent and divergent validity
Key tests of validity of measurement involve assessing correlations with theoretically related constructs measured independently. Convergent validity implies that theoretically linked measures ought to correlate highly. Divergent validity implies that correlations should be smaller with variables that are not clearly linked theoretically.

Observed physical disorder is correlated highly with those constructs measured in both the community survey (described earlier) and the independent sources (census data, official police records) most theoretically linked to it. Thus, we see (Table 5–4) that a substantial correlation (r = .71) emerges with perceptions of social disorder as measured in the community survey. SSO physical disorder is also moderately strongly correlated with the survey measures of social cohesion and social control (r = −.62 and r = −.55, respectively) in the direction expected. Physical disorder also correlates less strongly with those survey-derived constructs for which it has a weaker theoretical connection (e.g., anonymity, intergenerational ties, organizational density).

Turning next to construct validation with other independent sources, physical disorder is strongly related to census measures of concentrated poverty (r = .64) and less strongly with residential stability (r = −.25) and immigrant concentration (r = .36). (See Sampson et al. [1997] for further details of these census-based factors.) As expected, the observed physical disorder is significantly higher in neighborhoods characterized by

TABLE 5–4. Correlations of Systematic Social Observation (SSO) Scales with Theoretically Related Variables from the U.S. Census and Community Survey

	SSO	
	Physical Disorder	*Social Disorder*
I. Community survey		
Social disorder	.71	.65
Social cohesion	−.62	−.55
Social control	−.55	−.56
II. U.S. census		
Concentrated poverty	.64	.54
Residential stability	−.25	−.34
Immigrant concentration	.36	.21
III. Violence and crime		
Perceived violence	.54	.59
Crime victimization	.32	.33

poverty, instability, and areas undergoing ethnic transition. Furthermore, physical disorder measured in the SSO is positively and significantly correlated with survey perceptions of violence ($r = .54$) and aggregated reports of victimization ($r = .32$). These patterns conform to extant theory on urban disorder and crime (Taub et al., 1984; Taylor et al., 1985; Sampson and Groves, 1989; Skogan, 1990).

A similar pattern of correlations appears with respect to social disorder. In some cases the magnitude of the correlations is a bit smaller than those involving physical disorder, which may reflect the less sanguine behavior of the social disorder scale. Nonetheless, the SSO measure of social disorder has quite robust relationships with theoretically linked constructs—again whether derived from the neighborhood survey or census. Taken together, then, the multiple sources of data provide independent evidence of both the convergent and divergent validity of SSO measures of disorder.

CONCLUSION

As interest in the social sciences and public health turns increasingly to the integration of individual, family, and neighborhood processes, a potential mismatch arises in the quality of measures. Standing behind individual measurement are decades of research, producing measures that often have excellent statistical properties. In contrast, much less is known about measures of ecological settings such as neighborhoods, and the methodology needed to evaluate these measures is in its infancy. The aim of this chapter has been to adapt tools from psychometrics to improve the quality of ecometric measures.

An extension to the approach sketched in this chapter would take into account spatial autocorrelation. In this chapter neighborhood clusters have been treated as independent.[6] Ongoing work will build spatial associations into the models presented here. We expect information about spatial dependence to reduce standard errors of measurement, possibly substantially, and to make it possible to obtain reasonable measures of neighborhood ecology even for persons residing in areas sparsely assessed by direct observation. In the meantime, the results of the present analysis suggest that the survey and SSO approaches hold considerable promise for the reliable and valid assessment of neighborhood-level social processes.

ACKNOWLEDGMENTS

A more technical presentation of the methodology described here appears in Raudenbush and Sampson (1999). The research reported here was supported by the Project on Human Development in Chicago Neighborhoods (PHDCN), with funding from the National Institute of Justice and the John D. and Catherine T. MacArthur Foundation. We thank Felton Earls, Albert J. Reiss, Jr., and Steven Buka for their essential role in the design of PHDCN, and Richard Congdon for the programming of all computations. Meng-Li Yang checked the derivations and computed all results.

NOTES

1. Raudenbush and Bryk (2002, Chapter 5) describe in detail the differences between the a) within-group regression coefficient, b) the between-group coefficient, and c) the total coefficient.

2. Sampson, Raudenbush, and Earls (1997) used these measures to test theories about neighborhood collective efficacy and violence, violent victimization, and homicide. Raudenbush and Sampson (1999) developed methods for taking into account the measurement error at the neighborhood level in studying direct and indirect effects of such measures. Sampson, Morenoff, and Earls (1999) considered the spatial distribution of neighborhood resources for child development.

3. Between June and September 1995 observers trained by the National Opinion Research Center (NORC) drove a sport utility vehicle at a rate of five miles per hour down every street within the 80 sample NCs. As the NORC team drove down the street, a pair of video recorders, one located on each side of the vehicle, captured social activities and physical features of both face-blocks simultaneously. Also, at the same time, the two trained observers—one on each side of the vehicle—recorded their observations onto an observer log for each face-block.

Certain items were coded from videotapes while others were based on this observer log. See Raudenbush and Sampson (1999) for details. The overall sample sizes included 23,816 face-blocks and 80 neighborhood clusters.

4. Raudenbush and Sampson (1999) developed the statistical model for this example in some detail. This is a three-level model in which logit link function and a Bernoulli sampling model relate the level-1 outcome to the item effects plus a random intercept for each variable being measured. The intercepts vary between persons within neighborhoods and across neighborhoods at the next two levels according to multivariate normal distributions specified at each level. The authors also discuss problems of estimation theory and propose an accurate and computationally fast approximation to maximum likelihood. Sampson and Raudenbush (1999) used these data to assess theories about the relationship between physical evidence of disorder in urban neighborhoods and crime.

5. Indeed, subsequent analysis showed that the reliabilities of the physical disorder at the census tract level were nearly identical to those at the level of the NC, even though there are two to three tracts per NC.

6. This assumption is not entirely implausible in the case of the SSO, which involves a probability sample of 80 NCs from among 343 NCs in Chicago. Many of the sample NCs are not contiguous to other sample NCs. Nevertheless, a more complete treatment would model spatial dependence between NCs.

REFERENCES

Adler NE, Boyce T, Chesney MA, Folkman S, Syme SL (1993). Socioeconomic inequalities in health: No easy solution. *JAMA* 269: 3140–3145.

Berkman LF and Syme SL (1979). Social networks, host resistance, and mortality: A nine-year follow-up study of Alameda County Residents. *Am J Epidemiol* 109: 1886–2204.

House JS, Landis KR, Umberson D (1988). Social relationships and health. *Science* 241: 540–545.

House JS and Williams DR (1996). Psychosocial pathways linking SES and CVD. In *Report of the Conference on Socioeconomic Status and Cardiovascular Health and Disease*, November 6–7, 1995. National Institutes of Health, National Heart, Lung and Blood Institute, pp. 119–124.

Jencks C and Mayer SE (1990). The social consequences of growing up in a poor neighborhood. In Lynn LE and McGeary MFH, eds.: *Inner-City Poverty in the United States*. Washington, DC: National Academy Press, pp. 111–186.

Kaplan GA, Wilson TW, Cohen RD (1994). Social functioning and overall mortality: Prospective evidence from the Kuopio Ischemic Heart Disease Risk Factor Study. *Epidemiology* 5: 4985–5000.

Massey D and Denton N (1993). *American Apartheid: Segregation and the Making of the Underclass*. Cambridge, Mass: Harvard University Press.

National Opinion Research Center (1995). *PHDCN Project 4709: Systematic Social Observation Coding Manual, June 1995*. Chicago: NORC/University of Chicago.

Raudenbush SW and Bryk AS (2002). *Hierarchial Lines Notes: Applications and Data Analysis Methods*, Second Edition. Newbury Park, CA: Sage Publications.

Raudenbush SW and Sampson RJ (1999). Ecometrics: Toward a science of assessing ecological settings, with application to the systematic social observation of neighborhoods. *Sociological Methodology* 29: 1–41.

Sampson RJ, Morenoff JD, Earls F (1999). Beyond social capital: Spatial dynamics of collective efficacy for children. *American Sociology Review* 64: 633–660.

Sampson RJ and Groves W (1989). Community structure and crime: Testing Social-disorganization theory. *American Journal of Sociology* 94: 774–802.

Sampson RJ, Raudenbush SW, Earls F (1997). Neighborhoods and violent crime: A multilevel study of collective efficacy. *Science* 277: 918–924.

Skogan W (1990). *Disorder and Decline: Crime and the Spiral of Decay in American Neighborhoods.* Berkeley: University of California Press.

Taub R, Taylor DG, Dunham J (1984). *Paths of Neighborhood Change: Race and Crime in Urban America.* Chicago: University of Chicago Press.

Taylor RB, Gottfredson SD, Brower S (1984). Block crime and fear: Defensible space, local social ties, and territorial functioning." *Journal of Research in Crime and Delinquency* 21: 303–331.

Wilson JQ and Kelling G (1982). The police and neighborhood safety: Broken windows. Atlantic 127: 29–38.

Wilson WJ (1987). *The Truly Disadvantaged: The Inner City, the Underclass, and Public Policy.* Chicago: University of Chicago Press.

6

Neighborhood-Level Context and Health: Lessons from Sociology

Robert J. Sampson

A long-standing body of research supports the association of multiple health-related outcomes with the socioeconomic characteristics of neighborhoods and local communities. Why are so many health-related outcomes concentrated ecologically? A new generation of neighborhood-level research has emerged in recent years to address this question. The goal of this chapter is to highlight the implications of such research for our knowledge about the community-level context of public health and safety. In particular, I draw on recent lessons from sociological research to identify what it is about neighborhoods, above and beyond the status and attributes of the individuals who live there, that might lead to various health outcomes.

A Brief History of Community Research

The study of local community environments and health has a long lineage in both sociology and public health. In sociology, the urban ecological approach of the Chicago School brought neighborhood-centered research to the fore of the discipline during the early twentieth century. One influential element of this tradition was Shaw and McKay's (1942) theory of neighborhood social disorganization. Although focusing on delinquency, Shaw and McKay constructed a general framework for understanding how community processes relate to a wide range of outcomes, including health. Community social disorganization was conceptualized as the inability of a community structure to realize the common values of its residents and maintain effective social control. Social control refers to the capacity of a social unit to regulate itself according to desired principles and to realize collective goals (Janowitz, 1975). Typical common goals include the desire of residents to live in neighborhoods character- ized by economic sufficiency, good schools, adequate housing, freedom from predatory crime, and a healthy environment.

Shaw and McKay (1942) argued that delinquency was not an isolated phenomenon and showed in their research the association between com- munities and health. In particular, Chicago neighborhoods characterized by poverty, residential instability, and dilapidated housing were found to suffer disproportionately high rates of infant mortality, delinquency, crime, low birth weight, tuberculosis, physical abuse, and other factors detrimental to health. In another seminal study Faris and Dunham (1939) applied the concept of social disorganization to mental health, arguing that disorganized areas had disproportionately high rates of hospitaliza- tion for mental disorders. Interestingly, both Shaw and McKay and Faris and Dunham observed that high rates of adverse outcomes tended to per- sist in the same communities over time despite the movement of differ- ent population groups through them. From these findings the Chicago School sociologists concluded that neighborhoods possess relatively en- during features that transcend the idiosyncratic characteristics of partic- ular ethnic groups that inhabit them—so-called emergent properties. In any event, what makes the Chicago School framework relevant to con- temporary concerns is its theoretical emphasis on the characteristics of *places* rather than *people*.

Community environments were a focus of early epidemiologic re- search as well. An example of this tradition is the research of Goldberger and his colleagues on pellagra in southern villages. In a classic study of family income and the incidence of pellagra, Goldberger et al. (1920) found that the probability of contracting pellagra was related not only to individual-level socioeconomic status but also to the availability of nu- tritional foods in villages. They amassed an impressive array of both in- dividual- and village-level data relating to food supply and malnutrition that included village-level measures of the prevalence of retail grocery es- tablishments and home-provided foods and contrasts in the type of agri- culture in farm areas surrounding the villages.

Social characteristics continue to vary systematically across commu- nities along dimensions of socioeconomic status (e.g., poverty, wealth, oc- cupational attainment), family structure and life cycle (e.g., female-headed households, child density), residential stability (e.g., home ownership and tenure), and race–ethnic composition (e.g., segregation). In fact, the evi- dence shows that the ecological concentration of poverty and inequality increased in American neighborhoods during the 1980s and 1990s (Wil- son, 1987, 1996; Massey and Denton, 1993).

There is an unfortunate parallel in health regarding ecological concentration; the "comorbidity," or spatial clustering of homicide, infant mortality, low birth weight, accidental injury, and suicide, continues to the present day. In the period from 1995 to 1996, for example, data from Chicago revealed that census tracts with high homicide rates tended to be spatially contiguous to other tracts high in homicide. Perhaps more interesting, more than 75% of such tracts also contained a high level of clustering for low birth weight and infant mortality, and more than 50% for accidental injuries (Sampson, 2001). Suicide was more distinct, although even it showed that spatial clustering was significant. The ecological concentration of homicide, low birth weight, infant mortality, and injury indicates that there may be geographic "hot spots" for a number of unhealthy outcomes. The range of adolescent outcomes correlated with multiple forms of concentrated disadvantage is also quite wide and included teenage childbearing, low academic achievement and educational failure, maltreatment, and delinquency (see, e.g., Brooks-Gunn et al., 1997).

A growing body of research has examined community characteristics and *individual-level* health. Although the evidence is mixed and the magnitudes often small, a number of studies have linked health outcomes to neighborhood context even when individual attributes and behaviors are taken into account, including coronary risk factors and heart disease mortality, low birth weight, smoking, morbidity, all-cause mortality, and self-reported health (for a review see Robert, 1998, 1999). Of course, correlational and observational studies suffer well-known weaknesses with respect to making causal inferences. It may be that individuals with poor health selectively migrate to, or are left behind in, poor neighborhoods. If so, the observed correlations between community characteristics and health may simply be a reflection of the unmeasured processes through which individuals sort themselves into different neighborhoods (Manski, 1995).

To address this problem, researchers have begun to explore community-level effects on health outcomes with experimental and quasi-experimental research designs. One such example is found in the Moving to Opportunity (MTO) program, a series of housing experiments in five cities that randomly assigned housing project residents to one of three groups: an experimental group receiving housing subsidies to move into low-poverty neighborhoods, a group receiving conventional (Section 8) housing assistance, and a control group receiving no special assistance. A study from the Boston MTO site showed that children of mothers in the experimental group had significantly lower prevalences of injuries, asthma attacks, and personal victimization during follow-up. The move to low-poverty neighborhoods also resulted in significant improvements in the physical and mental health status of household heads (Katz et al., 1999). Because the experimental design was used to control individual-level risk factors, a reasonable inference is that an improvement in community socioeconomic environment leads to better health outcomes.

In summary, research in the social and behavioral sciences has established a reasonably consistent set of findings relevant to the community context of health. Although causality and magnitude are still at issue, there seems to be broad agreement that (1) considerable inequality exists between neighborhoods and local communities along multiple dimensions of socioeconomic status, (2) a number of health problems tend to cluster together in geographically defined ecological units such as neighborhoods or local community areas, (3) these two phenomena are themselves related—community-level predictors common to many health-related outcomes include concentrated poverty and/or affluence, racial segregation, family disruption, residential instability, and poor-quality housing—and (4) the relationship between community context and health outcomes—especially all-cause mortality, depression, and violence—appears to persist when controls are introduced for individual-level risk factors.

SOCIAL CAPITAL THEORY AND BEYOND

The spatial patterning of crime and health provides a potentially important clue in thinking about why it is that neighborhoods might matter for health. Namely, if multiple and seemingly disparate health outcomes are linked together empirically across communities and are predicted by similar structural characteristics, there may be common underlying causes or mediating mechanisms at the neighborhood level. For example, if "neighborhood effects" of concentrated poverty on health actually exist, they presumably stem from social processes that involve collective aspects of neighborhood life such as social cohesion, spatial diffusion, support networks, and informal social control. The theory of social capital addresses such social processes in a more rigorous manner than did the early Chicago School focus on disorganization.

Although he was not the originator of the idea, Coleman (1990) defined social capital as a resource stemming from the structure of social relationships, which in turn facilitate the achievement of specific goals. Such resources, be they actual or potential, are often linked to durable social networks (Bourdieu, 1986). Putnam defines social capital more expansively to include not only the networks themselves but also shared norms and mutual trust, which "facilitate coordination and cooperation for mutual benefit" (1993, p. 36). One form of social capital relevant to health is *reciprocal obligations* among neighbors, which create a source of "credit" that individuals can draw upon when in need of a favor (Coleman, 1990, pp. 306–310). A second form of social capital occurs when social relations are used to *exchange information.* Neighbors sometimes provide one another with advice, tips, and other types of information that might otherwise be costly to acquire. A third form is *intergenerational closure.* When parents know the parents of their children's friends, they have the potential to observe the children's actions in different circumstances, talk to one another about the children, compare notes, and establish rules (Coleman, 1988). Such intergenerational closure provides parents and children with social capital of a collective nature. Coleman also argued that *voluntary associations* can generate social capital, either intentionally, by generating community action around a specific purpose, or unintentionally, by creating new ties among people that are then used to facilitate other types of action.

Recent work bearing on public health has set out to clarify, extend, and operationalize the concept of social capital, a trend particularly evident in the fields of epidemiology, criminology, and urban sociology. In epidemiology the recent application of social capital to understanding variations in health has focused largely on norms that encourage cooperation and facilitate social cohesion. Drawing on Putnam (1993) perhaps more so than Coleman, Kawachi and Berkman (2000) argue that the core meaning of social capital is tied to the broader notion of *social cohesion,* which refers to the absence of social conflict coupled with the presence of strong social bonds and mutual trust. A small but intriguing body of research exists linking cohesion to health-related outcomes, although usually at higher levels of aggregation than a neighborhood. For example, measures of social cohesion and trust have been found to predict mortality rates at the state level. Kawachi et al. (1997) reported that the level of distrust (the percentage of residents in a state who agree that most people cannot be trusted) was strongly correlated with the age-adjusted mortality rate ($r = .79$, $p < .001$). Lower levels of trust were associated with higher rates of most major causes of death, including coronary heart disease, unintentional injury, and cerebrovascular disease. A negative association between levels of trust–cohesion and homicide rates was found at the state level as well (Kawachi et al., 1998). Kawachi et al. (1999) also found a relationship between state-level social capital and individual self-rated health. Specifically, controlling for individual risk factors (e.g., smoking, obesity, income, lack of access to health care), individuals living in states with low levels of social capital (low trust, reciprocity, and voluntary associations) exhibited a significantly greater risk of poor self-rated health.

A rich line of research on social networks in the fields of both health and urban sociology shares a natural affinity with the surge of interest in neighborhood social capital. Much evidence reveals that friendship ties and family social support networks promote individual health (Berkman and Syme, 1979; House et al., 1988). In addition, contrary to the popular belief that metropolitan life leads inexorably to the decline of personal ties, sociological research has shown that while urbanites may be exposed to more unconventionality and diversity, they retain a set of personal support networks just like their suburban and rural counterparts (e.g., Fischer, 1982). The difference is that the social ties of city dwellers tend to be more spatially dispersed. In other words, social ties are alive and well in American cities and appear to be a protective factor in health, even if these social ties are not as geographically concentrated as in the past.

At the same time, however, local social ties (whether urban or rural in nature) do not necessarily translate into high social capital at the neighborhood level. Wilson (1996) argued that many poor neighborhoods with strong social ties do not produce collective resources such as the social control of disorderly behavior. His research suggests that disadvantaged urban neighborhoods are places where dense webs of social ties among neighbors actually impede social organization: "(I)t appears that what many impoverished and dangerous neighborhoods have in common is a relatively high degree of social integration (high levels of local neighboring while being relatively isolated from contacts in broader mainstream society) and low levels of informal social control (feelings that they have little control over their immediate environment, including the environment's negative influences on their children)" (Wilson, 1996, pp. 63–64). Although members of such communities share strong social linkages with one another, they remain socially isolated, in Wilson's terms, because their network ties do not extend beyond immediate social environs to include *non*–community members and institutions. The limits of tight-knit social bonds were recognized earlier in Granovetter's (1973) seminal essay on the strength of "weak ties" in obtaining job referrals. Whether or not weak ties promote health is unknown.

Collective Efficacy

The research on cohesion and social ties reveals something of a paradox. First, many urbanites have an abundance of friends and social support networks that are not organized in a parochial, local fashion. Second, urbanites whose "strong ties" *are* tightly restricted geographically may actually produce an environment that discourages collective responses to local problems. To address this seeming anomaly, Sampson et al. (1997, 1999) have proposed a focus on mechanisms that facilitate social control without requiring strong ties or associations. As Warren (1975, p. 50) noted, the common belief that neighborhoods have declined in importance as social units "is predicated on the assumption that neighborhood is exclusively a primary group and therefore should possess the 'face-to-face,' intimate, affective relations which characterize all primary groups." Sampson et al. (1997) reject this outmoded assumption and highlight, instead, working trust and the shared willingness of local residents to intervene in support of public order. Personal ties notwithstanding, it is the linkage of mutual trust and shared expectations for intervening on behalf of the common good that defines the neighborhood context of what Sampson et al. (1997) term *collective efficacy*. Just as individuals vary in their capacity for efficacious action, they argue that so, too, do neighborhoods vary in their capacity to achieve common goals. Moreover, just as self-efficacy is situated rather than global (one has self-efficacy relative to a particular task or type of task), neighborhood efficacy exists relative to collective tasks, such as maintaining public order.

Sampson et al. (1999) thus view social capital as referring to the resources or potential inherent in social networks, whereas collective efficacy is a task-specific construct that refers to shared expectations and mutual engagement by residents in local social control. Moving away from a focus on private ties, the term *collective efficacy* signifies an emphasis on shared beliefs in a neighborhood's conjoint capability for action to achieve an intended effect, and hence an active sense of engagement on the part of residents. As Bandura (1997) argues, the meaning of efficacy is captured in expectations about the exercise of control, elevating the "agentic" aspect of social life over a perspective centered on the accumulation of "stocks" of social resources. This conception of collective efficacy is consistent with the redefinition of social capital by Portes and Sensenbrenner in terms of "expectations for action within a collectivity" (1993, p. 1323).

The theory of collective efficacy was tested in a survey of 8782 residents of 343 Chicago neighborhoods in 1995. A five-item Likert-type scale measured shared expectations about "informal social control." Residents were asked about the likelihood that their neighbors could be counted on to take action if: (1) children were skipping school and hanging out on a street corner, (2) children were spray-painting graffiti on a local building, (3) children were showing disrespect to an adult, (4) a fight broke out in front of their house, and (5) the fire station closest to home was threatened with budget cuts. "Social cohesion/trust" was measured by asking respondents whether they agreed (or disagreed) that "People around here are willing to help their neighbors"; "This is a close-knit neighborhood"; "People in this neighborhood can be trusted"; "People in this neighborhood generally don't get along with each other"; and "People in this neighborhood do not share the same values." Social cohesion and informal social control were strongly related across neighborhoods and thus combined into a summary measure of "collective efficacy."

Collective efficacy was associated with lower rates of violence, controlling for concentrated disadvantage, residential stability, immigrant concentration, and a set of individual-level characteristics (e.g., age, sex, socioeconomic status, race–ethnicity, home ownership). Whether measured by official homicide events or violent victimization as reported by residents, neighborhoods high in collective efficacy had significantly lower rates of violence. This finding held up controlling for earlier neighborhood violence that may have depressed later collective efficacy (e.g., because of fear); a two standard-deviation elevation in collective efficacy was associated with a 26 percent reduction in the expected homicide rate (Sampson et al., 1997, p. 922). The association of disadvantage and stability with violence was also reduced when collective efficacy was controlled. In particular, collective efficacy appears to be undermined by the concentration of disadvantage, racial segregation, family disruption, and residential instability (Sampson et al. 1997, 1999). The cross-sectional nature of the data and the likelihood of reciprocality (e.g., crime may reduce collective efficacy) mean that causal effects could not be reliably determined. Nonetheless, these patterns are consistent with the notion that neighborhood characteristics influence violence in part through collective efficacy.

Institutions and Public Control

A theory of social capital and collective efficacy should not ignore institutions, or the wider political environment in which local communities are embedded. Communities can exhibit intense private ties and shared expectations yet still lack the institutional capacity to achieve social control (Hunter, 1985; Woolcock, 1998). The institutional component of social capital is the resource stock of neighborhood organizations and their linkages with other organizations, both within *and* outside the community (Sampson, 2001). When the links among institutions within a community are weak, the capacity to defend local interests is weakened. Similar to the idea of "bridging" social capital, Bursik and Grasmick (1993) also highlight the importance of *public* control, defined as the capacity of local community organizations to obtain extra-local resources (e.g., police services, fire protection; block grants; health services) that help sustain neighborhood stability and control. Hunter (1985) identifies the dilemma of public control in a civil society. According to Hunter (1985), local communities must work together with forces of public control to achieve social order, principally through interdependence among private (family), parochial (neighborhood), and public (State) institutions, such as the police and schools.

Caveat

Any discussion of social capital needs to acknowledge its potential downside. After all, social networks can be drawn upon for negative as well as positive goals—the same strong social ties that benefit members of one particular group can be used to exclude others outside the group from sharing in those resources (Portes, 1998, p. 15). As but one example, racial exclusion is not desirable, yet dense social networks have often been used to facilitate segregation. Social capital (and by implication, collective efficacy) may thus be said to have a valence depending on the goal in question (Sandefur and Laumann, 1998, p. 493). Recognizing the valence of social capital, Sampson et al. (1999) apply the nonexclusivity requirement of a social good (Coleman, 1990, pp. 315–316) to judge whether neighborhood structures serve the collective needs of residents. Resources such as neighborhood safety and healthy environments produce positive externalities (Coleman, 1990, pp. 250–251) that are consensually desired but problematically achieved, owing in large part to variabilities in structural constraints. However, even if health and safety are consensually desired, there may be conflicts over the setting of priorities when resources are limited. For example, in some contexts disagreement over whether a violence-reduction program or a toxic waste cleanup deserves priority would lead to paralysis and not to collective action. As with the existence of strong ties, consensus on ultimate goals does not automatically lead to enhanced outcomes. Social capital and collective efficacy should therefore not be viewed as some all-purpose elixir but as normatively situated and endogenous to specific structural contexts (Sampson et al., 1999).

RECENT DEVELOPMENTS IN NEIGHBORHOOD RESEARCH

Research on the political economy of American cities has shown that the stratification of places is shaped, both directly and indirectly, by the extralocal decisions of public officials and businesses. For example, the decline of many central-city neighborhoods has been facilitated not only by individual preferences, as manifested in voluntary migration patterns, but by governmental decisions on public housing that concentrate the poor, incentives for suburban sprawl in the form of tax breaks for developers and private mortgage assistance, highway construction, economic disinvestment in central cities, and haphazard land use zoning (Logan and Molotch, 1987).

The embeddedness of neighborhoods within the larger system of citywide spatial dynamics is equally relevant (Sampson et al., 1999). Recent research on population change shows that population abandonment is driven as much by spatial diffusion processes (e.g., changes in proximity to violent crime) as by the internal characteristics of neighborhoods (Morenoff and Sampson, 1997). In particular, housing decisions are often made by assessing the quality of neighborhoods relative to what is happening in surrounding areas. Parents with young children appear quite sensitive to the relative location of neighborhoods and schools in addition to their internal characteristics. Spatial diffusion processes for dimensions of social capital are even more likely, mainly because social networks and exchange processes unfold across the artificial boundaries of analytically defined neighborhoods. A neighborhood-level perspective on health cannot afford to ignore the relative geographic position of neighborhoods and how that bears on internal dimensions of social capital. The importance of spatial externalities is shown by the finding that ecological proximity to areas high in collective efficacy bestows an advantage above and beyond the structural characteristics of a given neighborhood (Sampson et al., 1999).

A concern with community ecology suggests another often-overlooked mechanism in discussions of neighborhood effects—how land use patterns and the ecological structure of daily routine activities bear on well-being. The location of schools, the mix of residential with commercial land use (e.g., strip malls, bars), public transportation nodes, and large flows of nighttime visitors, for example, are relevant to organizing how and when children come into contact with other peers, adults, and nonresident activity. The "routine activities" perspective in criminology provides the important insight that predatory violence requires the intersection in time and space of motivated offenders and suitable targets and the absence of capable guardians (Cohen and Felson, 1979). The routine activity approach assumes a steady supply of motivated "offenders" and focuses instead on how targets of opportunity and guardianship combine to explain criminal events. This strategy has appeal in thinking about a range of adolescent health behaviors, such as drinking, early sexual behavior, and smoking, that reflect natural desires yet can yield negative outcomes both personally and for others (e.g., teenage childbearing, low birth weight, low achievement, poor health). For example, not only do mixed-use neighborhoods offer greater opportunities for expropriative crime, they offer increased opportunity for children to congregate outside the home in places conducive to peer-group influence (Sampson, 2001).

In short, because illegal and "deviant" activities feed on the spatial and temporal structure of routine legal activities (e.g., transportation, work, entertainment, and shopping), the differential land use of neighborhoods affects the ecological distribution of situations and opportunities conducive to a wide range of potentially adverse behaviors. In particular, the location of bars, liquor stores, strip-mall shopping outlets, and subway stops plays a direct role in the distribution of high-risk situations. The ecology of routine activities is not usually thought of in the "neighborhood effects" literature, much less as a mechanism. However, it holds promise as an explanatory factor, especially in combination with a theory of social capital. For instance, decisions to locate high-risk businesses are often targeted precisely to lower-income communities known to lack the organizational capacity to resist. Thus, one arena in which collective efficacy is likely to matter is in the differential ability of neighborhoods to organize against local threats such as disorderly bars, licensing of new liquor stores, and the mixing of strip malls with schools.

CHALLENGES FOR NEIGHBORHOOD-LEVEL RESEARCH

Despite promising leads from existing research, several limitations must be addressed if scientific knowledge on neighborhoods and health is to progress. First, aside from the experimental designs discussed above, neighborhood research has been largely silent on the issue of differential residential selection of individuals. This selection issue raises not only a methodological challenge to causal inference but also important substantive questions about how individuals sort themselves into neighborhoods. This sorting process surely has a bearing on how social capital gets produced. Closely related is the issue of "endogeneity" bias—for example, does social capital affect health, or does health status determine the need and capacity for a neighborhood to produce social capital?

Second, health environments are not limited to geographical communities. Families, the workplace, religious institutions, and peer groups, for example, generate their own collective properties that bear on health. As noted earlier, for example, friendship ties and family social support networks have been found to promote individual health (Berkman and Syme, 1979). In addition, the relevant health environments are not limited to urban settings and areas of disadvantage. Most of the United

States's population lives in suburban areas, and the relationship of socioeconomic status to health holds at the upper end of the socioeconomic distribution as well as the lower end (Robert, 1999). Nevertheless, much of the extant research literature is limited to the study of poverty in inner-city communities, underscoring the need to assess suburban and rural contexts.

Third, there is a need to further develop multilevel methodologies for contextually based research. Health data collected at nested levels of aggregation (e.g., neighborhood, city, state) pose important challenges to the standard analytic procedures that are prevalent among health researchers. In particular, the use of multilevel models has yet fully to incorporate the analysis of spatial interdependence. If social capital is a public good, then there is reason to believe that its benefits may diffuse over arbitrary neighborhood boundaries. Spatial processes may also influence some health-related behaviors, such as drug use and use of health services. A methodological challenge is thus to integrate multilevel methods with spatial dynamics.

A fourth research frontier is to build strategies for the direct measurement of social mechanisms and collective properties hypothesized to predict health (Mayer and Jencks, 1989). As Raudenbush (2003) argues in Chapter 5, while interest in the social sciences has turned to an integrated scientific approach that emphasizes individual factors in social context, a mismatch has arisen in the quality of measures. Decades of psychometric research have produced individual-level measures that often have excellent statistical properties. By contrast, much less is known about measures of ecological settings. Neighborhood level research is dominated by poverty and other demographic characteristics drawn from census data or other government statistics that do not provide information on the collective properties of administrative units. A major research frontier is thus the science of ecological assessment ("ecometrics") of social environments relevant to health (for further discussion see Raudenbush, 2003).

CONCLUSION

Consideration of the collective properties of neighborhood environments promises a deeper theoretical understanding of the etiology of health outcomes. The field of public health can also capitalize on sociological theory in pragmatic fashion by designing prevention strategies from the perspective of collective efficacy. Traditional thinking about disease has emphasized behavioral change among individuals as a means to reduce disease risk. For example, smoking interventions have targeted smokers and include hypnosis, smoking cessation programs, and nicotine patches. Environmental approaches look instead to macrolevel factors such as taxation policies, regulation of smoking in public places, and restriction of advertising in places frequented by adolescents. Such approaches appear to have yielded notable reductions in aggregate cigarette consumption in the United States. Community-level prevention that attempts to change places and social environments rather than people (e.g., "building community," targeting of "hot spots") may yield similar payoffs that complement traditional individual and disease-specific approaches. (For elaboration see Minkler and Wallerstein, 1988; Hope, 1995; Skogan and Hartnett, 1997; Israel et al., 1998; Robert, 1999; Yen and Syme, 1999; and Sampson and Morenoff, 2000).

ACKNOWLEDGMENTS
This is a condensed and revised version of a paper by Robert J. Sampson and Jeffrey Morenoff, "Public Health and Safety in Context: Lessons from Community-level Theory on Social Capital," presented at the conference Capitalizing on Social Science and Behavioral Research to Improve the Public Health, Institute of Medicine, Atlanta, February 3–4, 2000.

REFERENCES

Bandura A (1997). *Self Efficacy: The Exercise of Control.* New York: W.H. Freeman
Berkman L and Syme SL (1979). Social networks, host resistance, and mortality: A nine-year follow-up study of Alameda County residents. *Am J Epidemiol* 109: 186–204.
Bourdieu P (1986). The forms of capital. In Richardson J, ed.: *Handbook of Theory and Research for the Sociology of Education.* New York: Greenwood Press, pp. 241–258.
Brooks-Gunn J, Duncan GJ, Aber L, eds. (1997). *Neighborhood Poverty: Policy Implications in Studying Neighborhoods.* New York: Russell Sage.
Bursik RJ and Grasmick H (1993). *Neighborhoods and Crime: The Dimensions of Effective Community Control.* New York: Lexington.
Cohen L and Felson M (1979). Social change and crime rate trends: A routine activity approach. *Am Sociol Rev* 44: 588–608.
Coleman JS (1988). Social capital in the creation of human capital. *Am J Sociol* 94: S95–S120.
Coleman JS (1990). *Foundations of Social Theory.* Cambridge, Mass: Harvard University Press.
Faris R and Dunham WH (1965). *Mental Disorders in Urban Areas: An Ecological Study of Schizophrenia and Other Psychoses,* 2nd ed. Chicago: University of Chicago Press.
Fisher C (1982). *To Dwell Among Friends: Personal Networks in Town and City.* Chicago: University of Chicago Press.
Goldberger J, Wheeler GA, Sydenstrycker E (1920). A study of the relation of fam-

ily income and other economic factors to pellagra incidence in seven cotton mill villages of South Carolina in 1916. *Public Health Rep* 35: 2673–2714.

Granovetter M (1973). The strength of weak ties. *Am J Sociol* 78: 1360–1380.

Hope T (1995). Community crime prevention. In Tonry M and Farrington D, eds.: *Building a Safer Society*. Chicago: University of Chicago Press, pp. 21–89.

House JS, Umberson D, Landis KR (1988). Structures and processes of social support. *Annu Rev Sociol* 14: 293–318.

Hunter A (1985). Private, parochial and public social orders: The problem of crime and incivility in urban communities. In Suttles G and Zald M, eds.: *The Challenge of Social Control*. Norwood, NJ: Ablex, pp. 230–242.

Israel BA, Schulz AJ, Parker EA, Becker AB (1998). Review of community-based research: Assessing partnership approaches to improve public health. *Annu Rev Public Health* 19: 173–202.

Janowitz M (1975). Sociological theory and social control. *American J Sociol* 81: 82–108.

Katz L, Kling J, Liebman J (2001). Moving to opportunity in Boston: Early impacts of a housing mobility program. *Quarterly J Economics* 116(2): 607–654.

Kawachi I and Berkman L (2000). Social cohesion, social capital, and health. In Berkman L and Kawachi I, eds.: *Social Epidemiology*. New York: Oxford University Press.

Kawachi I, Kennedy BP, Glass R (1999). Social capital and self-rated health: A contextual analysis. *Am J Public Health* 89: 1187–1193.

Kawachi I, Kennedy B, Lochner K, Prothrow-Smith D (1997). Social capital, income inequality, and mortality. *Am J Public Health* 87: 1491–1498.

Logan J and Molotch H (1987). *Urban Fortunes: The Political Economy of Place*. Berkeley, Calif: University of California Press.

Manski C (1995). *Identification Problems in the Social Sciences*. Cambridge, Mass: Harvard University Press.

Massey DS (1996). The age of extremes: Concentrated affluence and poverty in the twenty-first century. *Demography* 33: 395 412.

Massey DS and Denton N (1993). *American Apartheid: Segregation and the Making of the Underclass*. Cambridge, Mass: Harvard University Press.

Mayer SE and Jencks C (1989). Growing up in poor neighborhoods: How much does it matter? *Science* 243: 1441–1445.

Minkler M and Wallerstein N (1988). Improving health through community organization and community building: A health education perspective. In *Community Organization and Community Building for Health*. New Brunswick, NJ: Rutgers University Press, pp. 30–54.

Morenoff J and Sampson RJ (1997). Violent crime and the spatial dynamics of Neighborhood transition: Chicago, 1970–1990. *Social Forces* 76: 31–64.

Portes A (1998). Social capital: Its origins and applications in modern sociology. *Annual Review of Sociology* 24: 1–24.

Portes A and Sensenbrenner J (1993). Embeddedness and immigration: Notes on the social determinants of economic action. *Am J Sociol* 98: 1320–1350.

Putnam R (1993). The prosperous community: Social capital and community life. *American Prospect* 35: 42.

Raudenbush S (2003). The quantitative assessment of neighborhood social environments. In Kawachi I and Berkman L, eds.: *Neighborhoods and Health*. New York: Oxford University Press, forthcoming.

Robert S (1998). Community-level socioeconomic status effects on adult health. *J Health Soc Behav* 39: 18–37.

Robert S (1999). Socioeconomic position and health: The independent contribution of community socioeconomic context. *Annu Rev Sociol* 25: 489–516.

Sampson RJ (2001). How do communities undergird or undermine human development? Relevant contexts and social mechanisms. In Booth A and Crouter N, eds.: *Does It Take a Village? Community Effects on Children, Adolescents, and Families.* Mahwah, NJ: Lawrence Erlbaum.

Sampson RJ, Raudenbush S, Earls F (1997). Neighborhoods and violent crime: A multilevel study of collective efficacy. *Science* 277: 918–924.

Sampson RJ, Morenoff J, Earls F (1999). Beyond social capital: Spatial dynamics of collective efficacy for children. *Am Sociol Rev* 64: 633–660.

Sampson RJ and Morenoff J (2000). Public health and safety in context: Lessons from community-level theory on social capital. Presented at the conference Capitalizing on Social Science and Behavioral Research to Improve the Public Health, Institute of Medicine, Atlanta, Ga., 3–4 February 2000.

Sandefur R and Laumann EO (1998). A paradigm for social capital. *Rationality and Society* 10: 481–501.

Skogan W and Hartnett S (1997). *Community Policing, Chicago Style.* New York: Oxford University Press.

Shaw C and McKay H (1969). *Juvenile Delinquency and Urban Areas*, 2nd ed. Chicago: University of Chicago Press.

Warren D (1975). *Black Neighborhoods: An Assessment of Community Power.* Ann Arbor, Mich: University of Michigan Press.

Wilson WJ (1987). *The Truly Disadvantaged: The Inner City, the Underclass, and Public Policy.* Chicago: University of Chicago Press.

Wilson WJ (1996). *When Work Disappears.* New York: Knopf.

Woolcock M (1998). Social capital and economic development: Toward a theoretical synthesis and policy framework. *Theory and Society* 27: 151–208.

Yen IH and Syme SL (1999). The social environment and health: A discussion of the epidemiologic literature. *Annu Rev Public Health* 20: 287–308.

7

Geocoding and Measurement of Neighborhood Socioeconomic Position: A U.S. Perspective

Nancy Krieger
Sally Zierler
Joseph W. Hogan
Pamela Waterman
Jarvis Chen
Kerry Lemieux
Annie Gjelsvik

Where do you live? Take a moment to visualize your neighborhood. Ask yourself: What are its class composition and boundaries? What kinds of data would you use to characterize neighborhood conditions, let alone explore their connections to health?

Ask any of these questions, and you immediately engage with core issues of geocoding and measurement of neighborhood socioeconomic position for public health research and practice. In this chapter we focus on conceptual and methodologic issues germane to public health monitoring in the United States. Many of the concepts, methods, and questions, however, are likely to be relevant to other countries (Gordon, 1995; Lee et al., 1995; Hankins et al., 1998; Cadum et al., 1999; da Silva et al., 1999; Mustard et al., 1999; Pringle et al., 1999) as well as to etiologic studies of neighborhood effects on health and other aspects of well-being (Brooks-Gunn and Duncan, 1997; Diez-Roux, 1998; MacIntyre and Ellaway, 2000).

GEOCODING AND MONITORING SOCIAL
INEQUALITIES IN HEALTH: OPPORTUNITIES
AND OBSTACLES—A U.S. PERSPECTIVE

Public health interest in delimiting the boundaries and socioeconomic
composition of the neighborhoods in which people live dates back nearly
two centuries. At issue is the extent to which neighborhood data are informative about—and relevant to the health of—their inhabitants. In 1826,
for example, Louis René Villermé (1782–1863), one of the leading public
health professionals in France, used area-based economic data and mortality rates to demonstrate empirically, for the first time, that social
conditions—and not just the "natural environment"—played a decisive
role in patterning mortality among neighborhoods of Paris (Villermé,
1828; Coleman, 1982). Specifically, he found that death rates were highest in areas whose residents paid the least in "untaxed rents," a type of
tax paid only by the wealthy. By contrast, no correlations existed between
neighborhood mortality rates and altitude, distance from the Seine, tem-
perature, and other environmental features. Subsequently, in 1845,
Friedrich Engels cited data in his classic text, *The Condition of the Working
Class in England*, indicating that mortality rates depended on both "class
of street" as well as "class of house" (Engels, 1958 (1845); Davey Smith,
1997). Thus, among people who lived in worse homes, mortality was
higher for those residing in poorer compared to more affluent neighborhoods. More recently, a revived concern about social inequalities in health
in the United States and other countries (Townsend et al., 1990; Evans et
al., 1994; Braveman, 1996; Krieger et al., 1997a; Pamuk et al., 1998; Mann
et al., 1999; Berkman and Kawachi, 2000; Kim et al., 2000), coupled with
new advances in geographic information system (GIS) technologies
(Moore and Carpenter, 1999; Richards et al., 1999; Yasnoff and Sondik,
1999), have led to new interest in analyzing population health in relation
to neighborhood characteristics, the theme of this book.

In the United States, however, still another factor spurs current interest in using area-based socioeconomic measures: the relative paucity,
if not absence, of socioeconomic data in most U.S. public health databases,
as reviewed below (Krieger and Fee, 1996; Krieger et al., 1997b). From a
public health standpoint, augmenting U.S. vital statistics and other public health surveillance systems with socioeconomic data is especially important because these data provide the fundamental basis for routinely
monitoring population burdens of disease and death, along with births
and their attendant joys and sometimes sorrow (Institute of Medicine,
1988, 1997). Absent adequate socioeconomic data, we cannot monitor—
or gauge progress or setbacks in rectifying—socioeconomic disparities in

health, let alone assess the contribution of socioeconomic position to equally troubling racial/ethnic inequalities in health (U.S. Department of Health and Human Services, 1991; Krieger et al., 1993; Williams and Collins, 1995; Krieger et al., 1997a; Freeman, 1998). Beyond this, routine public health data documenting social inequalities in health are vital to shaping the analyses, aspirations, and actions of social movements and governments in their efforts to create healthy public policies, at the local, national, and global levels, to reduce social disparities in health (Fox, 1989; Townsend et al., 1990; Braveman, 1996; Krieger et al., 1997b; Mann et al., 1999; Shaw et al., 2000).

The Problem: Paucity or Absence of Socioeconomic Data in U.S. Vital Statistics

Despite more than two centuries of international vital statistics documenting that people subjected to poorer living and working conditions live shorter, less healthy lives (Antonovsky, 1967; Fox, 1989; Townsend et al., 1990), it was only in 1989 that reporting of birth and death data stratified by educational level became routine in the United States (Tolson et al., 1991)—60 years after the last American attempt, in the 1930s, to produce national mortality data stratified by social class (Whitney, 1934; Krieger and Fee, 1996). Even so, as revealed by a 1997 survey of all U.S. state health departments, although 100% of states now collect information on education of mother and father and decedent, only 7% of cancer registries, 4% of tuberculosis (TB) registries, and no AIDS registries collect data on education (Krieger at al., 1997b). Moreover, although all states collect data on occupation of decedent, and 80% do so for their cancer registries, only 12% and 9%, respectively, break out these data by occupation. Other sources fare worse: only half the states collect—and none publish—birth data in relation to occupation of mother or father, and occupational data in state TB and AIDS registries distinguish only between health care and non–health care occupations. None of these public health databases obtain information on income or other relevant socioeconomic data.

These gaps in data at the state level are reflected at the national level. Before 1998, the annual federal report, *Health, United States*, contained little socioeconomic data (National Center for Health Statistics, 1996; Krieger et al., 1997a; National Center for Health Statistics, 1997). In 1998, however, this report included its first-ever chartbook on "Socioeconomic Status and Health," drawing on data from birth and death records plus the National Health Interview Survey (Pamuk et al., 1998). An absence of socioeconomic data in other databases, however, meant critical public health

problems, such as cancer, TB, and HIV/AIDS, could not be included. The
1999 issue unfortunately reverted to earlier practice, with socioeconomic
data once again appearing in only ten of the report's seventy-three tables
on "Health Status and Determinants" (National Center for Health Statistics, 1999). Moreover, fully 70% of the 467 U.S. public health objectives
for the year 2010 lack quantitative targets for reducing socioeconomic disparities in health, given a lack of baseline data (U.S. Department of Health
and Human Services, 2000), nor will this problem be rectified by better
national surveys. First, as acknowledged by the National Center for
Health Statistics, such surveys offer sparse or no data at the local level,
the principal locale for most public health planning and programs (Meri-
wether 1996; Pollack and Rice, 1997; U.S. Department of Health and Human Services, 2000). Second, most surveys are not designed to provide
routine data on diverse and relatively small racial/ethnic populations
(e.g., subpopulations of Asians and Pacific Islanders, Hispanics, and
American Indians) (U.S. Department of Health and Human Services, 1991;
Williams and Collins, 1995; Nolan et al., 1996; Krieger et al., 1997b).

Geocoding and Area-Based Socioeconomic Measures: A Potential Solution

Fortunately, the problem is not intractable. In fact, tracts are likely to be
part of the solution. This is because we can use census-derived, area-based
data to characterize persons in both public health databases and the total population, thereby permitting ascertainment of population-based
incidence or prevalence rates stratified by area-based socioeconomic position (Krieger et al., 1992, 1997a). The key to this strategy is the methodology of geocoding.

   Geocoding refers to the process of identifying an address's latitude,
longitude, and assigned geographic codes, which in the United States include its census-defined state, county, census tract, and block-group
codes, along with codes for political jurisdictions (e.g., congressional districts), economic regions, plus post office–defined ZIP codes (Kaplan and
Van Valey 1980; U.S. Department of Commerce 1990; U.S. Bureau of the
Census, 1991). As shown in Figure 7–1, the basic geographic building
blocks in the United States are literally the census blocks, with an average population of 85, nested within the census block-group (average population of 1,000), in turn nested within the census tract (average population of 4,000) (Kaplan and Van Valey, 1980; U.S. Department of
Commerce, 1990). Census tracts were first demarcated in New York City
in 1910 and were assigned to several major U.S. cities by 1940; as of 1990
block-group codes were assigned nationwide (Shevky and Bell, 1955;

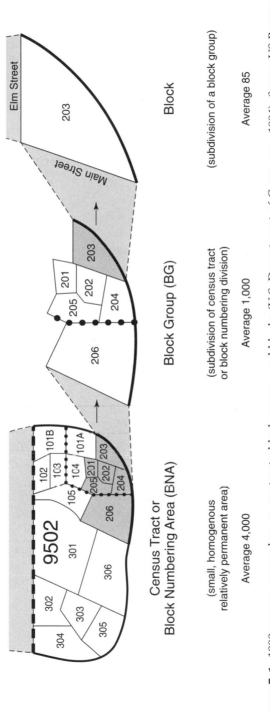

FIGURE 7–1. 1990 census geography: census tracts, block groups, and blocks (U.S. Department of Commerce, 1994). *Source:* US Bureau of the Census. Geographical areas reference manual. Washington, D.C.: US Department of Commerce, 1994.

Kaplan and Van Valey, 1980). These areas are intended to contain populations reasonably homogeneous with regard to socioeconomic composition. Block-groups constitute the smallest unit for which area-based socioeconomic measures are feasible, because, to protect confidentiality, no socioeconomic data are released at the block level (U.S. Department of Commerce, 1990; U.S. Bureau of the Census, 1991). By contrast, ZIP codes typically contain upwards of 30,000 people, are intended to facilitate delivery of mail, often cut across census tract and block-group boundaries, and are not designed to be economically homogeneous (Kaplan and Van Valey, 1980; U.S. Bureau of the Census, 1991; U.S. Post Office, 2000).

Three strengths of using area-based socioeconomic measures for monitoring social inequalities in health are that they (1) can be appended to any database with addresses, as is the case for key vital statistics and other public health surveillance databases (Krieger et al., 1997a, 1997b; Yasnoff and Sondik, 1999; Thrall, 1999a), (2) provide data for determining contextual as well as compositional neighborhood effects on health, above and beyond effects that are due to individual-level socioeconomic position (Diez-Roux, 1998; MacIntyre and Ellaway, 2000), and (3) can be applied equally to all persons, regardless of age, gender, and employment status (Krieger et al., 1997a; Krieger, 1992; Carstairs and Morris 1989). This methodology thereby avoids well-known problems associated with individual-level education and occupation data, that is, how to classify people who have not completed their education or who are not in the paid-labor force (children, housewives, househusbands, unemployed, or retired persons) (Carstairs and Morris, 1989; Sorensen, 1994; Krieger et al., 1997a, 1999). Three drawbacks are (1) they can be misconstrued as only a "proxy" for individual-level socioeconomic data (rather than seen as complementary data that, in fact, can be analyzed together with individual-level data in multilevel models), (2) they reflect socioeconomic context at the time of case ascertainment, not necessarily during the relevant etiologic period, and (3) they can be outdated, given the decennial nature of the U.S. census. Rendering this last objection moot, however, the U.S. is already shifting toward implementing the more frequent American Community Survey, which will generate data at the tract and block-group level (U.S. Census Bureau, 1999).

Given a wide array of census data, a variety of geographic levels (such as the census tract, block-group, and ZIP code), and a plethora of geocoding and other GIS software (Moore and Carpenter, 1999; Richards et al., 1999; Thrall, 1999b), the question then becomes: are there any standard, well-accepted area-based socioeconomic measures that have been validated for public health monitoring in the United States? Briefly stated, "No" (Krieger et al., 1997a; Lynch and Kaplan, 2000).

As of mid-2000, only seven U.S. public health studies have explored the validity of using area-based socioeconomic measures (Krieger, 1991, 1992; Cherkin, 1992; Greenwald et al., 1994; Krieger et al., 1996; Geronimus et al., 1996; Geronimus and Bound, 1998). Unfortunately, all used different census-derived socioeconomic variables and examined only a handful of health outcomes. All compared socioeconomic gradients in health detected by area-based and individual-level socioeconomic measures to assess the validity of using area-based measures to monitor socioeconomic gradients in health. Yielding results similar to the handful of comparable methodologic studies from the United Kingdom (Carr-Hill and Rice, 1995), Canada (Mustard et al., 1999) and Australia (Hyndman et al., 1995), five of the U.S. studies found that estimates of socioeconomic gradients in health produced with block-group or census tract socioeconomic measures were similar to, but often slightly less than, those produced with individual-level socioeconomic data (Krieger, 1991, 1992; Cherkin, 1992; Greenwald, 1994; Krieger et al., 1996); results were less consistent for the two studies that employed ZIP-code data (Geronimus et al., 1996; Geronimus and Bound, 1998; see also Krieger and Gordon, 1999; Davey Smith and Hart, 1999). Among these seven studies, four used differently categorized measures of neighborhood social class composition, educational and poverty level, and unemployment rate (Krieger, 1991, 1992; Krieger et al., 1996; Geronimus and Bound, 1998), two used measures of average annual family income (Greenwald et al., 1994; Cherkin et al., 1992), and two used data on median family income and educational level (Geronimus and Bound, 1996; Geronimus and Bound, 1998).

A profusion of measures is likewise apparent in the small but growing U.S. public health literature with demonstrated interest in using area-based socioeconomic measures. Employing an extremely eclectic array of census-derived variables at markedly different levels of geography, these investigations have focused on such diverse outcomes as births (Collins and David, 1997; O'Campo et al., 1997; Roberts, 1997; Wasserman et al., 1998), deaths (Kitagawa and Hauser, 1973; Hann et al., 1987; Davey Smith et al., 1996a, 1996b), cancer (Devessa and Diamond, 1980; Krieger, 1990; Greenwald et al., 1994; Liu et al., 1998; Prehn and West, 1998; Krieger et al., 1999; Morris, 1999; Arbes, 1999), cardiovascular disease (Casper et al., 1999; Iwashyna et al., 1999; Sayegh et al., 1999), AIDS and other infectious diseases (Zierler et al., 2000, Morse et al., 1991; Fife et al., 1992; Hu et al., 1994; Ellen et al., 1995; Simon et al., 1995; Chen et al., 1998), asthma (Wissow et al., 1988), mental health (Goldsmith et al., 1982), and violence and injuries (Collins and David, 1997; Harries, 1997; Anderson et al., 1998; Grisso et al., 1999; Hinton et al., 1999; Powell and Tanz, 1999). However, despite a common concern about socioeconomic inequalities in health, estimates of effect for socioeconomic position cannot readily be compared across these studies because of the lack of consistency in area-based socioeconomic measures. The sociologic literature is similarly rife with a heterogeneous assortment of measures developed over the past several decades, none systematically assessed for their relevance to health (Shevky and Bell, 1955; Rossi and Gilmartin, 1980; White, 1987; Brooks-Gunn et al., 1997). Moreover, with regard to government standards, the only federally designated demarcation is for "poverty area," defined as an area where 20% or more of the population lives below the poverty line (U.S. Bureau of Census, 1985; Jargowsky, 1997). By contrast, health research and government reports in the United Kingdom employ a small set of validated and well-established area-based measures of deprivation, with key ones—such as the Townsend index—explicitly developed for public health use (Townsend et al., 1988; Townsend, 1993; Carstairs, 1995; Gordon, 1995; Lee et al., 1995; see also Chapter 8).

In summary, in the United States, public health researchers and practitioners confront uncertainty about three important aspects of area-based socioeconomic measures: (1) validity, (2) content—including both which measures are included and how they are constructed, and (3) geographic level. No standard validated measure exists, whether for use by public health departments or by individual researchers.

GENERATING SOLUTIONS: A PROJECT TO DEVELOP VALID AREA-BASED SOCIOECONOMIC MEASURES FOR U.S. PUBLIC HEALTH DATABASES

To address this gap in U.S. public health research and practice, we are engaged in a project whose goal is to generate a valid, robust, easy to interpret, and easy to construct area-based socioeconomic measure that can readily be used by health departments anywhere in the United States, for any health outcome, from birth to death, whether for women or men, young or old, among any racial/ethnic group (Krieger et al., NIH Grant 1 R01 HD36865-01). Throughout, our guiding principle is to generate area-based socioeconomic measures that are grounded in sound statistical methodology yet whose meaning is readily evident to both data users and the public at large.

In presenting preliminary results of our project, five lessons stand out that are relevant to any project engaged with geocoding and/or using census-derived socioeconomic data. First, it is critical to ascertain the accuracy of geocoding software. Second, it is essential to develop protocols that protect confidentiality of the databases that are being geocoded. Third, it is important to evaluate the extent to which different databases can be geocoded to specified geographic levels. Fourth, it is necessary to be aware of how boundaries for different geographic regions are defined and may cross-cut one another. Fifth, it is imperative that analyses be conceptually grounded rather than algorithm-driven empirical exercises in data reduction.

Scope of Project

To evaluate the validity and feasibility of monitoring social inequalities in health using area-based socioeconomic measures, our project is using public health surveillance data from two states, Massachusetts and Rhode Island, along with 1990 census data from three geographic levels: census block-group (BG), census tract (CT), and ZIP code (ZC). The study's five main tasks are to (*1*) geocode the public health databases to the BG, CT, and ZC level, (*2*) at each geographic level generate the same set of area-based socioeconomic indicators, (*3*) within and across geographic levels examine patterns of associations between these variables and, where feasible, with individual-level socioeconomic data, (*4*) link the area-based socioeconomic measures to the geocoded health databases, and (*5*) estimate and compare socioeconomic gradients in health detected for each health outcome, using the same set of diverse area-based socioeconomic measures at each geographic level.

Public Health Databases: Eligibility and Confidentiality

For the purpose of our project, we defined as eligible all public health surveillance system databases in the states of Massachusetts and Rhode Island that included age, gender, race/ethnicity, and street address at the time of case ascertainment. Staff from the Massachusetts Department of Public Health and the Rhode Island Department of Health provided information on the eligibility of their surveillance system data for our project. Of the more than fifty surveillance systems surveyed, nine met eligibility criteria: birth, death, cancer, tuberculosis, sexually transmitted diseases, nonfatal gun and stab wounds, domestic violence, childhood lead screening, and the Health Interview Survey. Although HIV/AIDS surveillance systems also were eligible, we excluded them because the Massachusetts data were already being used in a pilot study conducted by two of our team's investigators (Zierler et al., 2000). In total, our project has health outcome data for 650,012 residents of Massachusetts and 324,078 residents of Rhode Island for the proposed years of monitoring surrounding the census year 1990, thus nearly 1 million records combined.

Confidentiality protocols were set by the respective health department's internal review boards, with input from the directors of each database and from project staff. To preserve confidentiality, for each database we created files for geocoding containing only each record's address, a dummy variable to identify the data source, and a newly generated unique identifier which the health department could then use to link the geocoded record back to the original database. Working with staff at each health department, we then created databases for analysis containing solely the relevant demographic and health data plus newly assigned geocodes. Thus, no street addresses are in any of our project's databases, except for the public domain death certificate data.

Selecting Geocoding Tools: Options and Accuracy

Recognizing that numerous companies and software products claim to geocode accurately, we decided to put the claims to the test (see Krieger et al., 2001, on p. 170). Although we located a few articles evaluating the capacity and user-friendliness of several commercial geocoding software products (Thrall, 1999b; Richards et al., 1999; Moore and Carpenter, 1999), we found none that explicitly compared the cost, timeliness, and accuracy of geocoding firms and software.

After searching the Internet to determine the range of services offered by commercial geocoding firms and ascertaining which software products were licensed to our workplace, we selected four firms and one software program. To each we submitted (1) information on the number of records we wanted to geocode (six submissions of 250,000 records each) and (2) seventy test addresses with known census tracts, consisting of fifty "incorrect" but geocodable addresses provided by a geocoding specialist at the Massachusetts Cancer Registry, which we supplemented with twenty telephone book addresses randomly selected from the local telephone book. The "incorrect" addresses contained various common errors, including out-of-range street addresses, abbreviated or misspelled street names, wrong street types (e.g., "avenue" instead of "street"), and correct towns but wrong zip codes. Census tracts of the fifty "incorrect" addresses were earlier verified by staff at the cancer registry; tracts of the twenty "telephone book" addresses were verified by project staff using the U.S. Bureau of the Census geocoding web site (U.S. Bureau of the Census, 2000).

Notably, the four firms and the software program varied dramatically in cost, timeliness, attitude, and, most importantly, accuracy. Estimated costs among the firms varied by a factor of two, ranging from $8,800 to $15,800. Project costs for the software program were lower ($1,460), but this price included only the cost of training two project staff members, not the cost of their labor for geocoding addresses nor the price of the software (which had been licensed to our university). If, however, we purchased the necessary software, costs would have increased by an additional $1,690 at the time of ascertaining this information for the test file. (At the time of preparing this chapter, however, the cost would have risen by an additional $11,190 due to increased expenses associated with upgrading or updating the software.)

Representatives for each firm and program estimated it would take one to two weeks to geocode the test file; actual turnaround time ranged from five hours to three weeks. Company A, the least expensive, friendliest, and suitably prompt geocoding firm did best, correctly geocoding 84% of the test addresses (80% of the "incorrect" addresses, 95% of the telephone book addresses). Company D, by contrast, despite costing twice as much, was the worst: it took 4 times as long, provided poor customer service, and correctly geocoded only 44% of the test addresses (36% of the "incorrect" addresses, 65% of the telephone book addresses).

Based on these results, we selected company A and sent them our files. Then, to evaluate the "real world" accuracy of the firm, we randomly selected 150 geocoded addresses from the public domain death certificate data. Our strategy was to compare company A's results to (1) the gold standard, defined as the census block-group maps generated by the U.S. Census Bureau, using actual maps and guides with street address ranges, (2) the U.S. Census Bureau Website (which permits geocoding one manually-entered record at a time, but only to the tract level) (U.S. Bureau of the Census, 2000) , and (3) the software program, which we nevertheless decided to use for its map-making abilities. We also drove by several of the selected addresses to ascertain their exact location. Company A continued to do an impressively accurate job, with the overall percentage of addresses geocoded correctly to the tract level equaling 96%, the same as that of the U.S. Census Bureau web site (95%). In doing this exercise, however, we also encountered one additional disturbing result: on several occasions the software program could accurately geocode an address but then mapped it to the wrong part of town.

The marked variability in accuracy of geocoding products accordingly raises several important issues. Notably, none of the public health studies we have seen using geocoded data have included their rationale for selecting a particular geocoding firm or software product, nor have any presented data on the accuracy of the selected geocoding methodology. Our results raise questions about the validity of the results of previously published studies using geocoding methodologies of unverified accuracy.

Selecting Census Data: Options and Boundaries

To obtain the original, uncompressed raw census data at the block-group and census tract level, we downloaded data from the U.S. Census Bureau

Summary Tape File (STF) 3A; the ZIP code data are in STF 3B (U.S. Bureau of the Census, 1991). We also obtained data from a menu-driven commercial product, which, although intended to be user-friendly, provided little documentation (Geolytics, 2000). Reassuringly, both sources provided identical data for a series of randomly selected block-groups, tracts, and ZIP codes.

In working with the ZIP code data, however, we learned that their boundaries stretch the geographic imagination and can pose interesting problems for geocoding projects (see Krieger et al., 2002, on pp. 170–171). First, unlike block-groups and census tracts, which are physically delimited geographic areas with official and public boundaries demarcated by the U.S. Census Bureau (U.S. Bureau of the Census, 1991; Kaplan and Van Valey, 1980), ZIP code boundaries are far more fluid. As described by staff at the U.S. Census Bureau, these boundaries "resemble spaghetti and follow delivery routes" (Stuber, 1999) and can also be "point locations (as in rural post office buildings)" (Nichols, 1999). Consequently, "most companies that make maps of ZIP codes interpolate where a boundary is by talking to local postmasters or using street and address databases to come up with some approximation" (Nichols, 1999), and "the imputed boundaries are not recognized or used by the U.S. Postal Service" (Stuber, 1999). Thus, without publicly available official ZIP code boundaries, ZIP code borders may vary by geocoding firm and software product (U.S. Post Office, 2000). Second, we also learned that because cross-county ZIP codes are not assigned state codes in the STF 3B files, selecting on ZIP codes by state can give misleading impressions of missing data, because neither cross-county nor cross-state ZIP codes will be selected.

Census-Derived Socioeconomic Measures: Conceptual and Operational Definitions

Before analyzing the actual census socioeconomic data, we mapped out six conceptual domains relevant to characterizing socioeconomic position (Krieger et al., 1997; Council of Economic Advisors for the President's Initiative on Race, 1998). Our intent was to think through which types of measures might be pertinent before using statistical methods to characterize relationships between these measures. We then operationalized each domain in terms of available census variables, as shown in Table 7–1. These domains and the relevant variables are

1. *Occupational class,* defined in terms of (*a*) percent of employed persons age 16 and older in working-class jobs, made up chiefly of nonsuper-

TABLE 7–1. Selected U.S. Census-Derived Area-Based Socioeconomic Measures: Conceptual and Operational Definitions

Variable: conceptual definition	Census Text Definition: numerator ÷ denominator	1990 Census Code Definition: numerator ÷ denominator
Working class: nonsupervisory employees	Σ (persons employed in the 8 working class census occupational categories) ÷ Σ (all 13 census occupational categories)	(P0780004 + … + P0780006 + P0780008 + P0780010 + … + P0780013) ÷ (P0780001 + … + P0780013)
Unemployment: persons actively seeking employment (as defined by the census)	# persons age 16+ in the labor force and unemployed ÷ # persons age 16+ in the labor force	(P0710003 + P0710007 + P0710011 + P0710015 + P0710019 + P0710023 + P0710027 + P0710031 + P0710035 + P0710039) ÷ (P0710002 + P0710003 + P0710006 + P0710007 + P0710010 + P0710011 + P0710014 + P0710015 + P0710018 + P0710019 + P0710022 + P0710023 + P0710026 + P0710027 + P0710030 + P0710031 + P0710034 + P0710035 + P0710038 + P0710039)
Low income: relative measure of poverty, set at half the national median income (European Union definition of poverty)	# households with income <$15,000 ÷ # households	(P0800001 + … + P0800005) ÷ (P0800001 + … + P0800025)
Median household income: income of households where half of households have income below this level and half have income above it	median household income	P080A
High income: income at least 5 times higher than the median income	# households with income $150,000 + ÷ # households	P0800025 ÷ (P0800001 + … + P0800025)

(continued)

TABLE 7–1. Selected U.S. Census-Derived Area-Based Socioeconomic Measures: Conceptual and Operational Definitions (Continued)

Variable: conceptual definition	Census Text Definition: numerator ÷ denominator	1990 Census Code Definition: numerator ÷ denominator
Presence of poverty: persons or households whose household income is below the threshold to cover basic needs, definedin relation to food (US census definition)	# persons for whom ratio of (1989 household_income/U.S. poverty line) is <0.5 ÷ # persons for whom poverty status is determined	P1210001 ÷ (P1210001 + . . . + P1210009)
	# persons with 1989 household income <U.S. poverty line ÷ # persons for whom poverty status is determined	(P1170013 + . . . + P1170024) ÷ (P0170001 + . . . + P0170024)
	# households with 1989 income <U.S. poverty line ÷ # households	(P1270016 + . . . + P1270030) ÷ (P1270001 + . . . + P1270030)
Absence of poverty: persons whose household income is two times more than the poverty line	# persons for whom ratio of (1989 household_income/US poverty line) is ≥2 ÷ # persons for whom poverty status is determined	P1210009 ÷ (P1210001 + . . . + P1210009)
Low assets: assets sufficient to own only housing stock of very low value	# housing units valued at <$50,000 ÷ # specified owner-occupied housing units	(H0610001 + . . . + H0610008) ÷ (H0610001 + . . . + H0610020)
High assets: sufficient assets to own a home at about 4× the median U.S. value of owner-occupied homes	# housing units valued at $300,000+ ÷ # specified owner-occupied housing units	(H0610018 + H0610019 + H0610020) ÷ (H0610001 + . . . + H0610020)
Less than high school: adults with low educational attainment	# persons aged 25+ with no high school diploma ÷ # persons aged 25+	(P0570001 + P0570002) ÷ (P0570001 + . . . + P0570007)
College: adults with high educational attainment	# persons aged 25+ with 4+ years of college ÷ # persons aged 25+	(P0570006 + P0570007) ÷ (P0570001 + . . . + P0570007)
Crowding: at household level, more people than rooms	# occupied housing units with >1 person per room ÷ # occupied housing units	(H0690002 + H0690003 + H0690005 + H0690006 + H0690008 + H0690009 + H0690011 + H0690012) ÷ (H0690001 + . . . + H0690012)

visory employees, represented by eight of the thirteen census-defined occupational categories (Krieger et al., 1997a; Wright, 1997; Wright et al., 1982) and (*b*) percent of persons age 16 and older who are unemployed;

2. *Income,* defined in terms of (*a*) median annual household income, (*b*) low income, referring to the percentage of households with annual income below half the annual median income, a measure of poverty commonly used in the European Union (Gordon and Spicker, 1999) and equivalent to an annual household income below $15,000 in 1989, and (*c*) high income, referring to the percentage of households with an annual income of $150,000 or higher, the highest income category reported by the U.S. Census;

3. *Poverty,* defined in terms of (*a*) the percentage of persons with household incomes below the U.S. federal poverty line, a threshold that varies by size and age composition of the household, and on average equaled $12,647 for a family of four in 1989 (U.S. Bureau of the Census, 1991), (*b*) extreme poverty, referring to the percentage of persons in households below 50% of the poverty line, and (*c*) not impoverished, referring to the percentage of persons with household incomes at least 200% higher than the poverty line;

4. *Wealth,* defined in terms of (*a*) high assets, referring to the percentage of owner-occupied homes valued at $300,000 or more and (*b*) low assets, referring to the percentage of owner-occupied homes valued at less than $50,000;

5. *Education,* defined in terms of (*a*) low education, referring to the percentage of adults age 25 and older who have not completed high school and (*b*) high education, referring to the percentage of adults age 25 and older who have completed at least 4 years of college education; and

6. *Crowding,* defined in terms of (*a*) household crowding, referring to the percentage of households with more than one person per room and (*b*) population density, a contextual variable.

We also considered two additional variables—lack of car ownership and percentage of rented households—because they are used as indicators of deprivation in the United Kingdom (Lee et al., 1995). Emphasizing the importance of context, however, we found neither variable to be consistently associated with either poverty or median household income, given the much higher rates of car and home ownership in the U.S.

Additionally, to explore characteristics of selected socioeconomic indexes employed in other studies, we created several measures incorporating data on one or more of the single-variable census measures. These included

1. *U.S. versions of two U.K. area-based deprivation indexes*, the Townsend and Carstairs indexes, which combine data on such characteristics as unemployment, lack of car ownership, household crowding, rented households, and low social class (Lee et al., 1995; Carstairs, 1995; Townsend, 1993);
2. *Two measures of income inequality*: (*a*) the Gini coefficient, and (*b*) the ratio of the median income of the top fifth to the bottom fifth of the income distribution (Bernstein et al., 2000);
3. *The Index of Local Economic Resources* employed in the recent Centers for Disease Control (CDC) atlas on cardiovascular mortality, which combines data on the percentage of persons unemployed, in white collar jobs, and median family income (Casper et al., 1999).

We also combined several of the single census indicators into several theoretically driven *a priori composite indicators*, that is, a measure classifying areas simultaneously in terms of occupational class, wealth, and poverty levels. The final step was then to generate all of the specified variables at each level of geography (BG, CT, and ZC). Once accomplished, we then did a visual "reality check" on our constructs by visiting several Boston block-groups represented in the Massachusetts death certificate data and identified by our data as being poor, middle-income, or affluent.

PRELIMINARY RESULTS: GEOCODING AND PATTERNS OF ASSOCIATION AMONG SOCIOECONOMIC DATA

Importantly, from the standpoint of the feasibility of using area-based socioeconomic measures for monitoring social inequalities in health, the success rate of geocoding the administrative surveillance databases was suitably high. As shown in Table 7–2, of the nearly 1 million records we submitted for geocoding, fully 92% were geocoded successfully to the census block-group level. Another 6% could not be geocoded to the block-group level but were successfully geocoded to the census tract level, whereas only 0.2% could be geocoded only to the ZIP code level. Among all the addresses submitted, only 1.8% could not be geocoded. Although these percentages varied somewhat among the thirteen surveillance systems and one survey database, the median percentage of addresses geocoded to at least the census tract level equaled 97.2%.

Our data analysis strategy is comprised of three parts: data exploration, model building, and confirmatory analyses. In this section we provide detailed results of our exploratory analysis of census variables. Data exploration focuses on understanding important features of variable distributions at each aggregation level from both the census and surveillance

TABLE 7–2. Feasibility of Geocoding Public Health Surveillance System Databases

| Database | N | % Geocoded to: | | | % Not Geocoded |
		BG	CT only	ZIP only	
Total	**970,086**	**92%**	**6%**	**0.2%**	**1.8%**
Massachusetts					
Birth	267,724	95	5	0	0
Death	162,071	92	8	0	1
Cancer	170,004	92	8	0	0
Gun/stab wounds	7,723	83	10	0	7
TB + STDs	42,490	75	23	0	2
Rhode Island					
Birth	106,443	94	3	1	2
Death	28,942	90	5	0	5
Cancer	21,392	92	8	0	0
Domestic violence	15,222	94	5	0	0
TB	576	91	3	0	7
STDs	9,353	88	1	1	10
Lead	135,567	91	1	0	9
HIS	2,579	75	0	7	18

*Years vary for each database, with years selected: (a) to be temporally proximal to the 1990 census, and (b) to ensure adequate sample size for calculation of stable rates.

TB, tuberculosis; STDs, sexually transmitted diseases; HIS, health interview survey; BG, block-group; CT, census tract; ZC, zip code.

data. For the census data we review analyses that involve both numerical and graphic summaries, stratified by level of aggregation and by state. These include univariate summaries, bivariate associations, and associations between individual census variables and the selected existing area-based socioeconomic indexes. Univariate summaries indicate whether census variables cluster around a particular value or set of values, identify possibly outlying observations and the extent of missing data, and provide information useful for identifying potentially meaningful cut-points or functional transformations (e.g., log or square root) needed for statistical modeling. They also permit comparisons of variability and distribution across levels of aggregation.

Figure 7–2 shows the distribution of several selected census variables using box and whisker plots. Heavy right skewness is evident is several variables, such as those related to poverty and wealth. The majority of

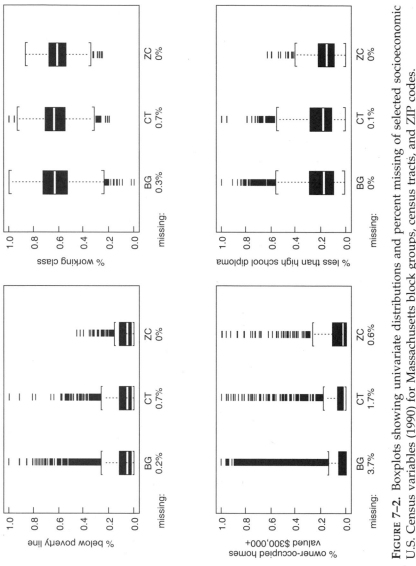

FIGURE 7–2. Boxplots showing univariate distributions and percent missing of selected socioeconomic U.S. Census variables (1990) for Massachusetts block groups, census tracts, and ZIP codes.

variables show little appreciable difference in either shape or central tendency across levels of aggregation. Specifically, quantiles defining the middle 50% of the distribution remain relatively constant across aggregation unit. As the aggregation units get larger, however, some "smoothing" is evident, reflected by attenuation of the minimum and maximum values in larger aggregation units. This phenomenon occurs because larger aggregation units encompass the smaller ones and average their values. It is interesting, however, to compare the observed range of values in poverty and wealth: although many block-groups and census tracts have poverty rates in excess of 50%, the maximum poverty rate in ZIP codes is 46%. By contrast, the full range of values for wealth appears largely to be preserved across levels of aggregation. Thus, aggregation by ZIP code preserves the full range of values for indicating extreme wealth, but extreme poverty appears to be "smoothed out."

We used Spearman's rank correlations and two-way scatterplots to summarize associations between individual census variables at each aggregation level. (Rank correlations are preferred due to skewed distributions.) The goals of the association analysis are to understand whether patterns of association are consistent across level of aggregation and whether groups of variables tend to cluster together to delineate underlying, latent area-level characteristics. The second goal can and will be addressed more formally using factor analysis (Bartholomew and Knott, 1999, Chapter 3).

Table 7–3 lists pairwise correlations by level of aggregation; the boldface is used to indicate clusters of variables with high pairwise correlation (e.g., greater than 0.7 in absolute value). Although correlation is relatively constant across aggregation level, the clusters tend to emerge with greater definition at higher levels of aggregation. The first cluster characterizes economic resources in relation to income (or lack thereof) and includes all the selected income and poverty measures. A second cluster, slightly more difficult to discern, captures aspects of wealth and social class and includes variables pertaining to class composition, assets, and educational level. Importantly, for both clusters the direction of association remains the same across levels of aggregation, even as the degree of association sometimes changes.

The third component of our exploratory analysis examines the nature of association between individual census variables and the selected existing area-based socioeconomic indexes. This analysis is undertaken to help understand the extent to which existing indexes reflect variation in important census indicators. As an illustration, Figure 7–3 shows scatterplots of poverty rate versus three area-based socioeconomic indexes: the Townsend index, the Gini coefficient of income inequality, and the CDC's

TABLE 7–3. Spearman Rank Correlation Matrix of Selected Socioeconomic U.S. Census Variables (1990) for Massachusetts Census Tracts, Showing Two Clusters of Highly Correlated Variables*

	Working Class (%)	Unemployed (%)	Median Household (HH) Income	<50% Median HH Income	HH Income ≥$150,000	Persons < Poverty (%)	Persons ≥200% Poverty (%)	Owner-Occupied Homes ≥$300,000 (%)	Adults < High School (%)	Adults ≥ 4 yrs College (%)	Crowded HH (%)
% unemployed	*0.614*										
Median household (HH) income	**−0.686**	**−0.650**									
<50% median HH income	**0.622**	**0.638**	**−0.938**								
HH income ≥ $150,000	**−0.711**	−0.576	**0.691**	**−0.615**							
% persons < poverty	0.522	**0.617**	**−0.857**	**0.882**	−0.557						
% persons ≥ 200% poverty	**−0.625**	**−0.654**	**0.936**	**−0.919**	**0.643**	**−0.921**					
% owner-occupied homes ≥ $300,000	**−0.684**	−0.487	**0.602**	−0.523	**0.702**	−0.470	0.545				
% adults < high school	*0.774*	0.693	−0.768	0.755	−0.682	0.670	−0.742	−0.658			
% adults ≥ 4 yrs college	*−0.906*	−0.670	0.668	−0.608	0.707	−0.503	0.605	0.702	−0.826		
% crowded HH	0.463	0.531	−0.608	0.579	−0.482	**0.668**	**−0.674**	−0.416	0.545	−0.438	
Population per square mile	0.216	0.347	−0.490	0.519	−0.345	0.593	−0.549	−0.293	0.395	−0.203	0.523

*Correlations >0.6 highlighted in bold identify a cluster of varibales pertaining to economic resources, in relation to poverty and income.

Correlations >0.6 highlighted in italics identify a cluster of variables related to social class, education, and wealth.

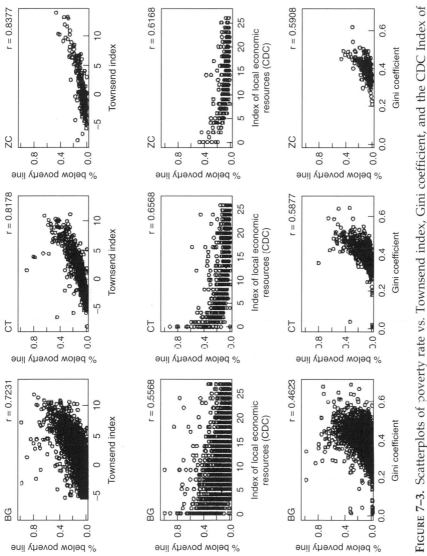

FIGURE 7-3. Scatterplots of poverty rate vs. Townsend index, Gini coefficient, and the CDC Index of Local Economic Resources, for Massachusetts block groups, census tracts, and ZIP codes using 1990 U.S. Census data.

Index of Local Economic Resources. Two features are readily apparent. First, as expected, the variability of each index at a fixed percentage of poverty (i.e., vertical variation in the plot) decreases as the area of aggregation increases. Second, at any given level of poverty, the variability in each index is quite substantial, even at the extremes, and especially for the CDC index. The high variation in the CDC index across fixed levels of poverty may indicate that it is not aptly named. The Gini coefficient also exhibits considerable variability at fixed poverty levels, but this is to be expected because the Gini coefficient measures economic disparity within an area and not per se (i.e., an area with uniform poverty can have the same Gini coefficient as does one with uniform wealth). This may be obvious but points to why a given measure may have different utility at different levels of aggregation: given economic segregation, the Gini coefficient and other measures of economic inequality are likely to be informative only at higher levels of aggregation (Jargowsky, 1997; Soobader and LeClere, 1999).

Our next steps involve both model building and confirmatory analyses. Building on our correlation analyses, we use factor analysis to identify subsets of variables that cluster in particular domains and use information on latent factors in our eventual construction of the index (Bartholomew and Knott, 1999, pp. 42 ff.). We also address two important issues that make our analysis slightly more complex than simply applying factor analysis to the census variables. First, census variables for adjacent geographic areas are likely to be spatially correlated, and incorporating this correlation is likely to improve our estimation of area-specific factors (Clayton and Kaldor, 1987; Moore and Carpenter, 1999). Second, especially at the ZIP code level, census data are derived from differently sized populations, making it necessary to incorporate appropriate weights.

Having obtained factor scores in addition to our single-variable socioeconomic measures and other existing indexes, we turn to the question of socioeconomic gradients in health outcomes. A standard approach for addressing this question is Poisson regression, appropriately generalized to deal with potential spatial correlation (e.g., Breslow and Clayton, 1993), in which the dependent variable is the number of events in an area (standardized by the population size) and the independent variables include various area-based socioeconomic measures. This modeling approach permits evaluating the utility of our various socioeconomic measures, both within and across levels of geography and across the different health outcomes on the bases of predictive accuracy, relevance to public health monitoring, transparency of meaning, and ease of use by government agencies that eventually will use these measures.

CONCLUSION

In conclusion, we believe our project affords an example of why it is useful to remember the basic fact that we each live in neighborhoods and that data on socioeconomic characteristics of these neighborhoods— whether compositional or contextual—can be useful for describing and monitoring social inequalities in health. This insight is not new: the first peer-reviewed U.S. public health studies using census tract socioeconomic data to augment vital statistics appeared shortly after World War II, more than a half-century ago (Terris, 1948; Cohart, 1954; Ellis, 1968). The seemingly obvious utility of area-based socioeconomic measures to overcome the absence of socioeconomic data in U.S. public health databases, however, is belied by the still scant research on what measures to use at which level of geography. Perhaps now, with the end the cold war; with renewed discussion of economic inequality, social class, and health; and with new challenges to individualistic frameworks arising from reinvigorated social movements for social justice and human rights (Copenhagen, 1995; Braveman, 1996; Krieger and Birn, 1998; Mann et al., 1999; Shaw et al., 1999; Berkman and Kawachi, 2000; Kim et al., 2000), plus new technologies like GIS (Thrall, 1999a, 1999b; Richards et al., 1999b; Yasnoff and Sondik, 1999; Moore and Carpenter, 1999), it will finally be possible in the United States, to put social inequalities in health on the proverbial map.

Recent Findings from the Public Health Disparities Geocoding Project

Since preparation of this chapter, empirical and methodological analyses of the described study—since named the *Public Health Disparities Geocoding Project*—have been published in scientific journals. Highlights and citations are provided below.

Analytic findings
Our central finding is that census tract (CT) and block group (BG) area-based socioeconomic measures (ABSMs) performed similarly, detecting gradients expected based on the extant literature, whereas ZIP code (ZC) measures are more problematic, at times generating effect estimates substantially smaller than, larger than, and sometimes in even the opposite

direction of, those generated with BG and CT measures. Additionally, measures of economic deprivation (e.g., percent of persons below poverty) consistently detected the expected gradients, whereas measures pertaining to occupation, education, and wealth often were less sensitive. One implication is that, from a monitoring perspective, measures of economic deprivation may be best for public health surveillance systems; from an etiologic perspective, however, it may be useful to employ diverse ABSMs to elucidate relevant pathways by which socioeconomic conditions affect the specified health outcomes. For further discussion, see the following

- Krieger N, Chen JT, Waterman PD, Soobader M-J, Subramanian SV, and Carson R (2002). Geocoding and monitoring US socioeconomic inequalities in mortality and cancer incidence: Does choice of area-based measure and geographic level matter?—*The Public Health Disparities Geocoding Project. Am. J. Epidemiol.* 156: 471–482.
- Krieger N, Chen JT, Waterman PD, Soobader M-J, Subramanian SV, and Carson R (in press). Choosing area-based socioeconomic measures to monitor social inequalities in low birthweight and childhood lead poisoning—*The Public Health DIsparities Geocoding Project* (US). *J. Epidemiol. Community Health.*
- Krieger N, Chen JT, Waterman PD, Soobader M-J, Subramanian SV (in press). Monitoring socioeconomic inequalities in sexually transmitted infections, tuberculosis, and violence: geocoding and choice of area-based soecioconomic measures—*The Public Health Disparities Geocoding Project* (US). *Public Health Reports.*

Methodologic studies

These studies: (1) documented the need for ensuring accuracy of geocoding for public health research (since accuracy across several geocoding firms ranked from as low as 44% to up to 96%), and (2) provided empirical evidence of bias introduced by the potential mismatch between census-defined and ZIP code-defined geographic areas (e.g., for colon cancer, the socioeconomic gradient observed using ZC ABSMs was in the opposite direction of the expected gradient that was observed with the BG and CT ABSMs). For further discussion, see the following:

- Krieger N, Waterman PD, Lemieux K, Zierler S, Hogan JW (2001). On the wrong side of the tracts? Evaluating accuracy of geocoding for public health research. *Am J Public Health* 91:1114–1116.
- Krieger N, Waterman PD, Chen JT, Soobader M-J, Subramanian SV, and Carson R (2002). ZIP code caveat: bias due to spatiotemporal mis-

matches between ZIP codes and US census-defined areas—*The Public Health Disparities Geocoding Project. Am J Public Health* 92:1100–1102.

ACKNOWLEDGMENTS
We gratefully acknowledge our collaborators at the Massachusetts Department of Public Health and the Rhode Island Department of Health, listed below, along with the helpful guidance of our project's initial advisory board: Peter Townsend and David Gordon (University of Bristol), and Michael White and Andrew Foster (Brown University).

Massachusetts Department of Public Health: Daniel J. Friedman, PhD, Assistant Commissioner; Alice Mroszczyk, Program Coordinator for 24A/B/111B Review Committee; *Weapon Related Injury Surveillance System (WRISS):* Victoria Ozonoff, PhD, Project Director; Beth C. Hume, MPH, Data Manager/Analyst; Laurie Janelli, Site Coordinator; Patrice R. Cummings, MPH, Epidemiologist; *Cancer Registry:* Susan Gershman, PhD, Director; Mary Mroszczyk, Geocoding/Special Projects Coordinator; Ann R. MacMillan, Data Analyst; *Bureau of Communicable Disease Control:* Alfred DeMaria, Jr., MD, Assistant Commissioner; Yuren Tang, MD, MPH, Chief, Surveillance Program; *Registry of Vital Records and Statistics:* Elaine Trudeau, Registrar of Vital Records; Charlene Zion, Public Information Office.

Rhode Island Department of Health: Jay Buechner, PhD, Chief; *Health Interview Survey:* Janice Fontes, MA, Principal Systems Analyst; *Vital Statistics:* Roberta Chevoya, State Registrar of Vital Records; *Division of Disease Prevention and Control:* John Fulton, PhD, Associate Director; Ted Donnelly, RN, MPH, Senior Public Health Epidemiologist; *Violence Against Women Prevention Program:* Wendy Verhoek-Oftedahl, PhD, Epidemiologist; Joyce Babcock, MAT, Assistant Epidemiologist; *Lead:* Bob Vanderslice, PhD, Chief; Susan Feeley, MPH, Epidemiologist.

We also thank Ichiro Kawachi for sharing the program that calculates Gini coefficients based on census-defined income categories. Research for this chapter was supported by NIH grant #1 R01 HD36865-01 ("Area-based socioeconomic measures for health data," Principle Investigator, Nancy Krieger).

REFERENCES

Anderson CL, Agran PF, Winn DG, Tran C (1998). Demographic risk factors for injury among Hispanic and non-Hispanic white children: An ecologic analysis. *Injury Prevention* 4: 33–38.

Antonovsky A (1967). Social class, life expectancy and overall mortality. *Millbank Mem Fund Q* 45: 31–73.

Arbes SJ, Jr, Olshan AF, Caplan DJ, Schoenbach VJ, Slade GD, Symons MJ (1999). Factors contributing to the poorer survival of black Americans diagnosed with oral cancer (United States). *Cancer Causes Control* 10: 513–523.

Barholomew DJ and Knott M (1999). *Latent Variable Models and Factor Analysis*, 2nd ed. New York: Oxford University Press.

Berkman L and Kawachi I, eds. (2000). *Social Epidemiology*. New York: Oxford University Press.

Bernstein J, McNichol EC, Mishel L, Zahradnik R (2000). *Pulling Apart: A State-by-State Analysis of Income Trends*. Washington, DC: Center on Budget and Policy Priorities, Economic Policy Institute.

Braverman P (1996). *Equity in Health and Health Care: A WHO/SIDA Initiative*. Geneva: World Health Organization.

Brooks-Gunn J, Duncan GJ, Lawrence Arber J, eds. (1997). *Neighborhood Poverty, Volume II: Policy Implications in Studying Neighborhoods.* New York: Russell Sage Foundation Press.

Brooks-Gunn J, and Duncan GJ (1997). *Consequences of Growing Up Poor.* New York: Russell Sage Foundation Press.

Breslow NE and Clayton DG (1993). Approximate inference in generalized linear mixed models. *J Am Stat Assoc* 88: 9–25.

Cadum E, Costa G, Biggeri A, Martuzzi M (1999). Deprivation and mortality: A deprivation index suitable for geographical analysis of inequalities. *Epidemiologia e Prevenzione* 23: 175–187.

Carr-Hill R and Rice N (1995). Is enumeration district level an improvement on ward level analysis in studies of deprivation and health? *J Epidemiol Community Health* 49(suppl 2): S28–S29.

Carstairs V (1995). Deprivation indices: Their interpretation and use in relation to health. *J Epidemiol Community Health* 49(suppl 2): S3–S8.

Carstairs V and Morris R (1989). Deprivation and mortality: An alternative to social class? *Communitiy Med* 11: 210–219.

Casper ML, Barnett E, Halvorson JA, Elmes GA, Brahan VE, Majeed ZA, Bloom AS, Stanley S (1999). *Women and Heart Disease: An Atlas of Racial and Ethnic Disparities in Mortality.* Morgantown, WV: Office for Social Environment and Health Research, West Virginia University.

Chen FM, Breiman RF, Farley M, Plikaytis B, Deaver K, Cetron MS (1998). Geocoding and linking data from population-based surveillance and the U.S. Census to evaluate the impact of median household income on the epidemiology of invasive *Streptococcus pneumoniae* infections. *Am J Epidemiol* 148: 1212–1218.

Cherkin DC, Grothaus L, Wagner EH (1992). Is magnitude of co-payment effect related to income? Using census data for health services research. *Soc Sci Med* 34: 33–41.

Clayton DG and Kaldor J (1987). Empirical Bayes estimates of age-standardized relative risks for use in disease mapping. *Biometrics* 43: 671–681.

Cohart EM (1954). Socioeconomic distribution of stomach cancer in New Haven. *Cancer* 7: 455–461.

Coleman W (1982). *Death Is a Social Disease: Public Health and Political Economy in Early Industrial France.* Madison, Wis: University Wisconsin Press, pp. 149–180.

Collins JW, Jr, and David RJ (1997). Urban violence and African-American pregnancy outcome: An ecologic study. *Ethnicity Disease* 7: 184–190.

Copenhagen Declaration on Social Development (1995). World Summit for Social Development, 6–12 March 1995. URL: http://www.icsw.org/copenhagen_imp...ground_information/copenhagen.html

Council of Economic Advisors for the President's Initiative on Race (1998). *Changing America: Indicators of Social and Economic Well-Being by Race and Hispanic Origin.* URL: http://www.whitehouse.gov/WH/EOP/CEA/html/publications.htm

da Silva LM, Paim JS, Cost M da C (1999). Inequalities in mortality, space and social strata. *Revista de Saude Publica* 33: 187–197.

Davey Smith G (1997). Down at heart—The meaning and implications of social inequalities in cardiovascular disease. *J R Coll Physicians Lond* 31: 414–424.

Davey Smith G and Hart C (1999). Use of census-based aggregate variables to proxy for socioeconomic group: Evidence from national samples (letter). *Am J Epidemiol* 150: 996–997.

Davey Smith, G, Neaton JD, Wentworth D, Stamler R, Stamler J (1996a). Socioeconomic differentials in mortality among men screened for the Multiple Risk Factor Intervention Trial: I. White men. *Am J Public Health* 86: 486–496.

Davey Smith G, Wentworth D, Neaton JD, Stamler R, Stamler J (1996b). Socioeconomic differentials among men screened for the Multiple Risk Factor Intervention Trial: II. Black men. *Am J Public Health* 86: 497–504.

Devesa SS and Diamond EL (1980). Association of breast cancer and cervical cancer incidence with income and education among whites and blacks. *J Natl Cancer Inst* 65: 515–528.

Diez-Roux AV (1998). Bringing context back into epidemiology: Variables and fallacies in multilevel analysis. *Am J Public Health* 88: 216–222.

Ellen JM, Kohn RP, Bolan GA, Shiboski S, Krieger N (1995). Socioeconomic differences in sexually transmitted disease rates among black and white adolescents, San Francisco, 1990 to 1992. *Am J Public Health* 85: 1546–1548.

Ellis JM (1968). Socioeconomic differentials in mortality from chronic diseases. In Jaco EG, ed.: *Patients, Physicians, Illness*. Glencoe, Ill: Free Press, pp. 30–37.

Engels F (1845 [1958]). *The Condition of the Working Class in England*, transl Henderson WO and Chaloner WH). Stanford, Calif: Stanford University Press, pp. 120–121.

Evans RG, Barer ML, Marmor TR, eds. (1994). *Why Are Some People Healthy and Others Not? The Determinants of Health of Populations.* New York: Aldine de Gruyter.

Fife D and Mode C (1992). AIDS incidence and income. *J Acquir Immune Defic Syndr Hum Retrovirol* 5: 1105–1110.

Fox J, ed. (1989). *Health Inequalities in European Countries.* Aldershot, UK: Gower.

Freeman HP (1998). The meaning of race in science—Considerations for cancer research: concerns of special populations in the National Cancer Program. *Cancer* 82: 219–225.

Geolytics Inc. (2000). *Census CD+*. East Brunswick, NJ. URL: http://www.geolytics.com

Geronimus AT and Bound J (1998). Use of census-based aggregate variables to proxy for socioeconomic group: Evidence from national samples. *Am J Epidemiol* 148: 475–486.

Geronimus AT, Bound J, Neidert LJ (1996). On the validity of using census geocode data to proxy individual socioeconomic characteristics. *J Am Statist Assoc* 91: 529–537.

Goldsmith HF, Lee AS, Rosen BM (1982). *Small Area Social Indicators.* National Institutes of Mental Health, Mental Health Service System Reports Series BN, No. 3, DHHS Pub. No. (ADM) 82-1189. Washington, DC: U.S. Government Printing Office.

Goldstein H (1995). *Multilevel Statistical Models,* 2nd ed. New York: Oxford University Press.

Gordon D (1995). Census based deprivation indices: Their weighting and validation. *J Epidemiol Community Health* 49(suppl 2): S39–S44.

Gordon D and Spicker P, eds. (1999). *The International Glossary on Poverty.* London: Zed Books.

Greenwald JP, Polissar NL, Borgatta EF, McCorkle R (1994). Detecting survival effects of socioeconomic status: Problems in the use of aggregate data. *J Clin Epidemiol* 47: 903–909.

Grisco JA, Schwarz DF, Hirschinger N, Sammel M, Brensinger C, Santanna J, Lowe

RA, Anderson E, Shaw LM, Bethel CA, et al. (1999). Violent injuries among women in an urban area. *N Engl J Med* 341: 1899–1905.

Haan M, Kaplan GA, Camacho T (1987). Poverty and health: Prospective evidence from the Alameda County Study. *Am J Epidemiol* 125: 989–998.

Hankins C, Tran T, Hum L, Laberge C, Lapointe N, Lepine D, Montpetit M, O'Shaughnessy MV (1998). Socioeconomic geographical links to human immunodeficiency virus seroprevalence among childbearing women in Montreal, 1989–1993. *Int J Epidemiol* 27: 691–697.

Harries K (1997). Social stress and trauma: Synthesis and spatial analysis. *Soc Sci Med* 45: 1251–1264.

Hinton RY, Lincoln A, Crockett MM, Sponseller P, Smith G, (1999). Fractures of the femoral shaft in children: Incidence, mechanisms, and sociodemographic risk factors. *J Bone Joint Surg* 81: 500–509.

Hu DJ, Frey R, Costa SJ, et al. (1994). Geographical AIDS rates and sociodemographic variables in Newark, New Jersey, metropolitan area. *AIDS Public Policy J* 9: 20–25.

Hyndman JCT, D'Arcy D, Holman J, Hockey RL, Donovan RJ, Corti B, Rivera J (1995). Misclassification of social disadvantage based on geographical areas: Comparison of postcode and collector's districts analyses. *Int J Epidemiol* 24: 165–176.

Institute of Medicine Committee for the Study of the Future of Public Health (1988). *The Future of Public Health.* Washington, DC: National Academy Press.

Institute of Medicine Committee on Using Performance Monitoring to Improve Community Health (1997). *Improving Health in the Community: A Role for Performance Monitoring.* Washington, DC: National Academy Press.

Iwashyna TJ, Christakis NA, Becker LB (1999). Neighborhoods matter: A population-based study of provision of cardiopulmonary resuscitation. *Ann Emergency Med* 34: 459–468.

Jargowsky PA (1997). *Poverty and Place: Ghettos, Barrios, and the American City.* New York: Russell Sage.

Kaplan CP and Van Valey TL (1980). *Census '80: Continuing the Fact Finding Tradition.* Washington, DC: U.S. Government Printing Office.

Kim JY, Millen JV, Irwin A, Gershman J (2000). *Dying for Growth: Global Inequality and the Health of the Poor.* Monroe, Maine: Common Courage Press.

Kitagawa EM and Hauser PM (1973). *Differential Mortality in the United States: A Study in Socioeconomic Epidemiology.* Cambridge, Mass: Harvard University Press.

Krieger N (1992). Overcoming the absence of socioeconomic data and medical records: Validation and application of a census-based methodology. *Am J Public Health* 82: 703–710.

Krieger N (1990). Social class and the black/white crossover in the age-specific incidence of breast cancer: A study linking census-derived data to population-based registry records. *Am J Epidemiol* 131: 804–814.

Krieger N (1991). Women and social class: A methodological study comparing individual, household, and census measures as predictors of black/white differences in reproductive history. *J Epidemiol Community Health* 45: 35–42.

Krieger N and Birn AE (1998). A vision of social justice as the foundation of public health: Commemorating 150 years of the spirit of 1848. *Am J Public Health* 88: 1603–1606.

Krieger N, Chen JT, Ebel G (1997b). Can we monitor socioeconomic inequalities in health? A survey of U.S. health departments' data collection and reporting practices. *Public Health Reports* 112: 481–491.

Krieger N, Chen JT, Selby JV (1999a). Comparing individual-based and house-hold-based measures of social class to assess class inequalities in women's health: A methodological study of 684 U.S. women. *J Epidemiol Community Health* 53: 612–623.

Krieger N and Fee E (1996). Measuring social inequalities in health in the United States: An historical review, 1900–1950. *Int J Health Serv* 26: 391–418.

Krieger N and Gordon D (1999). Re: "Use of census-based aggregate variables to proxy for socioeconomic group: Evidence from national samples" (letter). *Am J Epidemiol* 150: 892–896.

Krieger N, Quesenberry, Jr, C, Peng T, Horn-Ross P, Stewart S, Brown S, Swallen K, Guillermo T, Suh D, Alvarez-Martinez L, Ward F (1999b). Social class, race/ethnicity, and incidence of breast, cervix, colon, lung, and prostate cancer among Asian, black, Hispanic, and white residents of the San Francisco Bay area, 1988–92 (United States). *Cancer Causes Control* 10: 525–537.

Krieger N, Rowley D, Hermann AA, Avery B, Phillips MT (1993). Racism, sexism, and social class: Implications for studies of health, disease, and well-being. *Am J Prev Med* 9(suppl): 82–122.

Krieger J, Song L, Solet D (1996). Use of social status measures in community assessment. Paper presented at the American Public Health Association 124th annual meeting, New York , 18–21 November 1996.

Krieger N, Williams DR, Moss NE (1997a). Measuring social class in U.S. public health research: Concepts, methodologies, and guidelines. *Annu Rev Public Health* 18: 341–378.

Lee P, Murie A, Gordon D (1995). *Area Measures of Deprivation: A Study of Current Methods and Best Practices in the Identification of Poor Areas in Great Britain.* Birmingham, UK: Centre for Urban and Regional Studies, University of Birmingham.

Liu L, Deapen D, Bernstein L (1998). Socioeconomic status and cancers of the femal breast and reproductive organs: A comparison across racial/ethnic populations in Los Angeles County, California (United States). *Cancer Causes Control* 9: 369–380.

Lynch J and Kaplan G (2000). Socioeconomic position. In Berkman L and Kawachi I, eds.: *Social Epidemiology.* New York: Oxford University Press, pp. 13–35.

MacIntyre S and Ellaway A (2000). Ecological approaches: Rediscovering the role of the physical and social environment. In Berkman L and Kawachi I, eds.: *Social Epidemiology.* New York: Oxford University Press, pp. 332–348.

Mann JM, Gruskin S, Grodin MA, Annas GJ, eds. (1999). *Health and Human Rights.* New York: Routledge.

Merriwether RA (1996). Blueprint for a National Public Health Surveillance System for the 21st century. *J Public Health Management Practice* 2: 16–23.

Moore DA and Carpenter TE (1999). Spatial analytic methods and geographic information systems: Use in health research and epidemiology. *Epidemiol Rev* 21: 143–161.

Morse DL, Lessner L, Medvesky MG, Glebatis DM, Novick LF (1991). Geographic distribution of newborn HIV seroprevalence in relation to four sociodemographic variables. *Am J Public Health* 81(suppl): 25–29.

Mustard DL, Derksen S, Berthelot JM, Wolfson M (1999). Assessing ecologic proxies for household income: A comparison of household and neighbourhood
level income measures in the study of population health status. *Health Place* 5:
157–171.

National Center for Health Statistics (1996). *Health, United States 1995.* Hyattsville,
Md: Public Health Service.

National Center for Health Statistics (1997). *Health, United States, 1996–97, and Injury Chartbook.* Hyattsville, Md: U.S. Department of Health and Human Services.

National Center for Health Statistics (1999). *Health, United States, 1999, with Health
and Aging Chartbook.* Hyattsville, Md: U.S. Department of Health and Human
Services.

Nichols M (1999). Personal communication via e-mail. Products and Service Staff,
Geography Division, U.S. Census Bureau, 13 December 1999.

Nolan LJ, Freeman WL, D'Angelo AJ (1996). Local research: Needed guidance for
the Indian Health Service's urban mission. *Public Health Reports* 320: 111.

O'Campo P, Xue X, Wang MC, Caughy M (1997). Neighborhood risk factors for
low birthweights in Baltimore: A multilevel analysis. *Am J Public Health* 87:
1113–1118.

Pamuk E, Makuc D, Heck K, Reuben C, Lochner K (1998). *Socioeconomic Status
and Health Chartbook.* Health, United States, 1988. Hyattsville, Md: National
Center for Health Statistics.

Pollack AM and Rice DP (1997). Monitoring health care in the United States—A
challenging task. *Public Health Reports* 112: 108–113.

Powell EC and Tanz RR (1999). Child and adolescent injury and death from urban firearm assaults: Association with age, race and poverty. *Injury Prevention*
5: 41–47.

Prehn AW and West DW (1998). Evaluating local differences in breast cancer incidence rates: A census-based methodology (United States). *Cancer Causes Control* 9: 511–517.

Pringle DG, Walsh J, Hennessy M, eds. (1999). *Poor People, Poor Places: A Geography of Poverty and Deprivation in Ireland.* Dublin: Oak Tree Press.

Richards TB, Croner CM, Rushton G, Brown CK, Fowler L (1999). Geographic information systems and public health: Mapping the future. *Public Health Reports* 114: 359–373.

Roberts EM (1997). Neighborhood social environments and the distribution of low
birthweight in Chicago. *Am J Public Health* 87: 597–603.

Rossi RJ and Gilmartin KJ (1980). *The Handbook of Social Indicators: Sources, Characteristics, and Analysis.* New York: Garland STPM Press.

Sayegh AJ, Swor R, Chu KH, Jackson R, Gitlin J, Domeier RM, Basse E, Smith D,
Fales W. Does race or socioeconomic status predict adverse outcome after out
of hospital cardiac arrest: A multi-center study. *Resuscitation* 40: 141–146.

Shaw M, Dorling D, Gordon D, Davey-Smith G (1999). *The Widening Gap: Health
Inequalities and Policy in Britain.* Bristol, UK: University of Bristol Press.

Shevsky E and Bell W (1955). *Social Area Analysis: Theory, Illustrative Application,
and Computational Procedures.* Stanford, Calif: Stanford University Press.

Simon PA, Hu DJ, Diaz T, Kerndt PR (1995). Income and AIDS rates in Los Angeles County. *AIDS* 9: 281–284.

Soobader M-J and LeClere FB (1999). Aggregation and the measurement of income inequality: Effects on morbidity. *Soc Sci Med* 48: 733–744.

Sorensen A (1994). Women, family, and class. *Annual Review of Sociology* 20: 27–47.

Stuber C (1999). Personal communication via e-mail. U.S. Bureau of Census, 13 December 1999.

Terris M (1948). Relation of economic status to tuberculosis mortality by age and sex. *Am J Public Health* 38: 1061–1070.

Thrall GI (1999a). The future of GIS in public health management and practice. *J Public Health Management Practice* 5: 75–82.

Thrall SE (1999b). Geographic information system (GIS) hardware and software. *J Public Health Management Practice* 5: 82–90.

Tolson GC, Barnes JM, Gay GA, Kowaleski JL (1991). The 1989 revision of the U.S. standard certificates and reports. National Center for Health Statistics. DHHS Pub. No. PHS 91-1465. *Vital Health Stat* 4 (28).

Townsend P (1993). *The International Analysis of Poverty.* New York: Harvester/ Wheatsheaf.

Townsend P, Davidson N, Whitehead M (1990). *Inequalities in Health: The Black Report and the Health Divide.* London: Penguin Books.

Townsend P, Phillimore P, Beattie A (1988). *Health and Deprivation: Inequality and the North.* London: Croom Helm.

U.S. Bureau of the Census (2000). The Census Tract Street Locator. URL: http://tier2.census.gov/ctsl/ctsl.htm

U.S. Bureau of the Census (1991). *Census of Population and Housing, 1990: Summary Tape File 3 Technical Documentation.* Washington, DC: Bureau of the Census.

U.S. Bureau of the Census (1985). *Poverty Areas in Large Cities, PC80-2-8D: 1980 Census of Population, Vol. 2, Subject Reports.* Washington, DC: U.S. Government Printing Office.

U.S. Bureau of the Census (1999). *American Community Survey: Questions and Answers.* Washington, DC: U.S. Department of Commerce. URL: http://www. census.gov/acs/www

U.S. Department of Commerce (1990). *Census '90 Basics.* Washington, DC: U.S. Government Printing Office.

U.S. Department of Health and Human Services (1991). *Health of Minorities and Low Income Groups*, 3rd ed. Washington, DC: U.S. Government Printing Office.

U.S. Department of Health and Human Services (2000). *Healthy People 2010 (Conference Edition, in Two Volumes).* Washington, DC. URL: http://www.health. gov/healthypeople

U.S. Post Office (2000). URL: http://www.framed.usps.com/ncsc/lookups/ zip_faqs.htm

Villermé LR (1828). Mémoire sur la mortalité en France dans la classe aisée et dans la classe indigente. *Mémoires de l'Académie royale de medicine* 1: 51–98.

Wasserman CR, Shaw GM, Selvin S, Gould JB, Syme SL (1998). Socioeconomic status, neighborhood social conditions, and neural tube defects. *Am J Public Health* 88: 1674–1680.

White MJ (1987). *American Neighborhoods and Residential Differentiation.* New York: Russell Sage Foundation.

Whitney JS, ed. (1934). *Death Rates by Occupation Based on Data of the U.S. Census Bureau 1930.* New York: National Tuberculosis Association.

Williams DR and Collins C (1995). U.S. socioeconomic and racial differences in health: Patterns and explanations. *Ann Rev Sociol* 21: 329–386.

Wissow LS, Gittelsohn AM, Szklo M, Starfield B, Mussman M (1988). Poverty, race, and hospitalization for childhood asthma. *Am J Public Health* 78: 777–782.

Wright EO (1997). *Class Counts: Comparative Studies in Class Analysis.* Cambridge: Cambridge University Press.

Wright EO, Costello C, Hachen D, Sprague J (1982). The American class structure. *Am Sociol Rev* 47: 709–726.

Yasnoff WA and Sondik EJ (1999). Geographic information systems (GIS) in public health practice and the new millennium. *J Public Health Management Practice* 5(4): viii–xi.

Zierler S, Krieger N, Tang Y, Coady W, Siegfried E, DeMaria A, Auerbach J (2000). Economic deprivation and AIDS incidence. *Am J Public Health* 90:1064–1073.

8

Area-Based Deprivation Measures—a U.K. Perspective

DAVID GORDON

In Britain poverty, deprivation, and health statistics have been collected for many centuries. For example, since the sixteenth century details on the circumstances in which and age at which people died have been collected. In London in the 1530s, parish clerks were required to submit weekly reports on the number of plague deaths. These details were written up as "bills of mortality," which informed the authorities when public health measures should be taken against epidemics. The first summary of these reports was published as the *London Bills of Mortality* by the Company of Parish Clerks in 1604 (Brakenridge, 1755).

Similarly, information on the numbers and circumstances of paupers dates back to the early 1600s and was a result of the passing of Queen Elizabeth I's "Poor Law" in 1599–1601. Analysis of eighteenth-century mortality data reveals strong gradients in child mortality by socioeconomic status. Table 8–1 shows that, on average, 20% of the children of British dukes died before their fifth birthday compared with 24% of the children of fairly prosperous Bedfordshire peasants and 39% of the children of the relatively poorer Lincolnshire peasants. A similar social class gradient was also evident in the eighteenth century in the mortality rates of those under 21 years of age. Similar analysis of early data shows geographic differences in health, as shown in Table 8–2.

During the nineteenth century people in rural areas had lower mortality than did those in urban areas—life expectancy in rural Rutland was higher than in most urban areas—among all social classes. Indeed, the life expectancy of laborers and artisans living in basements in the inner city areas of Liverpool, Manchester, and London was less than 20 years (Chadwick, 1842). The nineteenth-century pioneers of public health medicine in Britain had no doubt that the high mortality and morbidity of the

TABLE 8–1. Mortality of Infants and Young People (1739–1779)

	Deaths among Recorded Baptisms (%)	
	Under 5 Years	Under 21 Years
British dukes (Hollingsworth, 1965)	20	27
Bedfordshire peasants (fairly prosperous) (Tranter, 1966)	24	31
Lincolnshire peasants (Chambers, 1972)	39	60

Source: Drever and Whitehead (1997).

poorest was, in large part, a consequence of the deprivations they suffered. The causal association between the geography of deprivation and ill health has been studied in the United Kingdom since then.

The systematic analysis and mapping of poverty in Britain was made possible by the invention of the basic statistical techniques we now take for granted (such as the five bar gate),[1] which enabled accurate census counts. Fletcher (1849) published standardized maps of pauperism in England and Wales for 1844. These were based on census and administrative data on the numbers receiving "indoor" and "outdoor" "relief" under the "new" Poor Law. There was a clear north–south divide, with high rates of pauperism in the rural southern counties.

Today's poverty maps also show a strong north–south divide. Now, however, there is much more poverty in the north than in the south, and this is particularly concentrated in the northern conurbations. Figure 8–1

TABLE 8–2. Longevity of Families, by Class and Area of Residence (1838–1841)

District	Gentry and Professional	Farmers and Tradesmen	Laborers and Artisans
Rural			
Rutland	52	41	38
Urban			
Bath	55	37	25
Leeds	44	27	19
Bethnal Green	45	26	16
Manchester	38	20	17
Liverpool	35	22	15

Source: Drever and Whitehead (1997).

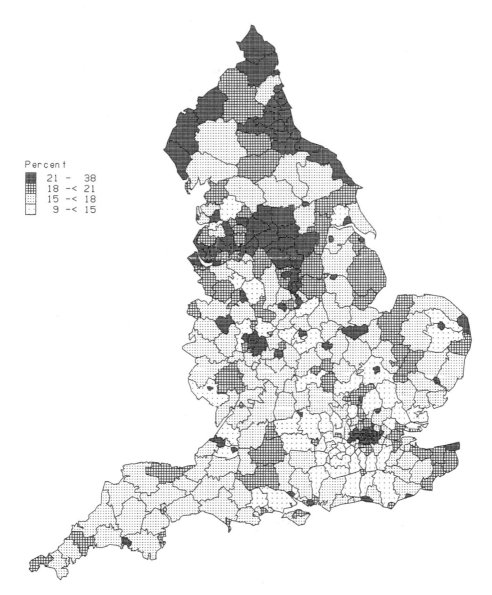

Figure 8–1. *Breadline Britain* poverty estimates for England at local authority level.

shows the estimated percentage of poor households in the 366 Local Authority Districts of England (Gordon and Forrest, 1995). The districts have been divided into approximate quartiles (the poorest 25% of authorities, the next 25%, and so forth), and a clear pattern is evident on the map. There are high numbers of poor households living in Tyneside, Merseyside, Greater Manchester, and into Yorkshire and inner London. Poor households are also found in the major cities and in rural districts of Cornwall, East Anglia, Kent, Cumbria, and Northumberland.

There is a very strong causal relationship between premature death, ill health, and poverty. Figure 8–2 shows a quartile map of the Standardised Limiting Long Term Illness Ratio for the 366 Local Authority Districts in England as recoded in the 1991 census. The map of standardized illness is effectively identical to the map of poverty shown in Figure 8–1. The areas with the highest rates of poverty have the highest rates of ill health after adjusting for age and sex.

Neighborhoods, Areas, and Health

One of the most high-profile government policies designed to tackle the problem of inequalities in health was the establishment of area-specific Health Action Zones (HAZ) in England in April 1998. John Denham (U.K. minister for health) has stated that "Health among the poor must improve at a faster rate than the general population. This means tackling ill health that results from poverty where poverty occurs [and that] Health Action Zones are a key part of the Government's drive in tackling health inequalities" (DoH, 1999).

However, area-based policies such as these action zones have a long history of limited success or even outright failure (Barnes and Lucas, 1975; CDP, 1977; Townsend, 1979; Robson et al, 1994; Glennerster et al, 1999). An area-based rather than people-based approach to attacking problems of health inequality, poverty, and deprivation can only provide help to a relatively small minority of people because most "poor areas" contain only a minority of "poor" households and a majority of "nonpoor" households (Lee et al, 1995). Similarly, the majority of "sick" people in Britain do not live in "unhealthy neighborhoods" (Davey Smith and Gordon, 2000). These problems have been understood for a long time; in 1975 the Education Priority Area (EPA) schools program was criticized because "For every two disadvantaged children who are in EPA schools five are outside them" (Barnes and Lucas, 1975) Similarly, in 1979 Peter Townsend argued in *Poverty in the UK* that, "An area strategy can never be the cardinal means of dealing with poverty or 'under privilege'. . . . However

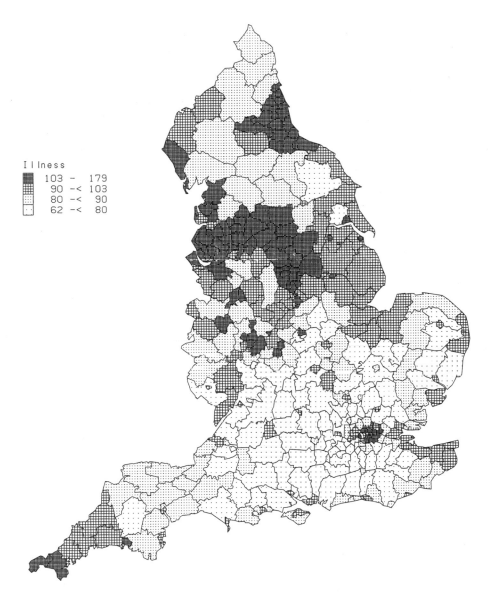

Illness
103 – 179
90 –< 103
80 –< 90
62 –< 80

FIGURE 8–2. Standardized illness ratio for England at local authority level.

we care to define economically or socially deprived areas, unless we include over half the areas in the country, there will be more poor persons or poor children living outside them." Similarly, Robinson et al. (1994) in their massive review of the effectiveness of urban area–based policies designed to reduce inequality and deprivation argued that "the consensus was that places had been the typical mode of targeting in the past. However, many argued that, in future, programmes would need to focus as much upon target population groups as on deprived areas. The view that targeting areas automatically benefited the people living within them was clearly challenged."

Inequalities in health are a national problem that requires national solutions. The root cause of inequalities in health is poverty, which area-based policies cannot tackle effectively or efficiently. Nevertheless, neighborhoods and area-based health policies are important when they form part of a national strategy. However, they are never likely to be very effective without national policies to back them up.

The existence of the National Health Service, with its U.K.-wide health focus, has given local-area public health policies and measures of deprivation a somewhat different emphasis than that in the United States. Public health discussions in the United States often focus on the biology and behavior of individuals and the appropriate health promotion strategy, whereas in the United Kingdom there is a greater tendency to focus on the health of populations. The health of populations is not just affected by people's behavior or biology but also by structural social causes like poverty. The health of populations also is not only the primary responsibility of individuals and the health service—it is also the responsibility of politicians. Therefore, much of the measurement of both deprivation and ill health in the United Kingdom, at small area level, has been by political geography (e.g., at parliamentary constituency, electoral ward, and district council level) rather than at the medical geography level (district health authority, etc.) or at the "homogeneous" neighborhood or community level. Politicians are responsible for the distribution of funds for health and other services. Therefore, knowledge of the political geography of sickness and poverty is crucial for resource allocation purposes.

DEFINITIONS

The word *poverty* means different things in the U.S. and U.K. scientific literature (Gordon and Spicker, 1999). In the United States when researchers talk about poverty they generally mean people/households with a low income, that is, below the poverty threshold. Poverty is defined solely in terms of low income. Orshansky (1965; 1969) used budget standard norms developed by the U.S. Department of Agriculture (USDA) to calculate basic food expenditures for different types of households. There were four such budgets; all sought to define a nutritionally adequate diet but differed in details and costs. It was decided by a political decision that the "economy food plan" should be used. This was designed for "temporary or emergency use when funds were low" (Fisher, 1992).

The poverty threshold is calculated for a family of any given size by multiplying the cost of the relevant economy food plan by 3 for families of three or more people and by 3.7 for families of two people. The multipliers of 3 and 3.7 are derived from the 1955 Household Food Consumption Survey. This survey showed that families of three or more typically spent a third of their after-tax income on food, and families of two typically spent 27% of their after-tax income on food. Thus, in 1965 the poverty line for an urban family of four was set at $3,000.

The poverty line is increased every year in relation to the Consumer Price Index but has not otherwise been changed in any major way.[2] This key characteristic makes it possible to draw conclusions about trends in poverty in a way that is not possible if a purely relative poverty line is used. However, this feature is also problematic. The gap between the average American household income and the poverty line has increased since the 1960s. Thus, in the 1990s living conditions among the poor deviated more from the average American lifestyle than in the 1960s. Even though the poverty line is adjusted in line with prices, it is not adjusted according to changes in the price relatives. For example, the percentage of income the average American household spends on food has decreased over time, indicating that the use of 3 as the multiplier of the food budget is inadequate (Harrington, 1984; Nolan and Whelan, 1996). Given these problems, many European academics would regard the official U.S. poverty line as a much better measure of low income or income inequality than of poverty.

There is also very little information about the population's income at small area level in Britain. Income information has never been collected in the U.K. Census, and despite considerable demand for the inclusion of an income question in the 2001 census (ONS, 1999), this proposal was eventually rejected due to fears that fewer people would respond if this question was added (Teague, 1999). Obtaining accurate and complete information on income from households has long been considered one of the most intractable problems facing British social researchers. Survey researchers often claim that "people are more willing to talk about their sexual behaviour than about their financial affairs and even if they are willing to talk they may not have the necessary knowledge to answer the questions" (Martin, 1990). This perception may, in part, be a historical truth resulting from class-based differences in discussing financial affairs within British society. In the past financial matters were considered to be a "proper" topic of conversation only between a suitor and his prospective father-in-law in upper- and upper-middle-class families. However, working-class households were often more forthcoming, and, indeed, the welfare state has always required disclosure of financial matters in order to claim means-tested benefits (Bradshaw et al., 1999).

National statistics on low income show that there has been a huge rise in the number of people living in households with incomes below half the average (the current de facto relative poverty threshold), as shown in Figure 8–3. During the 1960s the amount of income inequality in Britain remained fairly constant, with around 11% of the population living on incomes below half the average. The recession and "stagflation" of the early 1970s following the OPEC oil price increases caused the numbers living on less than half the average income to rise to a peak of slightly more than 13%. The government's relatively progressive social and economic policies in the mid-1970s resulted in poverty and inequality falling rapidly to a low of less than 8% of the population in 1977 and 1978. The 1979 election victory of the Conservative party under Margaret Thatcher's leadership brought a reverse in social and economic policies designed to promote equity and led to a rapid growth in poverty and inequality, which increased throughout the 1980s and early 1990s. The marginally more progressive social polices of the 1992 Conservative government (under John

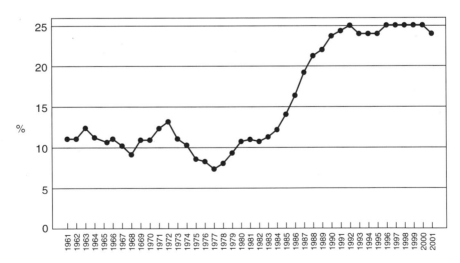

FIGURE 8–3. Percentage of the population below half average incomes after housing costs, 1961 to 2001. Source: Goodman and Webb (1994) and HBAI.

Major) resulted in a less rapid increase in inequality during the mid-1990s. However, by 2000 and 2001, the period for which we have the latest figures, 25% of the British population was living on incomes that were so low as to be below half the average income. The percentage of the British population living on low incomes more than trebled (from 8% to 25%) during the 1980s and early 1990s. By 2000 more than 14 million people in Britain were living in households with incomes below half the average (after the deduction of housing costs).

The geography of income in Britain can be estimated only from statistical models that use employment and administrative data (Gordon and Forrest, 1995). The richest areas are concentrated in the southeast, in the rural and semirural districts around London. Low-income areas do, in general, coincide with areas of high deprivation, but not always—there are some districts where the rich and poor live side by side, for example, in central London and some rural districts.

POVERTY IN EUROPE

Although there are very few "official" poverty lines in European countries, poverty is often defined in terms of both low income and deprivation, that is, a person or household in Britain is "poor" when they have both a low standard of living and a low income. They are "not poor" if they have a low income and a reasonable standard of living or if they have a low standard of living but a high income. Both low income and low standard of living can be accurately measured only relative to the norms of the person's or household's society.

A low standard of living is often measured by using a deprivation index (high deprivation equals a low standard of living) or by consumption expenditure (low consumption expenditure equals a low standard of living). Of these two methods deprivation indexes are more accurate because consumption expenditure is often measured over only a brief period and is obviously not independent of available income.

The 'objective' poverty line (or threshold) is shown in Figure 8–4. It can be defined as the point that maximizes the differences between the two groups ("poor" and "not poor") and minimizes the differences within the two groups.

This "scientific" concept of poverty can be made universally applicable by using the broader concept of "resources" instead of just monetary income. It can also be applied in developing countries where barter and income-in-kind can be as important as cash income. Poverty can then be defined as the point at which resources are so seriously below those com-

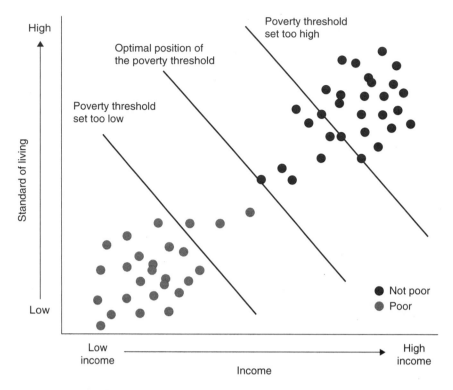

Figure 8–4. Definition of poverty in terms of income and standard of living.

manded by the average individual or family that the poor are, in effect, excluded from ordinary living patterns, customs, and activities. As resources for any individual or family diminish, there is a point at which a sudden withdrawal from participation in the customs and activities sanctioned by the culture occurs. The point at which societal withdrawal escalates disproportionately to falling resources can be defined as the poverty line or threshold (Townsend, 1979; Townsend and Gordon, 1989) (see Figure 8–5). A similar relationship has been demonstrated between ill health and low income in Britain. As income falls, there is a point of which ill health begins to increase disproportionately to falling resources (Blaxter, 1990).

In British poverty surveys, people and households with high incomes and high standards of living are defined as "not poor," whereas those with low incomes and a low standards of living are defined as "poor." However, two other groups of people and households that are "not poor" can also be identified in a cross-sectional (one point in time) survey, such as a census:

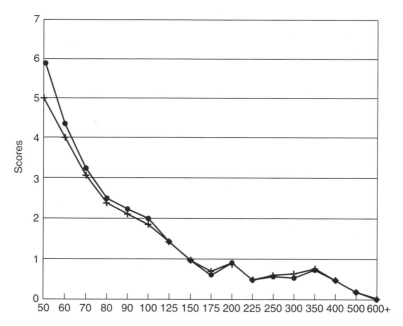

FIGURE 8–5. Relationship between equivalent household income and two deprivation index scores showing a clear poverty threshold at £150 per week. Source: Halleröd et al. (1997).

1. *People or households with low incomes but high standards of living.* This group currently is "not poor," but if their incomes remain low, they will become poor—they are currently sinking into poverty. This situation often arises when incomes fall rapidly (e.g., due to job loss) but people manage to maintain their lifestyles for at least a few months by drawing on their savings.
2. *People or households with high incomes but low standards of living.* This group is currently "not poor," and if their income remains high their standard of living will rise—they will have risen out of poverty. This group is in a situation opposite to the previous group. This situation can arise when the income of someone who is poor suddenly increases (e.g., due to getting a job). However, it takes time before they are able to buy the things that they need to increase their standard of living. Income can both rise and fall faster than the standard of living.

Poverty is, by definition, an extremely unpleasant situation in which to live, so it is not surprising that people go to considerable lengths to avoid it and try very hard to escape from it. Therefore, a cross-sectional poverty survey ought to find that the group of households sinking into poverty would be larger than the group escaping from poverty because, when income falls people try to delay the descent into poverty. If the income of a poor person increases, however, she will quickly try to improve her standard of living. Figure 8–6 illustrates these concepts.

Between Times 0 and 1 the household has both a high standard of living (dotted line) and a high income (solid line)—it is "not poor." At Time 1 there is a rapid reduction in income (e.g., due to job loss, the end of seasonal contract income, divorce, separation, etc). However, the household's standard of living does not fall immediately. It is not until Time 2 that the household's standard of living has fallen below the "poverty" threshold. Therefore, between Time 1 and Time 2, the household is "not poor" but is sinking into poverty (i.e., it has a low income but a relatively high standard of living). At Time 3 income begins to rise rapidly, although not as fast as it previously fell. This is because rapid income increases usually result from gaining employment, but there is often a lag between starting work and getting paid. Standard of living also begins to rise after a brief period as the household spends its way out of poverty. However, this lag means that there is a short period when the household has a high income but a relatively low standard of living. By Time 5 the household again has a high income and a high standard of living.

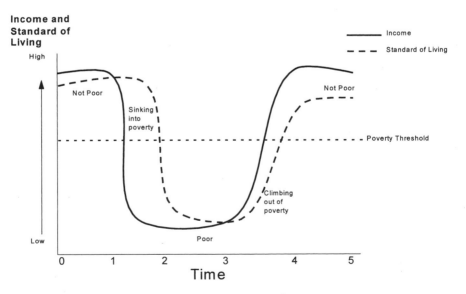

FIGURE 8–6. The dynamics of poverty.

THE DYNAMICS OF LOW INCOME IN EUROPE AND NORTH AMERICA

Britain and other European countries tend to use deprivation indexes as proxy poverty measures (rather than low-income data) when studying small areas. This is partly due to the lack of low-income data (at least in Britain, although not in Nordic countries), but also because at any given time there are a significant number of people and households with very low incomes who will not sink into poverty. This is because the low income period is a short lived, temporary, albeit unpleasant episode.

There are significant differences in the labor markets and effectiveness of the welfare states between Europe and North America. People on low incomes in Europe tend to manage to rise out of poverty much more rapidly than they do in North America. Table 8–3 shows that there are

TABLE 8–3. Poverty Rates and Transition out of Poverty for Families with Children

Country	Poverty Rate (% with Income Below 50% of Median Income of the Whole Population)	Transition Out of Poverty Rate (% per Year of the Poor Becoming Nonpoor)	Three-Year Poverty Rate (% of the Population with Incomes Below 50% of Median in All 3-Years of a 3-YearPeriod)
Europe			
France	4.0	27.5	1.6
Germany (all)	7.8	25.6	1.5
German residents	6.7	26.9	1.4
Foreign residents	18.0	20.0	4.0
Ireland	11.0	25.2	N/A
Luxembourg	4.4	26.0	0.4
Netherlands	2.7	44.4	0.4
Sweden	2.7	36.8	N/A
North America			
Canada	17.0	12.0	11.9
United States (all)	20.3	13.8	14.4
U.S. white residents	15.3	17.0	9.5
U.S. black residents	49.3	7.7	41.5

Poverty is defined as an equivalized income below 50% of the median income for the population.
Source: Modified from Duncan et al., 1993.

marked differences between European and North American countries in both the poverty rate (low income) and the likelihood of escaping from poverty. In Ireland, Luxembourg, the Netherlands and Sweden virtually no families with children lived continuously in poverty for the whole of a three-year period. In contrast, the majority of the poor in Canada and the United States remained in poverty for most of a three-year period. However, even in the United States, Bane and Ellwood (1986) found that about 60% of poverty spells lasted one or two years, and only around 14% lasted eight or more years. It must be noted that these are single spells, some of which would have been followed rapidly by subsequent periods of poverty.

DEPRIVATION INDEXES IN THE UNITED KINGDOM

The construction of census-based deprivation indexes in the United Kingdom is one of the most economically important uses of social statistics, as they form a key element in the allocation of both local government and health resources. The amount of money a district receives from central government can depend to a considerable extent on its deprivation score. However, none of the questions in the 1991 census was specifically designed to measure either poverty or deprivation, and no questions were asked about income. Therefore, any census-based index must be comprised of variables that are, at best, proxy indicators of deprivation rather than direct measures. It is, therefore, unsurprising that a bewildering array of indexes has been proposed, using different combinations of variables and different statistical methods.

The problems inherent to constructing census-based deprivation indexes were well understood by Holtermann (1975) in one of the first analyses of urban deprivation using the 1971 census. Holtermann concluded that there are two problems inherent in the use of census data in attempting to discover where the poor live. First, she referred to the ecological fallacy by identifying the problem of confusing multiply deprived areas with multiply deprived households and, second, she referred to the difficulties encountered when using census indicators as indirect measures when she posed the following question: "Is there a strong association between Census indicators and other aspects of deprivation not measurable from the Census?" (Holtermann, 1975, p. 44). Her methodological approach to the identification of the most deprived areas avoided the use of a composite index on the grounds that such an index ignored "the relative importance that deprived individuals themselves attach to the different dimensions of deprivation" and that composite scores involving arithmetical transformations "bear no relation to the relative importance of each aspect of deprivation in contributing to individuals' loss of welfare" (Holtermann, 1975, p. 34).

Holtermann therefore rejected the composite index approach in the measurement and identification of deprived areas. Instead, she took the spatial distribution (using Census Enumeration Districts) of a set of deprivation indicators and (arbitrarily) invoked a cut-off point at the distribution points of 1%, 5%, and 15%, observing the percentage of the phenomena being measured at each threshold. For example, she found that the worst 1% of urban Census Enumeration Districts in Great Britain had male unemployment rates of 24% or greater (Holtermann, 1975, p. 36).

Despite Holtermann's reservations, a number of deprivation indexes have been proposed since her work. These have been developed mainly on pragmatic rather than theoretical grounds—*some* method must be used to allocate resources. Eight census-based deprivation indexes have been fairly widely used: Jarman's (1983, 1984) Under Privileged Area Score UPA(8); the Department of the Environment's All Area Social Index (AASI); the Townsend Index (Townsend et al., 1988); the Scotdep Index of Carstairs and Morris (1989, 1991a, 1991b); the Scottish Development Department Index (SDD); the Matdep and Socdep Indices of Forrest and Gordon (1993); and, finally, the Department of the Environment's Index of Local Conditions (Department of Environment, 1994). The first five indexes were initially constructed using 1981 census variables, and the AASI was superseded by the Index of Local Conditions. This, in turn, was superseded by the Index of Local Deprivation (Department of the Environment, Transport and the Regions, 1998; Nobel et al., 1999).

Table 8–4 shows the variables used to construct these indexes (Bruce et al., 1995). Little agreement exists about which are the most important variables, and, with the exception of the Jarman UPA(8) Index, all the variables in all the indexes are given equal weight, that is, are considered to be equally important. This is, of course, nonsense. Some factors, such as not having access to a car, affect a large section of the population (36% in 1991), whereas others, such as lacking basic amenities, affect only 1% of the population. Similarly, the different social groups vary considerably in size and can overlap, for example, single-parent households and households with children under five.

Social scientists have been using deprivation surveys to study poverty in Britain for more than 100 years. All these surveys have shown that certain groups are more likely to suffer from multiple deprivation than are others—single parents and the unemployed are not equally likely to be living in poverty, and indexes that consider them to be are probably wrong. (See Gordon et al., 2000 for recent British poverty survey re-

Table 8-4. Variables Used to Construct British Census–Based Deprivation Indexes

Census Variables	Variable Type	UPA(8)	AASI	SDD	Townsend	Scotdep	Matdep	Socdep	ILC
Overcrowding	M	X	X	X	X	X	X		X
No car	M				X	X	X		X
Basic amenities	M		X				X		X
Not owner-occupied	M				X				
Not self-contained	M		X						
No central heating	M						X		
Below occupancy norm	M			X					
Children in unsuitable accommodation	M								
Unemployment	S	X		X	X	X		X	X
Youth unemployment	S			X				X	X
Single parent	S	X	X	X				X	
Low social class/unskilled	S	X		X		X			
Single pensioner	S	X						X	
Elderly household	S			X					
Dependants only	S, H							X	

New commonwealth	S			X	
Under five	S			X	X
Migrant	S			X	X
Educational Participation at 17	S	X			
Limiting long-term illness	H		X		
Children in low-earning holds	S	X			
Non-Census Variables					
SMRs	H	X			
Income support	S	X			
Low educational attainment (GCSEs)	S	X			
Long-term unemployed	S	X			
House contents insurance (crime)	S	X			
Derelict land	M	X			

M, material deprivation indicator; S, social deprivation indicator; H, health indicator; SMRs, standardised mortality ratios.

sults.) Therefore, census-based deprivation indexes that give equal weight to their component variables are likely to yield inaccurate results.

Because all census-based deprivation indexes are generally composed of surrogate, or proxy, measures of deprivation rather than direct measures, there are two basic requirements they should fulfill to ensure accuracy:

1. The components of the index should be weighted to reflect the different probability that each group has of suffering from deprivation, and
2. the components of the index must be additive, that is, if an index is composed of two variables, such as unemployment and single parenthood, then researchers must be confident that unemployed single parents are likely to be poorer than either single parents who are employed or unemployed people who are not single parents.

Weighted indexes also have the advantage that their results are often much easier to understand. For example, saying that in Inner London 25% of households are living in poverty has a much greater intuitive meaning than saying that Inner London has a Townsend Z-score of 7.86 or a Department of Environment Index of Local Conditions signed chi-squared score of 22.46.

The problems of weighting are general rather than specific to certain areas, although it is probable that different weightings should be applied in metropolitan districts compared with mixed urban/rural and remote rural regions. For example, access to a car is more of a necessity in a rural area with poor public transport than in Inner London, where traffic speed now averages 11 mph.

OBTAINING WEIGHTINGS FOR CENSUS-BASED POVERTY INDEXES

The easiest method of obtaining weightings for component variables in census-based poverty indexes is to use a survey (conducted at or around the same time as the census) specifically designed to measure poverty and deprivation. However, only two nationally representative surveys of poverty were conducted during the 1980s—the 1983 and 1990 surveys undertaken by Market and Opinion Research International (MORI) for the two *Breadline Britain* television series that were made for London Weekend Television. These are the only specific national surveys of poverty to be produced since the Royal Commission on the Distribution of Income and Wealth reported in 1978 (Mack and Lansley, 1985; Gordon and Pantazis, 1997; Bradshaw et al., 1998).

The 1983 *Breadline Britain* study pioneered what has been termed the "consensual," or "perceived deprivation," approach to measuring poverty. This methodology has since been widely adopted by other studies both in Britain and abroad (Gordon and Spicker, 1999; Gordon et al., 2000).

The consensual, or perceived deprivation, approach sets out to determine whether there are some people whose standard of living is below the minimum acceptable to society. It defines *poverty* from the viewpoint of the public's perception of minimum need (Mack and Lansley, 1985):

> This study tackles the questions 'how poor is too poor?' by identifying the minimum acceptable way of life for Britain in the 1980s. Those who have no choice but to fall below this minimum level can be said to be 'in poverty'. This concept is developed in terms of those who have an enforced lack of *socially perceived* necessities. This means that the 'necessities' of life are identified by public opinion and not by, on the one hand, the views of experts or, on the other hand, the norms of behaviour per se.

The 1983 *Breadline Britain* study used a relative criteria to define the "poor"—it assumed that "poverty is a situation where such deprivation has a multiple impact on a household's way of life affecting several aspects of living thus, a family which just about manages but to do so does without an annual holiday, is deprived by today's standards; in our judgement, however, it is not in poverty. Deprivation has to have a more pervasive impact to become poverty." Two criteria were identified for determining at what point multiple deprivation was likely to cause poverty.

1. The poverty line should be drawn where the overwhelming majority of those who lack necessities[3] have low incomes in the bottom half of the income range.
2. Their overall spending pattern should reflect financial difficulty rather than high spending on other goods.

By carefully examining a large number of tables, Mack and Lansley (1985) decided that "a level of lack of one or two necessities is largely enforced though not overwhelmingly . . . a level of lack of three or more necessities is, by contrast, overwhelmingly enforced".

The "three or more necessities lacked" poverty line was later confirmed by regression analysis.[4] Using this poverty threshold, Mack and Lansley showed that 14% of British households could be shown to be living in poverty in 1983, and by 1990 the number in poverty had increased to 20% of British households (Gordon and Pantazis, 1997).

Producing a Weighted Deprivation Index

It is possible to obtain weightings for the best subset of deprivation indicator variables that were measured in both the 1991 census and the *Breadline Britain* survey using a multivariate statistical technique of Logistic Regression (Gordon and Forrest 1995; Gordon, 1995). Eleven variables, which have been used in one or more census-based indexes, were examined:

1. unemployment
2. single parents
3. limiting long-term illness or disability
4. unskilled or low social class
5. no access to a car
6. living in rented accommodation (not owner occupied)
7. single pensioners
8. divorced people
9. widows
10. lacking or sharing basic amenities (indoor toilet, bath or shower)
11. non–self-contained accommodation

There was a considerable degree of overlap between single pensioners and widows, and both variables were excluded because they were not good predictors of poverty. Divorced people were excluded because of their high overlap with single parenthood, which was a better predictor of poverty. "Lacking basic amenities" and "non–self-contained accommodation" were dropped because they were found not to be additive.[5] For example, households that contained someone with a limiting long-term illness and also lacked basic amenities were not likely to be poorer than were households with an ill person but with basic amenities. The reason for this is that many poor disabled people live in Local Authority accommodations, which invariably have indoor toilets and bathrooms.

An estimate of the number of poor households in an area can be calculated as: 21.7% of the number of households with no access to a car, plus 20.3% of the number of households not in owner-occupied accommodations, plus 16% of the number of single-parent households, plus 15.9% of the number of workers in Social Classes IV and V, plus 10.8% of the number of households containing a person with a limiting long-term illness, plus 9.4% of unemployed workers.

THE RELIABILITY AND VALIDITY OF UK DEPRIVATION INDEXES

The term *reliability* often causes confusion because the common usage of the word differs from its scientific meaning. In common usage a reliable measurement is a correct measurement, that is, something that can be relied upon. However, in scientific terms a reliable measurement is not necessarily correct, it is just precise. For example, if you repeatedly measured an object with a "one-foot" ruler that in reality was only eleven inches long, you would produce a series of very similar measurements. This series of measurements would be highly reliable even though they would be completely inaccurate. Scientific reliability is about the consistency of a measurement, not its accuracy, and there are a number of statistics that can be used to measure the internal consistency (reliability) of scales such as deprivation indexes.

The reliability of the ten most-used 1991 census-based deprivation indexes was examined by Lee et al. (1995) using classical test theory. These included the eight widely used deprivation indexes shown in Table 8–4 and two additional deprivation indexes that had been used in the cities of Bradford and Oxford (Bradford MBC, 1983; Nobel et al., 1994). The Sample of Anonymised Records (SARs) provides complete census data for a 1% sample of households (215,789 households) in Britain (Marsh, 1993). These data can be used to test the reliability of the components of the ten deprivation indexes.

Nunnally (1981) has argued that

> in the early stages of research . . . one saves time and energy by working with instruments that have modest reliability, for which purpose reliabilities of 0.70 or higher will suffice . . . for basic research, it can be argued that increasing reliabilities much beyond 0.80 is often wasteful of time and funds, at that level correlations are attenuated very little by measurement error.

It can be seen from Table 8–5, that none of the census-based deprivation indexes comes close to being as reliable as Nunnally's criteria. This is unsurprising given that none of the questions in the census were designed to measure poverty or deprivation. However, they are not all equally bad.

TABLE 8–5. Reliability Analysis Results for British Census-Based
Deprivation Indexes

	Number of Variables in the Index	Cronbach's Coefficient Alpha	Correlation between the "True" Deprivation Score and the Index Score
Oxford	7	0.4746	0.69
Breadline	6	0.4352	0.66
Townsend	4	0.4287	0.65
Bradford	9	0.4162	0.64
Socdep	6	0.3254	0.57
DoE91	7	0.3229	0.57
Matdep	4	0.2629	0.51
Scotdep	4	0.1670	0.41
DoE81	6	0.0909	0.30
Jarman	8	0.0495	0.20

The four most reliable indexes (Oxford, *Breadline*, Townsend, and Bradford) have reliabilities more than three times as large as the worst index
(Jarman's UPA(8) Score). This, again, is unsurprising, as Jarman's UPA(8)
Score is not designed to be used as a deprivation index (although it has
been used by others for this purpose). Rather, it is designed as an index
of general practitioners' workload and cannot be expected to be a reliable
measure of deprivation as well (Carr-Hill and Sheldon, 1991; Senior, 1991).
By contrast, the variables used in the four best indexes have all been chosen using theoretical and/or empirical models of poverty and/or deprivation and were specifically designed to measure these concepts. However, these low reliability scores mean that it is impossible to obtain an
accurate rankings of areas in Britain using census-based deprivation
indexes.

The validity of the ten deprivation indexes was tested using three
validating variables for the 10,500 electoral wards in Britain:

- estimated weekly earnings at electoral ward level
- standardized illness ratio at electoral ward level
- standardized mortality ration at electoral ward level

These variables are robust measures of validity because there is now overwhelming evidence that poverty and deprivation cause ill health

TABLE 8–6. Spearman's Rank Correlation Coefficients for SMR 0-64, Standardized Illness Ratio, and Estimated Average Weekly Earnings by the Ten Census Based Deprivation Indexes for the 10,500 Electoral Wards of Britain

Variable/Index	Meanearn	Illness	SMR 0-64
Meanearn	1.00	−.76	−.55
Illness	−.76	1.00	.64
SMR 0-64	−.55	.64	1.00
Scotdep	−.80	.81	.64
Breadline	−.73	.80	.64
Socdep	−.73	.85	.61
Bradford	−.72	.77	.63
Townsend	−.71	.76	.63
Oxford	−.70	.77	.63
Matdep	−.67	.72	.61
DoE91	−.67	.70	.59
DoE81	−.64	.72	.59
Jarman	−.65	.70	.59

(Townsend and Davidson, 1988; Whitehead, 1988; Independent Inquiry into Inequalities in Health, 1998; Gordon et al., 1999; Shaw et al., 1999) and that deprivation is caused by low income.

Table 8–6 displays the results of the validation analysis. It shows the Spearman's rank correlation coefficients between the ten census-based deprivation indexes and standardized illness ratio (illness), standardized mortality ratio (SMR 0-64), and the estimated average weekly earnings (meanearn).

It is clear from Tables 8–5 and 8–6 that the ten census-based deprivation indexes can conveniently be divided up into three groups:

1. Group 1 consists of Jarman, DoE81, DoE91 and Matdep. These are the least accurate (valid) indexes on all three validation criteria (standardized illness ratio, standardized mortality ratio, and estimated average weekly earnings). The Jarman and DoE81 indexes are also the least reliable. It is apparent that the DoE91 index appears to be both more valid (on average) and more reliable than does the DoE81 index. However, it still falls far behind the best indexes.
2. Group 2 consists of the Oxford, Townsend, and Bradford indexes. These are both reasonably valid on all three criteria and reasonably reliable.

3. Group 3 consists of Socdep, *Breadline*, and Scotdep. These three, on average, are the most valid (i.e., they have the highest correlations with the three validating criteria). Socdep is the most unusual, as it correlates very highly with standardized illness ratio but relatively poorly with standardized mortality ratio. It is obviously better at measuring some aspects of deprivation than others. This result is unsurprising because Socdep was designed to measure only "social" deprivation and not other aspects of deprivation (such as material deprivation) that are known to affect health. Scotdep is the most accurate index, displaying a slightly higher correlation with all three validating criteria than does the *Breadline* index. However, it is also the third most unreliable index of the ten. The *Breadline* index appears to be the best compromise between validity and reliability (Lee et al., 1995). It has also been independently validated by researchers at the Universities of York (Burrow and Rhodes, 1998) and Kent (Saunders, 1998).

A number of conclusions can be drawn from these results that should aid researchers when trying to choose the most appropriate index. If the research problem demands the highest possible levels of accuracy, such as when trying to measure how many poor wards there are in a region (or large city), then Scotdep is the best index. However, if the problem requires both a valid and a reliable result, such as when trying to rank the poorest wards in a region, then *Breadline* is clearly the best index. If the research problem is to look at just specific aspects of deprivation, such as the effects of social deprivation on morbidity, then Socdep is the best index to use.

DOES LOW INCOME OR DEPRIVATION CAUSE ILL HEALTH?

This chapter has described how the practice of measuring poverty at small area level in Britain differs significantly from that in the United States. In Britain deprivation indexes tend to be used, whereas in the United States low-income thresholds are preferred. The key question for health researchers is which is the most significant for studies of ill health and mortality. This debate cannot be resolved here, but studies such as MRFIT in the United States (Davey-Smith et al., 1996a; 1996b) have demonstrated that a clear and continuous gradient exists between mortality and income at ZIP code level.

Studies in the United Kingdom, however, have also shown high levels of association between deprivation indexes and morbidity and mortality at various geographical levels. For example, Figure 8–7 shows a scat-

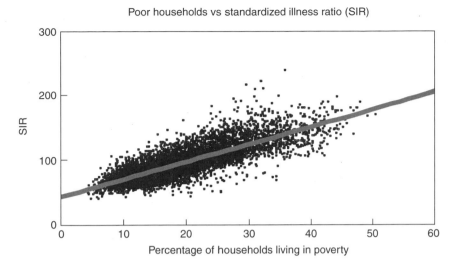

FIGURE 8–7. Percentage of poor households by standardized illness ratio.

ter plot of the estimated percentage of poor households against the standardized illness ratio for the 8,519 electoral wards of England. The regression line with a 95% confidence interval is also shown. There appears to be very good agreement between these two variables (Pearson's Product Moment Correlation 0.82). Many U.K. researchers would argue, on theoretical grounds, that it is not low income per se that causes ill health but the material and social deprivations caused by low income. For example, squalor makes you sick. However, there is no overwhelming evidence on either side of this debate at present.

NOTES

1. The five bar gate refers to the method of counting whereby I = 1, II = 2, III = 3, IIII = 4, and ~~IIII~~ = 5.

2. Although the Panel on Poverty and Family Assistance and the Census Bureau have suggested major changes (Citro and Michael, 1995; Betson et al., 1999; Short et al., 1999).

3. Lack of necessities refers to households that stated they did not have a necessity because they could not afford it and not to those households who lacked a necessity because they did not want it.

4. Desai M (1986). Drawing the line: on defining the poverty threshold. In Golding P, Ed.: *Excluding the Poor.* Child Poverty Action Group, London. See also Desai M and Shah A (1985). *An Econometric Approach to the Measurement of Poverty,* Suntory-Toyota International Centre for Economics and Related Disciplines, WSP/2, London School of Economics, London.

5. Standard statistical techniques were used to establish additivity. First-order interaction plots were produced using the Minitab v12 package, and fully saturated ANOVA and GLM models were used to examine higher-order interactions.

REFERENCES

Bane MJ and Ellwood D. (1986). Slipping into and out of Poverty: The Dynamics of Spells. *Journal of Human Resources* 21(1): 1–23.

Barnes J. and Lucas H. (1975). *Educational Priority*. London: HMSO.

Betson DM, Constance F, Citro M, Robert T. (2000). Recent developments for poverty measurement in U.S. official statistics. *Journal of Official Statistics* 16(2): 87–111.

Blaxter M. (1990) *Health and Lifestyle*. London: Tavistock.

Bruce A, Gordon D, Kessell J. (1995). Analysing Rural Poverty. *Local Government Policy Making* 22(1): 16–23.

Bradshaw J, Gordon D, Levitas R, Middleton S, Pantazis C, Payne S, Townsend P. (1998). *Perceptions of Poverty and Social Exclusion*. Bristol: Report to the Joseph Rowntree Foundation, Townsend Centre for International Poverty Research.

Bradford MBC. (1993). *Areas of Stress within Bradford District*. Chief Executive's Department, Bradford Metropolitan District Council.

Brakenridge W. (1755). A letter from the Reverend William Brakenridge, D.D. and F.R.S. to George Lewis Scot, Esq., F.R.S., concerning the London Bills of Mortality. *Philosophical Transactions of the Royal Society, London* 48: 788–800.

Burrows R and Rhodes D. (1998). *Unpopular Places? Area Disadvantage and the Geography of Misery in England*. Bristol: Policy Press.

Carr-Hill R and Sheldon T. (1991). Designing a deprivation payment for general practitioners: The UPA(8) Wonderland. *BMJ* 302: 393–396.

Carstairs V and Morris R. (1989). Deprivation: Explaining differences in mortality between Scotland and England and Wales. *BMJ* 299: 886–889.

Carstairs V and Morris R. (1991a). *Deprivation and Health in Scotland*. Aberdeen: Aberdeen University Press.

Carstairs V and Morris R. (1991b). Which deprivation index? A comparison of selected deprivation indexes. *J Public Health Med* 13(4): 318–326.

Chadwick E (1842). *Report on the Sanitary Conditions of the Labouring Population of Great Britain*. London.

Citro CF and Michael RT, eds. (1995). *Measuring Poverty. A New Approach*, Washington, D.C.: National Academy Press.

Community Development Project (1977). *Gilding the Ghetto: The State and the Poverty Experiments*. Nottingham: CDP & The Russell Press Limited.

Company of Parish Clerks (1604). *London Bills of Mortality*. London: Company of Parish Clerks.

Davey Smith G and Gordon D (2000). Poverty across the life-course and health. In Pantazis C and Gordon D eds.: *Tackling Inequalities: Where Are We Now and What Can Be Done?* Bristol: The Policy Press, pp. 141–158.

Davey Smith G, Neaton JD, Wentworth D, Stamler R, and Stamler J (1996a). Socioeconomic differentials in mortality risk among men screened for the Multiple Risk Factor Intervention Trial: Part I—Results for 300,685 white Men. *Am J Public Health* 86: 486–496.

Davey Smith G, Neaton JD, Wentworth D, Stamler R, and Stamler J (1996b). Socioeconomic differentials in mortality risk among men screened for the Multiple Risk Factor Intervention Trial: Part II—Results for 20,224 black Men. *Am J Public Health* 86: 497–504.

Department of Social Security (DSS) (1998). *Households Below Average Income 1979–1996/97*. London: Corporate Document Services.

Department of Environment (1994). *Index of Local Conditions: An Analysis based on 1991 Census Data*. London: Department of Environment.

Department of Environment, Transport and the Regions (1998). *1998 Index of Local Deprivation*. London: Department of Environment, Transport and the Regions.

Department of Health and Denham J (1999). Health Action Zones invited to apply for £4.5m funding for innovation and fellowship. Press Release 1999/0386, Friday 25 June.

Drever F and Whitehead M, eds. (1997). *Health Inequalities*. London: The Stationery Office.

Duncan GJ, Gustafsson B, Hauser R, Schmauss G, Messinger H, Muffels R, Nolan B, Ray JC (1993). Poverty dynamics in eight countries. *Journal of Population Economics* 6: 215–234.

Fisher GM (1992). The development and history of the poverty thresholds. *Social Security Bulletin* 55(4): 3–14.

Fletcher J (1849). Moral and educational statistics of England and Wales. *Journal of the Royal Statistical Society of London* 12(151–176): 189–335.

Flowerdew R (1992). Deprivation indices in standard spending assessment. In Spenser N and Janes H, eds.: *Uses and Abuses of Deprivation Indices*. Coventry: University of Warwick, pp. 45–56.

Forrest R and Gordon D (1993). *People and Places: A 1991 Census Atlas of England*. Bristol: SAUS.

Glennerster H, Lupton R, Noden P, Power A (1999). Poverty, social exclusion and neighbourhood: Studying the area bases of social exclusion. CASE Paper 22. London: London School of Economics.

Goodman A and Webb S (1994). For richer, for poorer: The changing distribution of income in the United Kingdom 1961–91. Institute of Fiscal Studies Commentary no 42. London: Institute of Fiscal Studies.

Gordon D (1995). Census based deprivation indices: Their weighting and validation. *J Epidemiol Community Health* 49 (Suppl 2): S39–S44.

Gordon D, Adelman L, Ashworth K, Bradshaw J, Levitas R, Middleton S, Pantazis C, Patsios D, Townsend P, Williams J (2000). *The Poverty and Social Exclusion Survey of Britain*. York: York Publishing Services and Joseph Rowntree Foundation.

Gordon D, Davey Smith G, Dorling D, Shaw M, eds. (1999). *Inequalities in Health: The Evidence Presented to the Independent Inquiry into Inequalities in Health*. Bristol: The Policy Press.

Gordon D and Forrest R (1995). *People and Places Volume II: Social and Economic Distinctions in England—A 1991 Census Atlas*. Bristol: SAUS and the Statistical Monitoring Unit.

Gordon D and Pantazis C, eds. (1997). *Breadline Britain in the 1990s*. Aldershot: Ashgate.

Gordon D and Spicker P, eds. (1999). *The International Glossary on Poverty*. London: Zed Books.

Harrington M (1985). *The New American Poverty*, London: Firethorn Press.

Holtermann S (1975). Areas of urban deprivation in Great Britain: An analysis of 1971 Census Data. *Social Trends* no. 6, pp. 33–47.

Independent Inquiry into Inequalities in Health (1998). *Report of the Independent Inquiry into Inequalities in Health*. London: The Stationery Office.

Jarman B (1983). Identification of underprivileged areas. *BMJ* 286: 1705–1709.

Jarman B (1984). Underprivileged areas: Validation and distribution of scores. *BMJ* 289: 1587–1592.

Lee P, Murie A, Gordon D (1995). *Area Measures of Deprivation: A Study of Current Methods and Best Practices in the Identification of Poor Areas in Great Britain*. Birmingham: University of Birmingham.

Mack J and Lansley S (1985). *Poor Britain*. London: Allen and Unwin.

Marsh C (1993). The sample of anonymised records. In Dale A and Marsh C, eds.: *The 1991 Census Users Guide*. London: HMSO.

Martin J (1990). Asking about money: ESRC survey methods seminar series. *Joint Centre for Survey Methods Newsletter* 10(2): 2.

Nobel M, Smith G, Avenell D, Smith T, Sharpland E (1994). *Changing Patterns of Income and Wealth in Oxford and Oldham*. Oxford: Oxford University Press.

Nobel M, Penhale B, Smith G, Wright G (1999). *Measuring Multiple Deprivation at the Local Level: Index of Deprivation 1999 Review*. Oxford: Oxford University Press. (See http://index99.apsoc.ox.ac.uk/ for latest updates.)

Nolan B and Whelan CT (1996). *Resources, Deprivation and Poverty*. Oxford: Clarendon Press.

Nunnally JC and Bernstein IH (1994). *Psychometric Theory*. 3rd ed. New York: McGraw-Hill.

Office for National Statistics (1999) *The 2001 Census of Population*, Cm4253. London: The Stationery Office. (Also available at http://www.statistics.gov.uk/nsbase/census2001)

Orshansky M (1965). Counting the poor: Another look at the poverty profile. *Social Security Bulletin* 28: 3–29.

Orshansky M (1969). How poverty is measured. *Monthly Labor Review* 92: 37–41.

Pantazis C and Gordon D, eds. (2000). *Tackling Inequalities: Where Are We Now and What Can Be Done?* Bristol: The Policy Press.

Phillimore P, Beattie A, Townsend P (1994). Widening inequality of health in Northern England, 1981–91. *BMJ* 308: 1125–1128.

Robson B, Bradford M, Deas I, Hall E, Harrison E, Parkinson M, Evans R, Garside P, Harding A., Robinson F (1994). *Assessing the Impact of urban Policy*. London: HMSO.

Saunders J (1998). Weighted Census-based deprivation indices: Their use in small areas. *J Public Health Med* 20(3): 253–260.

Senior ML (1991). Deprivation payments to GPs: Not what the doctor ordered. *Environment and Planning C: Government and Policy* 9: 79–94.

Shaw M, Dorling D, Gordon D, Davey Smith G (1999). *The Widening Gap: Health Inequalities and Policy in Britain*. Bristol: The Policy Press.

Short K, Garner T, Johnson D, Doyle P (1999). Experimental poverty measures: 1990 to 1997. US Census Bureau, Current Population Reports, Series P60-205. Washington, DC: U.S. Government Printing Office. (See also http://www.census.gov/hhes/www/povmeas.html)

Teague A (1999). Income data for small areas. Summary of response to consultation. Census Advisory Group Paper AG (99)19, Office of National Statistics, London. http://www.statistics.gov/uk/census2001/pdfs/ag9919.pdf

Townsend P (1979). *Poverty in the United Kingdom*. London: Allen Lane and Penguin.

Townsend P and Davidson N (1988). *Inequalities in Health: The Black Report*, 2nd ed. London: Penguin Books.

Townsend P and Gordon D (1991). What is enough? New evidence on poverty allowing the definition of a minimum benefit. In Alder M, Bell C, Clasen J, Sinfield A, eds. *The Sociology of Social Security*. Edinburgh: Edinburgh University Press, pp. 35–69.

Townsend P, Phillimore P, Beattie A (1988). *Health and Deprivation, Inequality and the North*. London: Croom Helm.

Whitehead M (1988). *Inequalities in Health: The Health Divide*, 2nd ed. London: Penguin Books.

II

NEIGHBORHOODS AND HEALTH OUTCOMES

9

Neighborhoods and Infectious Diseases

Mindy Thompson Fullilove

Infectious diseases are spread through human populations by a large number of routes that vary according to the well-known triad of agent, host, and environment. The study of neighborhoods and infectious disease provides an opportunity to examine the intersection between ecological setting and human behaviors. Given the number of infectious organisms, the number of ecological settings, and the variations in the ways people organize their settlements, the number of possible permutations and combinations of such intersections is very large.

Because all these factors shift constantly, understanding patterns of settlement, particularly as they relate to patterns of infectious disease, depends on a sound knowledge of basic science and a great deal of field investigation. Thus, the Centers for Disease (CDC) Control Epidemiological Investigation Service is a vital part of the infectious disease surveillance system for the United States. The extraordinary laboratories of the CDC are called on many times a year to figure out the precise nature of an infectious agent and to advise on methods of control. However, despite miracles of laboratory science, disease control routinely bumps up against social issues that structure the spread of disease and create the circumstances within which we try to control it.

This chapter focuses on a series of neighborhood-level social/structural processes that have influenced the spread of HIV, syphilis, gonorrhea, and tuberculosis in the United States. Specifically, through the lens offered by three highly social processes, I examine the ways in which fundamental causes of disease, in the sense proposed by Link and Phelan (1995), contribute to the propagation of infectious disease agents and cases of infection. For purposes of this paper, I focus on the local construction of sex and drug scenes, disruption in neighborhood cohesion, and the "redlining" of epidemics that are concentrated in marginalized communities.

Before starting with specific examples, I will revisit Link and Phelan's important construction of "fundamental" causes of disease. In their 1994 paper they challenged the proposition that "social conditions such as socioeconomic status are mere proxies for true causes lying closer to disease in the causal chain" (p. 80). They reviewed a large number of socioepidemiologic studies examining this issue and concluded that, quite the contrary, by focusing on "proximal" causes one may find an answer to the cause of a specific disease but fail to solve the problem of excess morbidity and mortality among less advantaged social groups.

Link and Phelan explained this seeming paradox by pointing out, "Thus studies of the association between SES [socioeconomic status] and disease over the past several decades reveal an important fact—the risk factors mediating the association have changed. As some risk factors were eradicated, others emerged or were newly discovered. As new risk factors became apparent, people of higher SES were more favorably situated to know about the risks and to have the resources that allowed them to engage in protective efforts to avoid them" (p. 86). Link and Phelan concluded that the fundamental causes of disease are those that put people "at risk for risks." Such causes act prominently through access to resources.

The understanding of fundamental causes of disease is made more difficult because we must avoid thinking simplistically in terms of linear models that link "cause" and "effect" through a series of intermediate factors. What we seek is a much more complex investigation of cause and effect in which we are challenged to think about the contexts of people's lives in order to understand their ability to adapt to shifting circumstances. It is this challenge that informs the issues discussed here.

UNDERSTANDING LOCAL SEX-DRUG SCENES

The spatial organization of life, circa 2000, is widely understood to be global. The increasing interdependence of all parts of the world is highlighted by the explosion of the internet as a new international marketplace of goods and ideas. The importance of the international, the dispersed, and the nonlocal appears to overshadow, and perhaps eliminate, the local. This perception has greatest salience for the international class of entrepreneurs and intellectuals who live much of their lives in the multinational centers of activity. Students in the Joseph L. Mailman School of Public Health of Columbia University, for example, routinely depict their personal geography as consisting of many centers in the United States and abroad. The international exchange of cultures, businesses, languages, peoples, exotic plants and animals, foods, and diseases is a major feature of daily life, underscoring the internationalization of the world.

Globalization does, indeed, reshape the local, but not in a way that eliminates its importance. In fact, globalization creates a strong gradient of desirability that has dramatic implications for the local. Viewed from the perspective of resources—and hence of fundamental causes of disease—globalization entails a distinctly unequal flow of resources, such that a small number of places are inordinately privileged while others are depleted. "Wastes" flow in the opposite direction from "goods" so as to intensify the localization of the toxic and dangerous in impoverished areas. People, too, are sorted such that people with skills, education, talent, and good health end up in the centers of wealth, while the weak, vulnerable, and unskilled end up at the margins.

Greenberg and Schneider (1994) studied this process of the concentration of negative objects in marginalized communities. They focused on the existence of TOADS, standing for "temporally obsolete abandoned derelict sites," and LULUs, standing for "locally unwanted land uses," in inner city areas. They noted that

> LULUS are dangerous or offensive because they may operate or are in operation. The hazards TOADS produce spring primarily from neglect. Both are being systematically concentrated in marginal areas where the vast majority of Americans can ignore them. TOADS in most poor areas are invaded by arsonists, crack dealers, homeless, midnight dumpers, and other parties interested in illegal or socially unacceptable activities. Some cities fuel these dangerous environments by withdrawing police, fire and medical services from TOADS areas. Left unchecked, the spread of TOADS and insertion of LULUs can destroy communities, leaving only the most marginal people to prey on each other. (p. 180)

The construction of privilege or deprivation at the neighborhood level, although at this point an international process, informs the social relationships that occur within each area. The fascinating observation that gonorrhea rates were correlated with neighborhood scores on a "broken windows" index may be read as evidence of a series of symbolic messages about "having" (Cohen et al., 2000). Homeowners work hard to create grass that is even and green, a symbol of "keeping it together," also read as "keeping it," or conversely as "not losing it." People with broken windows, by contrast, have "lost" something crucial in their control over the environment. The context of loss is at times a setting for a decrease in the influence of cultural proscriptions, which can lead to major shifts in drug-taking and sexual behavior, which, in turn, can facilitate the spread of sexually transmitted diseases.

Consider, for example, the construction of crack-related settings for sexual encounters that occurred across the United States in poor communities affected by the crack epidemic. These sex and drug scenarios played an important role in spreading syphilis, gonorrhea, and HIV. Crack, introduced to U.S. cities in the early 1980s, was a cheap cocaine derivative that was quick-acting and that produced an intense state of euphoria that was rated by many users as vastly superior to most other illicit drugs. As the brief high receded, an equally intense state of dysphoria set in, driving the user to procure another "hit." The joy of the intense high coupled with the need to avoid the painful crash drove users to take another hit, followed by another, and so on. In early reports users described that there was no "dose" of crack, as there was with a dose of heroin. "People take as much crack as they have money," a user explained. "If you have $200, you take that much crack. If you have $1,000, you take that much crack. If you have a house, you sell your house and then you smoke up the profit."

Crack defined a new era in drug taking, one in which the "dose-you-could-afford" was the driving factor. The craving for crack was nearly insatiable. Many users who had disposed of their worldly possessions turned to other sources of money. Not surprisingly, many began to sell their bodies. However, whereas an older generation of people addicted to heroin had developed a mannerly form of participation in commercial sex work, the bartering that developed in the context of the crack era was a no-holds-barred revision of what it meant to engage in sex work. Under the compulsion of addiction to crack, users had little ability to negotiate the niceties of place or price. Dealers quickly discovered that those addicted to crack would do nearly anything for the promise of a hit. The perhaps apocryphal stories that began to circulate described dealers making outrageous sexual demands—oral sex with five men or intercourse with a dog—in exchange for a small dose of the drug. Not only were the sexual acts outrageous by community standards, but the sexual encounters were often carried out in public or semipublic places such as alleys and hallways, violating existing conventions of public decorum.

While some of these stories are undoubtedly exaggerations, a seven-city study of sex-for-crack found ample evidence of altered social and sexual relationships in the context of crack use (Ratner, 1993). Some consistent patterns emerged from city to city. First, in the context of crack, and unlike during earlier drug epidemics, sexual favors were likely to be exchanged directly for drugs or for money to buy drugs. Often the actual amounts of money or drug were miniscule, undercutting the prices charged by other sex workers. Second, many kinds of acts could be included under the rubric of sex-for-drugs exchanges. These ranged from the casual sharing of drugs and sex by friends to the formal practices of crack houses, where women and drugs were available for money. Because individuals might engage in some or all of these practices, gradually the number of partners per individual grew, as did the set created by the function "partner of my partner is a member of my sexual lot." Additionally, the conditions of crack use contributed to the risk of exposure to infection with sexually transmitted diseases. For example, crack smoking caused burns on the lips and gums that might facilitate infection. Similarly, crack, although marketed as an aphrodisiac, actually inhibited orgasm in men, contributing to prolonged erection and intercourse that might irritate or tear the genitals of both men and women.

The seven-city study offered a glimpse into the structure of the institutions that formed the crack culture. First, and probably most important from the perspective of the spread of disease, was the crack house. The crack house was a location dedicated to the consumption of drugs. Crack houses often "supplied" women as well as drugs. They were a place for people to meet one another and to socialize while getting intoxicated. Crack houses were located in deserted buildings, apartments, houses, or any other location taken over by dealers for the purpose of selling drugs. In addition to the houses, which were the most formal locations, a second tier of homes existed where people gathered to smoke crack. Such crack spots were more informal places. Users provided the host with a share of the drug in exchange for the use of the location.

The complex and diffuse organization of crack use created a social geography of the crack culture. Unlike legal establishments, crack houses and crack spots were unstable. They might be closed by the police or destroyed in other ways. For example, in New York City a deserted building that served as a crack house burned down as a result of a dispute between two users. This constant alteration of the physical and social environment was one of the dominant features of crack culture.

Sex and drug settings emerge in many forms in marginalized communities. Gay men, for example, have invented a wide array of venues that shelter sexual encounters. Bathhouses, bars, clubs, and the party circuit are examples of the indoor scene, while wooded areas like the Ramble in Central Park, New York City, exemplify the outdoor scene. Describing these sex and drug settings requires careful ethnographic research. It is critical that experienced observers document the manner in which sexual behaviors are intertwined with drug use in particular locales, in a particular the drug subculture. In the mid-1990s James Inciardi, an ethnographer who has studied the drug culture, conducted observations of the reemerging bathhouse scene among gay men in Los Angeles (McCoy and Inciardi, 1995). He found that the bathhouses were a site where men took drugs (largely marijuana) and engaged in various kinds of sexual acts. Although the bathhouses offered condoms to clients and displayed AIDS prevention posters, Inciardi observed a variety of unsafe sex acts.

The careful study of sex and drug settings can be an important foundation for intervention. As one example of this proposition, consider an outbreak of syphilis reported in Chester, Pennsylvania, a once prosperous industrial town that had fallen on hard times (Hibbs and Gunn, 1991). In the mid-1980s crack arrived in Chester. The arrival of this epidemic led to an increase in prostitution by people interested in obtaining money for crack. The crack sex workers were located near the points where drugs were sold. In 1988 the health department noted a fivefold increase in cases of syphilis compared to 1987 in these areas.

Because the health department was aware of the structure of the sex and drug trade in Chester, they decided to try a novel approach by taking syphilis treatment to the high-risk areas. A screening program, conducted over a period of six days, reached 136 people and treated all who were sexually active. Twenty-five people were found to have syphilis. Among the intervention cases there was a higher percentage of early latent syphilis cases than among routinely reported patients. The health department noted a decline in cases after the intervention, suggesting that it may have played a role in halting the spread of infection.

Such scenes are created out of the local circumstances of people, including the drugs they have at their disposal, the settings they invent for taking drugs, and the linkages they create between drug use and sexual behavior. This is an intensely local process, yet, as the international drug trade and the gay circuit parties demonstrate, it is profoundly linked to actions and processes around the globe.

DISRUPTION IN NEIGHBORHOOD COHESION

Neighborhood cohesion depends upon the stability of the population and the sustainability of the habitat. Habitat disruption produced major shifts in the populations of U.S. cities in the aftermath of World War II. Major social, physical, and economic processes, including the massive building of highways to new suburbs, urban renewal that decimated older neighborhoods in city centers, and the economic shifts that undermined manufacturing in urban areas of the Northeast led to major population loss. This "shrinkage" of the cities led some to call for a "planned" process that would guide the downsizing of urban areas. In particular, it was proposed that poor neighborhoods be leveled, thereby spreading the population elsewhere in the city. As Roger Starr, a major proponent of this "planned shrinkage," wrote,

> This sort of *internal resettlement*—the natural flow out of areas that have lost general attraction—must be encouraged. . . . Gradually the city's population in the older sections will begin to achieve a new configuration, one consistent with a smaller population that has arranged itself at densities high enough to make the provision of municipal services economical. . . . The stretches of empty blocks may then be knocked down, services can be stopped, subway stations closed, and the land left fallow until a change in the economic and demographic assumptions makes the land useful once again. (quoted in Gratz, 1994, pp. 176–177, emphasis added)

"Planned shrinkage" was implemented through a variety of policy mechanisms, including diminished public transit, cutbacks in police and fire protection, reduced housing assistance programs, and curtailed sanitation services (Gratz, 1994, p. 186). This denial of services to specific areas was the equivalent, Gratz pointed out, of a government sponsored redlining program. The "internal resettlement" so desired by Starr and his colleagues was "encouraged" through a firestorm that swept through vulnerable New York City neighborhoods throughout much of the 1970s and 1980s.

"Planned shrinkage" was based on fallacious reasoning and produced powerful consequences, both intended and unintended. It led to disinvestment in weaker neighborhoods and increased investment in what Gratz called "choicer" areas. As neighborhoods like Harlem, the South Bronx, and Bedford Stuyvesant were burned, new construction—largely of middle-class and luxury housing—rose in such places as Roosevelt Island and Battery Park City. The decline in housing for the poor and working people of the city created a veritable "housing famine" that led to an epidemic of homelessness and a marked increase in the number of families living doubled- or tripled-up in the few remaining low-cost apartments.

The forced "internal resettlement"—like other experiences of massive displacement—sundered social relationships, undermined community life, and imposed heavy psychological burdens on the uprooted. The abrupt decline in social conditions created the potential for a series of epidemics that acted synergistically with one another to cause an explosive increase in morbidity and mortality. These epidemics further undermined social functioning. The series of assaults—first from displacement and

then from epidemics—led to disintegration of the social functioning of affected communities. In order to explore this issue further, I turn to the
seminal studies conducted by Rodrick Wallace.

The Desertification of New York

"Planned shrinkage" was applied to a number of New York City communities, among them the very poor area of the South Bronx. In particular, an area known as the "poverty spine" of the Bronx was subjected to
withdrawal of fire services beginning in 1971. That area had an aging
housing infrastructure and was overcrowded. The reduction in fire service led to a massive increase in fires, and the fires tended to be more de-
structive, causing more extensive damage and requiring more effort to
control and extinguish the fire. The fires moved in a contagious fashion
throughout the neighborhood, mimicking the contagious pattern of housing abandonment that Dear had observed in studies in North Philadelphia (Dear, 1976).

Specifically, the burning of one building on a block increased the
relative risk of a second fire in an adjacent building. As buildings burned
on a given block, the risk to buildings on adjacent blocks increased as
well. In general, the burning consumed a core area and radiated out-
ward. Over a relatively short period of time—between 1970 and 1978—
the sixty-two contiguous health areas that made up the "poverty spine"
lost between 50% and 80% of its housing stock, a destruction of housing previously unheard of during peacetime (Wallace, 1988). In fact, it
was not uncommon for observers to compare the South Bronx to the
heavily bombed city of Dresden as it had looked at the end of World
War II.

Wallace's ecological studies examined the impact of this contagious
housing destruction on the health of local residents. Through examination of pupil transfer records, he was able to establish that displaced residents moved to the areas immediately adjacent to the "poverty spine."
Using health area records, he was able to show an abrupt rise in a variety of health measures in the receiving areas. These included drug-related
deaths.

The transfer of addiction from one area to another would have been
unfortunate, but the displacement of the South Bronx population not only
moved the location of illnesses but also increased the number and types
of illnesses. Among the new illnesses was AIDS, which was apparently
seeded in the "poverty spine" and then "shotgunned" to the surrounding neighborhoods. Thus, the neighborhoods surrounding the "poverty
spine" that had received the refugees from the burned area were the same

communities that reported significant numbers of AIDS deaths from 1980 to 1985.

Addiction to crack cocaine was another illness that flared in the receiving neighborhoods. The emergence of the crack epidemic followed by a violence epidemic largely based on homicides related to the drug trade was closely linked to the disruption of the social community of the South Bronx. The loss of social cohesion meant there were fewer and weaker controls on individual behavior, making it easier—especially for adolescents—to become involved in illegal behavior. Further, the experience of displacement heightened the sense of alienation from the dominant culture and served to justify the adoption of behaviors defined by the larger society as "criminal."

The series of plagues acted in a synergistic manner, such that housing destruction increased drug use, which increased the incidence of AIDS, which decimated families, which led to a decrease in social control, more drug use, and more trauma, which undermined family strength, and on and on. Wallace called this "the synergism of plagues." In sum, the process of epidemics in a physically degraded environment contributed to community disintegration, which permitted more epidemics to enter the community. An extraordinary downward spiral was created that weakened communities in a painful, stepwise fashion.

"REDLINING" OF EPIDEMICS

Observations of epidemics in marginalized communities have revealed an unexpected finding: under some conditions, some epidemics will be ignored. The outbreak of multidrug-resistant tuberculosis in New York City in the mid-1990s was an exceptional event in that it was the one instance in the past twenty years when the full weight of the public health establishment was thrown behind solving an inner-city problem. On the heels of the identification of this threat, conferences were organized, public health experts flew in, resources were allocated, and changes were made. While the changes were, to a great extent, superficial, it was a lesson in the advantages of "having" for many working in impoverished inner-city communities.

In contrast—and the more usual case for inner-city epidemics—was the HIV/AIDS epidemic. The public health response to AIDS got off to a bad start when the disease was named "gay-related immune disorder," unleashing America's homophobia, on the one hand, and misconstruing the nature of risk, on the other. As a clearer picture of key risk groups emerged, the response to AIDS was slowed by its identification as a problem affecting *only* homosexuals, minorities, and drug users. Mann et al., (1992) proposed that those social and contextual factors that impede response to an epidemic create a form of "vulnerability" to disease. This vulnerability played out at the local level throughout the United States. Harlem, long recognized as one of the epicenters of the epidemic, finally got a van to tour the area and encourage HIV testing in the spring of 2000.

The redlining of the epidemic came to the fore in a remarkable way in a 1993 report from the National Research Council titled *The Social Impact of AIDS*. The report noted

> the limited responsiveness of institutions can in part be explained because the absolute numbers of the epidemic, relative to the U.S. population, are not overwhelming, and because U.S. social institutions are strong, complex, and resilient. However, we believe that another major reason for this limited response is the concentration of the epidemic in socially marginalized groups. The convergence of evidence shows that the HIV/AIDS epidemic is settling into spatially and socially isolated groups and possibly becoming endemic within them. Many observers have recently commented that, instead of spreading out to the broad American population, as was once feared, HIV is concentrating in pools of persons who are also caught in the "synergism of plagues" . . . many geographical areas and strata of the population are virtually untouched by the epidemic and probably never will be; certain confined areas and populations have been devastated and are likely to continue to be. (p. 7)

This was an extraordinary statement, as it both attacked redlining of the epidemic and justified its continuation. Based on the fallacious conflation of "concentration" with "containment," the report undermined efforts to destroy the symbolic construction of AIDS as an epidemic of "others."

The report reflects an assumption, pervasive in American society, that the "isms" that structure social relationships are immutable. Thus, residential segregation cannot be undone, acceptance of gays cannot be achieved, and overcoming the obstacles to AIDS action is an impossibility. This fatalism about action against hatred reflects an acceptance that "isms" are, in some way, true and permanent.

While there are many ways in which this presents itself in the discourse about change in the United States, one of the most remarkable features of this fatalism is how untrue it is. Racism and other "isms" are indeed pervasive in society, but these are constantly shifting frames. In the 1950s prejudice was a popular topic in social science, and many scales were created to measure prejudice and hatred. At that time it made perfect sense to ask white people how much, on a scale of 1 to 10, they hated black people. Such questions would be terribly ineffective in today's world, because the structure of discrimination and segregation that gave those beliefs validity no longer exists. Furthermore, many white people are horrified by the idea of racism and would not want to be associated with such ideas. This was hardly the case in the 1950s, when segregationists howled at little black children on their way to previously all-white schools.

The end result of the redlining of the AIDS epidemic was, first, an unnecessary burden of disease within marginalized groups and, second, an unnecessary burden of disease for all Americans. Wallace and Wallace have demonstrated what they call the "paradox of apartheid," that is, that rates of disease in society at large will be proportional to the rates in marginalized communities (Wallace and Wallace, 1995). It is this reality—the effects outside a redlined community of ignoring an infectious disease within it—that has not penetrated the consciousness of those who think "concentration" is equivalent to "containment."

CONCLUSION

I have chosen three perspectives on neighborhoods and infectious disease: the construction of the local, the problem of neighborhood disruption, and the problem of redlining epidemics. These perspectives inform a dynamic and ecological view of epidemics as local events with global connections. Neighborhoods are not stable creations. Rather, neighborhoods are constantly recreating themselves as people, goods, and institutions enter and exit. In this dynamic process vulnerability to infection will rise with the introduction of new infectious agents and new social problems but fall with the introduction of social and scientific resources to limit the spread of illness. The concentration of illness and the construction of neighborhoods that limit the free flow of resources will increase the burden of disease not just in the affected neighborhood but throughout the larger embedding society and perhaps throughout the world. The downside of globalization is that nothing is simply local anymore.

Perhaps the most serious problem is this: the communities impoverished by globalization are lost to sight. This distinctly visual metaphor follows directly from the view of these communities as "marginal," on the periphery, at the edge of our visual range or not in it at all. Greenberg and Schneider draw on this visual metaphor in the following manner:

> In truth, the United States is not going to reduce violence by focusing on stereotypical views of its main victims; Americans are going to have to face the reality that their economic and political systems have contributed to the construction of deadly marginal environments. When and

if that reality becomes widely accepted, the United States will face the sobering choice of whether to drive around marginal areas and pretend they do not exist or make an earnest effort to commit real resources to a more equitable landscape. (p. 186)

The words they selected are telling: facing reality versus pretending marginal areas do not exist. This is not hyperbole, however, as the process of globalization is a powerful force driving marginalization. If society does not face the distributive issues raised by globalization, then epidemics of infectious disease will spread at higher rates and through larger portions of society than would otherwise be the case. The lady or the tiger—what shall we choose?

REFERENCES

Dear MJ (1976). Abandoned housing. In Adams J, ed. *Urban Policy-Making and Metropolitan Development*. Cambridge: Ballanger.

Gratz RG (1994). *The Living City: How America's Cities Are Being Revitalized by Thinking Small in a Big Way*. Washington, DC: Preservation Press.

Greenberg M and Schneider D (1994). Violence in American cities: Young black males is the answer, but what was the question? *Soc Sci Med* 39: 179–184.

Hibbs JR and Gunn RA (1991). Public health intervention in a cocaine-related syphilis outbreak. *Am J Public Health* 81: 1259–1262.

Link BG and Phelan J (1995). Social conditionas as fundamental causes of disease, *J Health Soc Behavior* (extra issue): 80–94.

Mann J, Tarantola DJM, Netter TW, eds. (1992). *AIDS in the World: A Global Report*. Cambridge, Mass: Harvard University Press.

McCoy CB and Inciardi JA (1995). *Sex Drugs and the Continuing Spread of AIDS*. Los Angeles: Roxbury.

National Research Council (1993). *The Social Impact of AIDS in the United States*. Washington, DC: National Academy Press.

Patterat JJ, Rothenberg RB, Woodhouse DE, Muth JB, Pratts CI, Fogle JS II (1985). Gonorrhea as a social disease. *Sex Transm Dis* 12: 25–32.

Ratner MS (1993). *Crack Pipe as Pimp: An Ethnographic Investigation of Sex-for-Crack Exchanges*. New York: Lexington Books.

Wallace R (1988). A synergism of plagues: "Planned shrinkage," contagious housing destruction, and AIDS in the Bronx. *Environ Res* 47: 1–33.

Wallace R, Wallace D (1995). U.S. apartheid and the spread of AIDS to the suburbs: A multi-city analysis of the political economy of spatial epidemic threshold, *Soc Sci Med* 41(3): 333–345.

10
Infant Health: Race, Risk, and Residence

JAMES W. COLLINS, JR.
NANCY FISHER SCHULTE

Infant mortality is more than a discrete health indicator of the number of deaths that occur in the first year of life, it is a symbolic benchmark of how a nation cares for its future generations. By this standard the United States is seriously deficient (Guyer et al., 1999). Despite an advanced and expensive health care system, the U.S. ranking among industrialized countries has plummeted during the past forty years from 6th to 23rd (Table 10–1). Glaring and enduring disparities between African-American and white infants explain much of this international slippage. In 1998 the infant mortality rate (the number of deaths under one year of age per 1,000 live births) was 7.2, matching the all-time low set the previous year and more than 40% lower than in 1980, yet the comparative outcomes for African-American infants have worsened, with the relative risk of African-American to white infant mortality rising from 1.6 in 1960 to 2.0 in 1980 and 2.4 in 1998 (David and Collins, 1991; Guyer et al, 1997). African-American infants are more than twice as likely as white infants to die before their first birthday (14.1 per 1,000 vs. 6.0 per 1,000, respectively). Thus, some 6,000 infant deaths a year could be prevented if the infant mortality rate of African-Americans were lowered to the level of whites.

Birthweight is the other main measurement of infant health. It is not only a significant predictor of infant mortality but also closely linked to serious, long-term physical and mental disabilities. Unlike the infant mortality rate, the percentage of low birthweight babies, those weighing less than 2500 g, or 5 lbs, 8 oz, has risen steadily since 1984 (Chike-Obi, 1996). In 1997 the 7.5% of all births that were low birthweight accounted for 65% of all infant deaths (Guyer et al., 1999). Even more vulnerable are very low birthweight babies, those weighing less than 1500 g, or 3 lbs, 3 oz).

TABLE 10–1. Infant Mortality Rates for
Countries of > 2,500,000 Population

Country	Infant Mortality Rate
Sweden	3.6
Japan	3.7
Singapore	3.8
Hong Kong	4.0
Norway	4.1
Finland	4.2
Switzerland	4.5
Austria	4.7
Denmark	4.7
Spain	4.7
Germany	4.9
Netherlands	5.0
France	5.1
Australia	5.3
Italy	5.5
Canada	5.6
Czech Republic	5.9
United Kingdom	5.9
Belgium	6.1
Ireland	6.2
New Zealand	6.6
Greece	6.9
United States	7.2

Source: Guyer et al., 1999

One-half of all infant deaths were among the 1.4% very low birthweight infants (Guyer et al., 1999). Again, there are striking racial differences: African Americans have a twofold greater rate of low birthweight infants (13% vs. 6.6%) and almost a threefold greater rate of very low birthweight infants (3.1% vs. 1.2%) than do whites.

The overall decline in infant mortality rates reflects major advances in neonatal medicine, especially in caring for low birthweight infants. Unfortunately, this success has not been matched by a reduction in the percentage of low birthweight infants. Among African Americans in particular, this unfavorable birthweight distribution accounts for most of their excess infant mortality.

While the underlying causes of these persistent racial disparities have not been empirically established, we have made some progress in understanding the complicated issue of race and infant outcome. The challenge is to disentangle the effects of race and poverty. The prevalence of disadvantages among individual African Americans does not fully explain their poor birth outcomes, nor is there a biological vulnerability specific to African-Americans. In this chapter we look beyond individual attributes and explore where and how African-American women live in an effort to understand these enduring inequalities. We focus on our studies of the residents of Chicago, the third most segregated city in the United States.

RACE AND INDIVIDUAL RISK

For more than forty years the emphasis in epidemiologic studies of infant health and mortality has been to identify the individual characteristics of the mother that result in compromised births. A mother's age, education, income, marital status, prenatal care, interpregnancy interval, and personal behaviors (cigarette smoking, alcohol intake, and illicit drug use) are variables predictive of adverse outcomes (Kleinmen and Kessel, 1987; Kleinman et al., 1988; Collins and David 1990; Joyce, 1991; Kotelchuck, 1992; Schoendorf et al., 1992; Rawlings et al., 1995), yet these well-known risk factors fail to explain the racial disparity in infant birthweight (Kleinmen and Kessel, 1987; Kleinman et al., 1988; Collins and David, 1990; Schoendorf et al., 1992). Using national vital records from the early 1980's, Kleinmen and Kessel (1987) showed not only persistent but actually widening racial disparities in infant birthweight as socioeconomic risk declined. Furthermore, numerous studies have shown that prenatal care does not close the racial disparity in infant birthweight and neonatal mortality (Murray and Bernfield, 1988; Collins and David, 1992; Barefield et al., 1996; Collins et al., 1997a).

Could genetic factors underlie these pervasive racial disparities in infant birthweight? To answer this question we compared the births in Illinois from 1980 to 1995 for three groups of mothers: sub-Saharan African-born blacks, U.S.-born blacks, and U.S.-born whites (David and Collins, 1997). If genetics played a prominent role in birth size differentials, one would expect African-born women, having the purest racial ancestry, to bear the smallest babies. Instead, we found the opposite: regardless of socioeconomic status, the infants of black women who were born in Africa weighed more than the infants of comparable black women born in the United States. Furthermore, the birthweight patterns of infants of African-born black women and U.S.-born white women were more closely related to each other than to the birthweights of the infants of U.S.-born black women.

These results highlight the significance of a mother's birthplace on her infant's health and suggest that the early-life experiences of foreign-born black women may cushion the risks when their babies are born in disadvantaged neighborhoods in the United States. A study by Fang et al. (1999) of births in New York City between 1988 and 1994 found that within the same poor communities black mothers from Africa and the Caribbean islands were less likely to have low birthweight infants than were white mothers, even after controlling for maternal sociodemographic characteristics. Conversely, the influences of a mother's childhood environment may also have deleterious consequences that undermine the effects of adult-achieved beneficial characteristics (Emanuel, 1986; Sanderson, 1995; Coutino et al., 1997). What are these environmental factors that affect two generations? For African-American women, clues are found in their segregated neighborhoods.

RESIDENTIAL ENVIRONMENT AND RISK

Residential segregation is a distinguishing organizational feature of African-American life that profoundly affects its residents (National Advisory Commission on Civil Disorders; 1968; National Research Council, 1990; Massey and Denton, 1993). This pattern of geographic separation that confines African Americans because of their race to circumscribed and disadvantaged neighborhoods may explain racial disparities in birth outcomes that persist even with improving socioeconomic and health circumstances (see Chapter 12).

While segregated neighborhoods exist throughout the United States, the most extreme examples are in sixteen metropolitan areas that together account for more one-third of the total African-American population (Massey and Denton, 1993). New York City and Chicago are two of these "hypersegregated" areas. Yankauer published a seminal study of infant mortality, race, and residential segregation in 1950. He found that in New York City the rates of nonwhite (African-American and Puerto Rican) and white infant deaths rose as the percentage of nonwhite residents increased. Interestingly, the infant mortality rate of nonwhite infants who resided in predominately white neighborhoods was lower than that of white infants who lived in African-American ghettos. Because of the similar educational and occupational backgrounds of both groups, Yankauer suggested that the African-American ghetto environment itself negatively affected infant outcome.

Another study (LaViest 1989) revealed a similar association between the degree of racial segregation and the infant mortality rate of African Americans in 176 U.S. cities between 1981 and 1985. In an analysis of 38 large U.S. standard metropolitan areas (SMSA) with a total population of more than 1 million, Polednak (1991) showed that racial segregation was the most important predictor of the racial differential in infant mortality rates independent of median family income and poverty prevalence. In a subsequent study of trends in infant mortality rates from 1982 through 1991, Polednak (1996) found that high mortality rates persisted in the most segregated areas and contributed to the widening African-American to white rate ratio.

This led us to investigate the contribution of residential environment to the racial gap in birth outcomes in Chicago. We used median family income and the percentage of families living below the poverty level in the mother's census tract to measure ecologic risk (Collins and David, 1990; Collins and David, 1992; Collins et al., 1998a). Our studies showed that the vast majority of African-American infants were born to women who lived in high-risk communities, unlike the infants of white mothers who rarely resided in impoverished neighborhoods of Chicago. We found the same enduring racial disparities, especially among lower-risk African-American mothers. While African-American women were much more likely to live in the poorest areas, those who did live in higher-income neighborhoods still had low birthweight rates that exceeded those of whites who resided in low-income neighborhoods (Table 10–2). Furthermore, these rates were still twice those of whites regardless of a mother's age, education, and marital status.

TABLE 10–2. Percentage of Low Birthweight African-American and White Infants According to Census Tract Income

Annual Income	African American (N = 51,827)	White (N = 51,245)	Relative Risk (95% CI)
< $10,001	15%	8%	1.9 (1.6–2.2)
$10,001–$20,000	14%	6%	2.1 (2.0–2.2)
$20,001–$30,000	12%	5%	2.2 (2.0–2.4)
$30,001–$40,000	10%	5%	2.2 (1.4–3.5)

Source: Collins and David, 1990

Not surprisingly, we found that for both races the use of prenatal care varied by residential environment, with those living in the poorest neighborhoods least likely to receive adequate care (Collins and David, 1992; Collins et al., 1997a). For African-American women who received adequate prenatal care, those who lived in poor neighborhoods had a 60% greater low birthweight rate than did those who lived in nonpoor neighborhoods. Most strikingly, the racial differential in infant birthweight persisted among mothers who received adequate prenatal care and lived in moderate-income neighborhoods. However, the long arm of segregation extends into nonpoor African-American neighborhoods. An analysis of 1990 U.S. census data by the Chicago *Tribune* found that approximately 80% of middle-class African-American households were in predominantly African-American communities that were within four blocks of impoverished neighborhoods (Chicago *Tribune*, 1997). Thus, the large majority African-American mothers and their infants were subjected to the particular stresses of a segregated environment.

Even the prospects of normal birthweight babies are compromised by their surroundings. African-American infants that weigh more than 2,500g (5 lbs, 8 oz) are still twice as likely to die as are white infants of the same size. Most of these deaths occur in the postneonatal period, from 28 days to 1 year, when environmental factors are more influential than are medical ones. Sudden infant death syndrome (SIDS) and injuries are the leading preventable causes of postneonatal death. It appears that African-American communities have not fully benefited from the national education campaign stressing the importance of babies sleeping on their back (*Morbidity and Mortality Weekly Report*, 1998; Willinger, 2000). Intentional and unintentional injuries represent a combination of risk in the environment. The postneonatal mortality rate of African Americans is highest in the most segregated communities (LaVeist, 1990). Our preliminary research in Chicago showed the familiar pattern whereby residence in impoverished communities accounted for a significant percentage of postneonatal deaths among African Americans, but the racial disparity in mortality rates persisted in nonimpoverished communities as well (Papacek et al., 1999).

PUTATIVE PATHWAYS

The exact pathways of these environmental stressors are not clearly evident. Some are acute, others chronic, but they all involve real-life experiences and perceptions (McLean et al., 1993).

Neighborhood Stressors with a Demonstrated Racial Bias

A handful of studies suggest that residence in violent communities is a stressor that adversely affects pregnancy outcomes (Zapata et al., 1992; Ascherio et al., 1992; Savitz et al., 1993). This is especially significant for African Americans, who are more likely to live in violent communities independent of income (National Research Council, 1989). In a study of impoverished urban African Americans, we found that infants of mothers who resided in the most violent neighborhoods had a 50% greater low birthweight rate, and three-fold greater rate of intrauterine growth retardation (weight for gestation length less than the tenth percentile) than infants of mothers who lived in the least violent communities (Collins and David, 1997b). (See also Chapter 11 for discussion of association between exposure to neighborhood violence and another health outcome, asthma.)

Psychophysiological Reactions to Residential Environment

The human dimension, as reflected in subjective appraisal of one's community, should not be overlooked. Women's personal experiences and perceptions matter. We found that a greater percentage of African-American mothers of very low birthweight infants rated their neighborhoods unfavorably compared to African-American mothers of nonlow birthweight infants (Collins et al., 1998b) (Table 10–3). In addition, African-American mothers of very low birthweight infants were more likely to

TABLE 10–3. Percentage of Very Low Birthweight and Non–Low Birthweight Mothers Who Reported Unfavorable Ratings of Their Residential Environment

	Very Low Birthweight (n = 28)	Non–Low Birthweight (n = 52)	Odds Ratio (95% CI)
Police	55%	26%	3.2 (1.2–8.4)
Property	43%	23%	1.9 (1.1–3.4)
Personal safety	48%	25%	2.8 (1.0–7.4)
Friendliness	39%	20%	2.2 (0.8–5.8)
Services	29%	19%	1.7 (0.6–5.0)
Cleanliness	50%	28%	2.5 (1.0–6.4)
Quietness	61%	42%	2.1 (0.8–5.4)
Schools	28%	15%	2.8 (0.8–9.7)
Overall	46%	21%	3.2 (1.2–8.8)

Source: Collins et al., 1998

experience stressful life events during pregnancy than were African-American mothers of nonlow birthweight infants.

Perceived Exposure to Racial Discrimination

Unfortunately, residential segregation and racial discrimination are intimately woven into the cultural framework of U.S. society. In an exploratory study we found as association between low-income African-American mothers' self-reported episodes of racial discrimination and very low birthweight of their infants (Collins et al., 2000). Although the optimal model in pregnant women for stress brought about by societal patterns of racial discrimination has yet to be developed, this study points the way for what should be a fruitful area for investigation.

ACKNOWLEDGMENTS
This chapter was funded in part by Chicago Community Trust (to J. W. C.).

REFERENCES

Ascherio A, Chase R, Cote T, Dehaes G, Hoskins E, Laaouej J (1992). Effect of the Gulf War on infant and childhood mortality in Iraq. *N Engl J Med* 327: 931–936.

Barefield W, Wise P, Rust F, Rust K, Gould J, Gortmaker S (1996). Racial differences in outcomes in military and civilian births in California. *Arch Pediatr Adolesc Med* 150: 1062–1067.

Chicago Tribune, February 1, 1997.

Chike-Obi U, David R, Coutinho R, Wu S (1996). Birth weight has increased over a generation. *Am J Epidemiol* 144: 563–569.

Collins J, David R (1990). The differential effect of traditional risk factors on infant birthweight among blacks and whites in Chicago. *Am J Public Health* 80: 679–681.

Collins J, David R (1992). Differences in neonatal mortality by race, income, and prenatal care. *Ethnicity Dis* 2: 18–26.

Collins J, Wall S, David R (1997a). Adequacy of prenatal care utilization, maternal ethnicity, and infant birthweight in Chicago. *J Natl Med Assoc* 89: 198–203.

Collins J, David R (1997b). Urban violence and African-American pregnancy outcome: An ecologic study. *Ethnicity Dis* 7: 184–190.

Collins J, Schulte N, Drolet A (1998a). Differential effect of ecologic risk factors on the low birthweight components of African-American, Mexican-American, and non-Latino white infants in Chicago. *J Natl Med Assoc* 90: 223–232.

Collins J, David R, Symons R, Handler A, Wall S, Andes S (1998b). African-American mothers' perception of their residential environment, stressful life events, and very low birthweight. *Epidemiology* 9: 286–289.

Collins J, David R., Symons R, Handler A, Wall S, Dwyer L (2000). Low-income

African-American mothers' perception of exposure to racial discrimination and infant birthweight. *Epidemiology* 11(3): 337–339.

Coutinho R, David R, Collins J (1997). Relation of parental birth weight to infant birth weight among African-Americans and whites in Illinois: A transgenerational study. *American Journal of Epidemiology* 146: 804–809.

David R, Collins J (1991). Bad outcomes in black babies: Race or racism? *Ethnicity Dis* 1: 236–244.

David R, Collins J (1997). Differing birth weights among infants of US-born blacks, African-born blacks, and US-born whites. *N Engl J Med* 337: 1209–1214.

Emanuel I (1986). Maternal health during childhood and later reproductive performance. *Ann NY Acad Sci* 477: 27–39.

Guyer B, Strobino D, Ventura S, Singh G (1995). Annual summary of vital statistics–1994. *Pediatrics* 96: 1029–1039.

Iyasu S, Becerra J, Rowley D, Hogue C (1992). Impact of very low birth weight on the black–white infant mortality gap. *Am J Prev Med* 8: 271–277.

Joyce T (1990). The dramatic increase in the rate of low birthweight in New York City: An aggregate time-series analysis. *American Journal of Public Health* 80: 682–684.

Kleinman J, Pierre M, Madans J, Land G, Schramm W (1988). The effects of maternal smoking on fetal and infant mortality. *Am J Epidemiol* 127: 274–282.

Kotelchuck M (1994). The adequacy of prenatal care utilization: Its US distribution and association with low birth weight. *Am J Public Health* 84: 1486–1489.

LaVeist T (1989). Linking residential segregation to the infant mortality race disparity in U.S. cities. *Sociol Res* 73: 90–94.

LaVeist T (1990). Simulating the effect of poverty on the race disparity in postneonatal mortality. *J Public Policy* Winter: 463–473.

Massey D, Denton N (1993). *American Apartheid: Segregation and the Making of the Underclass.* Cambridge Mass: Harvard University Press.

McLean D, Hatfield-Timajehy K, Wingo P, Floyd R (1993). Psychosocial measurement: Implications for the study of preterm birth and delivery in black women. *Am J Prev Med* 9: 39–81.

Morbidity and Mortality Weekly Report (1998). Assessment of infant sleeping pattern-selected states, 1996. 47: 873–876.

Murray J, Bernfield M (1988). The differential effect of prenatal care on the incidence of low birth weight among blacks and whites in a prepaid health plan. *N Engl J Med* 74: 1003–1008.

National Research Council (1989). *A Common Destiny: Blacks and American Society.* Washington, DC: National Academy Press.

Papacek E, Drolet A, Schulte N, Collins J (1999). Disparate postneonatal mortality rates of African-American and Mexican-American infants: A challenge for epidemiologic research. *Pediatr Res* (abstract) 45: 611.

Polednak A (1991). Black–white differences in infant mortality in 38 standard metropolitan statistical areas. *Am J Public Health* 81: 1480–1482.

Polednak A (1996). Trends in U.S. urban black mortality by degree of residential segregation. *Am J Public Health* 86: 723–726.

Polednak A (1997). *Segregation, poverty, and mortality in urban African-Americans.* New York: Oxford University Press.

Rawlings R, Rawlings V, Read J (1995). Prevalence of low birth weight and preterm delivery in relation to the interval between pregnancies among white and black women. *N Engl J Med* 332: 69–74.

Sanderson M, Emanuel I, Holt V (1995). The intergenerational relationship between mother's birthweight, infant birthweight, and infant mortality in black and white mothers. *Paediatric and Perinatal Epidemiol* 9: 391–405.

Savitz D, Thang N, Swenson I, Stone E (1993). Vietnamese infant and childhood mortality in relation to the Vietnam war. *Am J Public Health* 83: 1134–1138.

Schoendorf K, Hogue C, Kleinman J, Rowley D (1992). Mortality among infants of black as compared to white college-educated parents. *N Engl J Med* 326: 1522–1526.

United States Commission of Civil Disorders (1968). *Reports of the National Advisory Commission on Civil Disorders*. New York: Bantam Books.

US Bureau of the Census (1989). *Statistical Abstract of the United States (1989)*. 110th ed. Washington, DC: Government Printing Office.

Willinger M, Ko C, Hoffman H, Kessler R, Corwin M (2000). Factors associated with caregivers choice of infant sleep position, 1994–1998: The National Sleep Study. *JAMA* 283: 2135–2142.

Yankauer A (1950). The relationship of fetal and infant mortality to residential segregation. *Am Sociol Res* 15: 644–648.

Zapata B, Reboilledo A, Atalah E, Newman B, King M (1992). The influence of social and political violence on the risk of pregnancy complications. *Am J Public Heath* 82: 685–690.

11

Putting Asthma into Context: Community Influences on Risk, Behavior, and Intervention

ROSALIND J. WRIGHT
EDWIN B. FISHER

The etiology of health problems is increasingly recognized as a complex interplay of influences operating at several levels, including the individual, the family, and the community. As part of this growing complexity, evidence supports the notion that connections between health and economic well-being are embedded within the larger context of people's lives (Williams 1990; Wagener et al. 1993). Findings reviewed throughout this book point to the potential influence on health of diverse community (or group-level) characteristics in addition to economic and individual characteristics.

Recently observed epidemiologic trends suggest that asthma may provide an excellent paradigm for understanding the role of community-level contextual factors in disease. Specifically, a multilevel approach that includes an ecological perspective may help us understand heterogeneities in asthma expression across socioeconomic and geographic boundaries that to date remain largely unexplained. Traditionally, asthma epidemiology has focused on individual-level risk factors and family factors. Far less attention has been given to the broader social context in which individuals live.

This chapter examines contextual factors related to the occurrence and risk of asthma, health behaviors, access to health care, and the design of effective interventions to reduce the burden of asthma. The latter is exemplified through the discussion of a specific community-based approach to asthma management, the Neighborhood Asthma Coalition.

Two limitations on the scope of this review should be noted. First, many novel interventions at the community level have been developed, some published in research journals and some not (Addington and Weiss, 1999; McElmurry et al., 1999). These are not reviewed exhaustively. Instead, the chapter highlights the range of community influences on asthma and their implications using specific examples. Second, the diversity and often the subtlety of community influences complicate research. With a few exceptions, however, the relevant methodological issues are beyond the scope of the present overview, but they can be reviewed elsewhere (Kaufman and Kaufman, 2001; Pickett and Pearl, 2001).

UNEXPLAINED EPIDEMIOLOGIC TRENDS

Asthma prevalence and associated morbidity are increasing worldwide (Pearce et al., 1998; Wright and Weiss, 2000). In the United States these trends disproportionately affect nonwhite children living in urban areas and children living in poverty (Lang and Polansky, 1994). Higher rates of asthma prevalence, hospitalizations, and mortality have also been described among poor individuals and members of minority groups worldwide (McElmurry et al., 1999). Data that are seemingly contradictory to this pattern include a number of British studies that report increased asthma prevalence among children and adolescents of higher socioeconomic status (SES) (Anderson et al., 1983; Kaplan and Mascie-Taylor, 1985; Lewis et al., 1995), which may be explained by diagnostic labeling bias related more to social class than to underlying disease (Littlejohns and Macdonald, 1993). This idea is supported by the fact that severe asthma, which is less susceptible to diagnostic labeling bias, is more common among lower social groups in the United Kingdom (Mitchell and Dawson, 1973; Kaplan and Mascie-Taylor, 1988), a pattern that is also seen in the United Staes (Mielck et al., 1996) and other countries (SIDRIA Collaborative Group, 1997).

Recent evidence suggests that the epidemiology of asthma is still more complex. In the United States, a graded association between SES and asthma prevalence, morbidity, and mortality has been documented (Mitchell et al., 1989; Weitzman, et al., 1990; Bor et al., 1993; Weiss et al., 1993; Chen et al., 2002). A relation between SES and childhood asthma severity has been found in both U.S. and international studies whereby lower SES is associated with higher rates of severe asthma (Chen et al., 2002). Moreover, data from the United States demonstrate significant geographic variations in asthma outcomes among large cities (Perrin et al., 1989) and neighborhoods within cities (Carr et al., 1992; Marder et al., 1992; Lang and Polansky, 1994). Carr and colleagues (1992) documented up to tenfold differences in asthma hospitalization and mortality rates among certain New York inner-city neighborhoods compared to national rates.

Notably, variation in asthma morbidity across urban neighborhoods cannot be explained by economic factors alone. For example, many New York City communities do not have elevated asthma morbidity despite the fact that they are comparably low on many economic indicators and have seemingly similar physical environmental exposures as do the high-risk neighborhoods. Among low SES neighborhoods those with predominantly minority, segregated populations seem especially burdened, however. In Harlem, a community with a high level of poverty and a majority of African-American and Latino residents, the asthma mortality rate among males is twice as high as in other New York communities (Ford et al., 1998). These findings indicate that other factors (e.g., minority group status, residential segregation) may mediate the effects of living in low SES neighborhoods

Racial–ethnic differences seem to exist independently of SES (Crain et al., 1994; Cunningham et al., 1996). In the United States asthma prevalence, hospitalization, and emergency room use declined with increasing income for nonblack but not for black children (Miller, 2000). Minority ethnic status has also been associated with higher rates of asthma and greater morbidity in New Zealand (Mitchell, 1991) and the United Kingdom (Partridge, 2000). For example, recent data from the United Kingdom show increased prevalence and morbidity among South Asian minorities (i.e., the largest ethnic minority in the nation) compared with white Europeans living in the same socioeconomically deprived areas (Moudgil et al., 2000). Jones and colleagues demonstrated that children of Asian origin were 3.6 times more likely to have exercise-induced bronchoconstriction than were white children living in the same inner-city region in Britain (Jones et al., 1996). Another U.S. study found that the lifetime prevalence of asthma was 2.1 times higher in blacks than in whites, despite the fact that subjects were of similar middle and higher economic status (Nelson et al., 1997). Although the authors propose that their findings may be attributable to biological differences based on race, several considerations argue against this explanation. Most notably, the observed increase in asthma and growing disparities documented between ethnic minorities and whites have occurred over one to three decades, which is too rapid to be plausibly attributed to genetic mutation or change. These data do suggest that other unique characteristics among minority populations, beyond simply economic well-being, may affect their health.

In summary, while the preponderance of epidemiologic evidence worldwide suggests that asthma morbidity is negatively related to lower economic status, the association is not universal but rather varies significantly across countries, cities, communities and neighborhoods, and subpopulations. Regardless of SES, ethnic minorities seem to be disproportionately burdened. The wide geographic and sociodemographic variation in asthma expression remains a paradox largely unexplained by known environmental risk factors, and it has led to reconsideration of the interplay among biological and social determinants in attempting to understand such disparities in the asthma burden (Wright et al., 1998a). The rest of this chapter emphasizes how this variation in asthma burden may be explained by community-level factors, including both physical environmental determinants of asthma, and the potential influence of social, cultural, and institutional structures.

NEIGHBORHOOD CONTEXTUAL FACTORS

Community-level variables are receiving increased attention for their potential role in determining health outcomes. These variables include the effects of income inequality on mortality (Haan et al., 1987; Kennedy et al., 1996; Wilkinson, 1996; Roberts, 1998; Kawachi and Kennedy, 1999), the links between residential segregation and black infant mortality (La Veist, 1993; see also Chapter 12), and the effect of neighborhood deprivation on coronary risk factors (Diez-Roux et al., 1997) and low birthweight (Roberts, 1997). Few studies have directly examined the influence of such contextual factors on asthma. Two recent studies have shown significant associations between greater neighborhood income inequality and higher childhood asthma hospitalization rates (Huang and Johnson, 1998; Watson et al., 1996). In New Zealand Salmond and colleagues (1999) used small area analysis to find a linear increase in twelve-month period prevalence of asthma with increasing area deprivation. In addition, a persistent independent effect for ethnicity was demonstrated. Asthma prevalence rates were 1.4 times (95% CI 1.3, 1.5) higher among Maori and 1.3 times (95% CI 1.1, 1.5) higher among the Pacific Island group compared with the mostly European reference group. Appropriate control for individual-level SES is a methodological concern in these studies (Kaufman and Kaufman, 2001; Pickett and Pearl, 2001).

The range of findings linking community-level variables to health outcomes and the initial studies indicating associations with asthma strongly support the importance of further research on such community- and neighborhood-level influences. Given the range of variables that may be considered, identifying pathways that may link community influences to asthma morbidity that are supported in existing research may be most informative. Plausible risk factors include (1) environmental exposures, (2) stress (3) health behaviors and psychological factors, and (4) access to health care. These categories constitute the focus of the following sections of this chapter, followed by an illustration of how they may be addressed through a community-oriented asthma management program.

ENVIRONMENTAL EXPOSURES

To date much of the literature has focused on the potential importance of physical environmental characteristics on asthma morbidity, including outdoor air pollution (Pierson and Koenig, 1992); crowding as it may predispose to viral respiratory illness (Schenker et al., 1983); and changing housing stock, which may increase exposure to indoor allergens (Dekker et al., 1991; Platts-Mills et al., 1991). In the last case it has been hypothesized that changes in housing construction, including insulated windows and central heating systems in industrialized countries, have predisposed to increased growth of dust mites and molds, thus increasing indoor allergen exposure. Other hypotheses have favored the increased likelihood of *in utero* and environmental tobacco smoke exposure among lower SES populations (Weiss et al., 1980). Notably, both outdoor air pollution (U.S. Environmental Protection Agency, 1998; Heinrich et al., 1998) and cigarette smoking (at least when examined at the individual level) (Fingerhut and Warner, 1997) have been decreasing during the period of increases in asthma morbidity, suggesting that they cannot, in and of themselves, explain these asthma trends. U.S. studies have shown a relatively small increase in the prevalence of smoking among young women with low educational background, but not at rates likely to be responsible for the significant increases in asthma. Similarly, there is no evidence of significant changes in home allergen levels over this period (Hirsch, 1999), nor does existing evidence support the notion that the differences in specific sensitization are related to differences in the exposure to specific allergens.

Future research may need to pay increased attention to social, political, and economic forces that result in marginalization of certain populations in disadvantaged neighborhoods that may increase exposure to these known environmental risk factors. We also need to better understand how the physical and psychological demands of living in a relatively deprived environment may potentiate an individual's susceptibility to such exposures (Brunner, 1997).

STRESS

There is a renewed interest in the influence of psychological stress on asthma (Busse et al., 1994; Wright et al., 1998a). This is a useful way to conceptualize community-level influences on health whether one considers the environment a social or a physical construct. Both physical and social factors can be a source of environmental demands that contribute to stress experienced by populations living in a particular area (Evans, 2001). Differential exposure to and perception of stress may, in part, explain the associations between SES and health (Adler et al., 1994). Various sociodemographic characteristics (e.g., lower social class, ethnic minority status, sex) may predispose individuals to particular forms of chronic life stress (Dohrenwend and Dohrenwend, 1969; McLean et al., 1993; Rabkin and Struening, 1976), which may be in turn significantly influenced by the characteristics of the communities in which they live (Taylor et al., 1997).

One type of chronic stress that has been investigated in relation to the well-being of U.S. urban populations is neighborhood disadvantage (ND), characterized by the presence of a number of community-level stressors, including poverty, unemployment, substandard housing, and high crime and violence rates (Attar et al., 1994). Such stress is chronic and can affect all subjects in a given environment regardless of their individual-level risks. For example, a person whose income is above the national median but who lives in a disadvantaged neighborhood may experience stress related to the community. Data exist to suggest that the health implications of low income are significantly different for individuals living in areas with high ND (Haan et al., 1989). In the United States, trends in social environmental factors over the past few decades have resulted in many urban communities being characterized by high ND (Wilson, 1987). As well, changes have occurred in the residential distribution of the U.S. population, resulting in the disproportionate concentration of minority groups in areas of concentrated poverty (Williams, 1998; see also Chapter 12).

Similar to ND are the constructs of social organization, "social capital," or "community assets" (Lochner et al., 1999; see also Chapter 6). Closely related to these are the physical features of the environment, such as crowding and noise. Research has linked these to stress, but few studies have evaluated their relationship to asthma outcomes (Evans, 2001).

The broad construct of ND, or low levels of community assets, subsume key exposures such as living in the presence of pervasive violence and crime. Violent crime undermines social cohesion (Sampson et al., 1997; Kennedy et al., 1998; Kawachi et al., 1999; see also Chapter 6) and is associated with the erosion of social capital and community resilience. Crime is most prevalent in societies that permit large disparities in the material standards of living of its citizens (Kawachi et al., 1999). Thus, in addition to direct impacts on community residents, crime and violence (or the lack of them) can be used as indicators of collective well-being, social relations, or social cohesion within a community and society.

Furthermore, the conditions known to be associated with exposure to violence are related to experienced stress (Breslau et al., 1991), and chronic exposure to violence has been conceptualized as a pervasive environmental stressor imposed on already vulnerable populations (Isaacs, 1992). Studies are beginning to explore the health effects of living in an environment with a chronic pervasive atmosphere of fear and the perceived threat of violence (Herman, 1988; Yach, 1988; Martinez and Richters, 1993; Boney-McCoy and Finkelhor, 1995; Zapata et al., 1992).

Exposure to violence has been associated with asthma in both the clinical (Wright and Steinbach, 2001) and research setting. In a population-based study in Boston lifetime exposure to violence was ascertained retrospectively through a parental report interview questionnaire administered to 416 caregivers and their children who were followed longitudinally for respiratory health outcomes, including asthma. Preliminary analyses suggest a link between high lifetime exposure to community violence and an increased risk of asthma and wheeze syndromes and prescription bronchodilator use among these inner-city children (Wright et al., 1997).

Minority group status may predispose individuals to pervasive chronic stressors (e.g., discrimination) and societal factors that link minorities and ND. For example, the broader political and economic forces that result in marginalization of minority populations in disadvantaged inner-city neighborhoods may lead to increased stress experienced by these populations and thus greater disease morbidity (Kawachi and Kennedy, 1999).

Future studies need to examine the links among ND, minority group status, low levels of social capital, violence exposure, and other social influences (and the heightened stress that they may elicit) as risk factors for childhood asthma analogous to physical environmental exposures (e.g., allergens, tobacco smoke, air pollution). Such studies are likely to further our understanding of the increased asthma burden on populations of children living in poverty in urban areas and other disadvantaged communities.

HEALTH BEHAVIORS AND OTHER PSYCHOLOGICAL FACTORS

Exposure to tobacco smoke is associated with childhood asthma (Weitzman et al., 1990; Martinez et al., 1992). Smoking can be viewed as a strategy to cope with negative affect or stress (Anda et al., 1990; Beckham et al., 1995; Acierno et al., 1996). Indeed, smoking has been associated with a variety of stressors and types of disadvantage, including unemployment, minority group status, family disorder, and violence as well as depression, schizophrenia, and other psychological problems (Fisher et al., in press). Stress in particular is associated with adolescent cigarette use (Castro et al., 1987), smokers' reported desire for a cigarette, and being unsuccessful at quitting (Cohen and Lichtenstein, 1990a, 1990b). These relationships among stress and smoking may be considered from a neighborhood perspective as well. Studies have demonstrated effects of neighborhood social factors on smoking behavior (Karvaonen and Rimpela, 1996; Kleinschmidt et al., 1997; Reijneveld, 1998). It has been hypothesized that neighborhood SES may be related to increased social tolerance and norms that support behavioral risk factors such as smoking (Curry et al., 1993).

In adult African-American populations the prevalence of smoking is higher than among whites. Evidence from the 1987 General Social Survey suggests that stress may be one factor that promotes the increased prevalence of smoking in these populations (Feigelman and Gorman, 1989). Romano and colleagues (1991) surveyed 1,137 African-American households and found that the strongest predictor of smoking was report of high-level stress, represented by an abbreviated hassles index. The hassles index was a ten-item scale based on items chosen to represent a dimension that community residents perceived to be especially relevant. Among the items were neighborhood-level factors, including concern about living in an unsafe area.

In addition to their influences on health behaviors such as smoking, evidence has linked community-level variables to key individual characteristics, such as perceived control. A large body of research indicates the importance of constructs such as perceived control (global feeling of the ability to deal with an event) over health as, for example, they mediate the relationship among illness experience, understanding, and compliance (Shagena et al., 1988). Three constructs that are closely related to perceived control are self-efficacy (belief in one's own ability to carry out tasks), locus of control (belief that events and outcomes are determined by internal or external forces), and learned helplessness (belief that positive as well as negative consequences are independent of one's own actions) (Bandura, 1977; Petermen, 1982). Perceived control has been found to correlate with many aspects of disease burden (Stein et al., 1988; Holden, 1991).

Evidence indicates that exposure to violence reduces perceived control. DuRant and colleagues (1995) examined the relationships between exposure to community violence and depression, hopelessness, and purpose in life among black urban youths. These authors found that higher current depression and hopelessness and lower purpose in life were significantly associated with the reported higher frequency of exposure to, or victimization by, violence in their lifetime. Thus, tying together several of the findings discussed here, exposure to violence or living in a community with a high occurrence of violence may lead to reduced perceived control, which may, in turn, be associated with poorer asthma management and outcomes.

An important methodological issue should be raised here. If increased exposure to tobacco smoke or reduced perception of control are a result of increased stress caused by the physical or social environment, then they should be considered mediators rather than confounders of the relationships between community-level variables and asthma outcomes. Inappropriate adjustment for such factors may result in the attenuation of a true effect (Evans, 2001; Kaufman and Kaufman, 2001).

ACCESS TO HEALTH CARE

A leading hypothesis states that the observed sociodemographic and geographic variation in asthma morbidity is due to differential access to and use of health care services (Weiss et al., 1992) and quality of health care (Wise and Eisenberg, 1989). Paradoxically, however, heightened asthma burden has been documented in urban populations residing in close proximity to major medical centers (Richards, 1989; Ernest et al., 1995). In the United States asthma mortality is higher in regions with more medical specialists (adjusting for region size), suggesting that the problem is not simply proximity to quality care but barriers to its use (Sly and O'Donnell, 1992).

National efforts in the United States to decrease asthma morbidity by reducing emergency department use and hospitalizations have focused on developing and disseminating national guidelines for patient education and self-management as well as clinical management of asthma (National Institutes of Health, 1991, 1997). These national guidelines recommend that persons with persistent (i.e., mild, moderate, or severe) asthma should receive long-term control medication (e.g., anti-inflammatory medication) in addition to quick-relief medications (e.g., beta-agonists) to manage asthma exacerbations. Underuse of anti-inflammatory medication within a community has been associated with higher hospitalization rates for asthma. Gottlieb and colleagues (1995) demonstrated that hospitalization rates across Boston areas (defined by ZIP codes) were inversely correlated with the ratio of inhaled anti-inflammatory and beta-agonist medication use. Use of beta-agonists alone has been associated with increased acute care visits and bronchial reactivity (Cockroft et al., 1995; Donahue et al., 1997), perhaps because medical providers in the community do not follow established guidelines for the management of asthma (Crain et al., 1998; Jatulis et al., 1998).

An alternative explanation for overuse of beta-agonist medications may be that asthma education programs do not adequately reach those patients suffering the greatest morbidity. Standard asthma education interventions have been found to be less effective among lower SES and ethnic minority groups (Apter et al., 1998; Moudgil and Honeybourne, 1998). A recent study in East Harlem, an area with one of the highest hospitalization and mortality rates for asthma in the United States, found that the use of anti-inflammatory medications varied among different ethnic groups that shared comparable SES and lived in the same community (Diaz et al., 2000). Among those with more severe asthma, Puerto Rican children were more likely to use anti-inflammatory medications on a daily basis than were African-American children or those from other ethnic groups.

Factors such as inadequate literacy have been shown to be related to a poor knowledge of both asthma and medication use (Williams et al., 1998). Recent immigrants may be more greatly affected, as they are more likely to encounter language barriers in accessing medical care and understanding asthma education guidelines (Guendelman and Schwalbe, 1986; Kirkman-Liff and Modragon, 1991). However, the failure to use medical care or understand guidelines despite the use of relevant ethnic dialects in some studies suggests that the problem does not simply reflect linguistic difficulties. The ethnicity of minority groups, including cultural practices and perspectives, may pose barriers to translation of health practices developed from a Western, middle-class perspective (Pachter and Weller, 1993; Ledogar et al., 2000).

Patients and their families may delay seeking care because of a lack of safe transportation or fear of safety in their communities. Fong (1995) reported the impact of violence on the management of hypertension in urban African Americans, noting that violence was a perceived barrier to keeping appointments and following prescribed exercise programs. This may lead to lapses in the use of prophylactic medications, delayed interventions, and consequently greater morbidity. Violence can also affect access to medical care indirectly by diverting limited funds away from primary care and specialty clinics, including those for asthmatics (Fleming et al., 1992; Robicsek et al., 1993).

Other barriers to adherence to prescribed asthma regimens include the lack of twenty-four–hour pharmacy availability in some communities. Even when open, pharmacy resources vary across neighborhoods and may be deficient. For example, in some New York communities with the highest asthma mortality rates, many pharmacies did not stock or sell medications or devices (e.g., spacers) that would facilitate compliance with accepted asthma guidelines (Ford et al., 1996). In contrast, the easy availability of over-the-counter inhalers (e.g., epinephrine) was likely to encourage the use of acute symptomatic relief, which is documented to increase the risk of morbidity.

In addition to these barriers to care, cultural factors such as beliefs and practices about health and health care may interfere with some groups' engagement with Western, middle-class approaches to health that emphasize preventing and curing disease and the *responsibility of the individual* in doing so (Dressler, 1991; Heurtin-Roberts and Reisin, 1992; Kumanyika, 1998; Anderson et al., 2000). In St. Louis substantial attitude and knowledge differences emerged between predominantly low-income African-American patients of a neighborhood health center compared to white middle-class patients from a suburban practice asthma clinic (Haire-Joshu et al., 1993). The African-American group rated asthma as less of a concern and indicated they were less careful to take their asthma medications, more satisfied with over-the-counter medications for asthma, and more likely to try to fight asthma attacks on their own, without medical help. Other studies (Mitchell et al., 1981; Blendon et al. 1989) indicate generally reduced contact with and use of formal and professional health services among certain ethnic minorities.

Thus, the paradox of deficient care among those who live in the shadows of leading urban medical centers reflects the themes of this chapter. Community-based barriers of violence, ethnicity, limited neighborhood resources such as well-stocked pharmacies, and education programs not well designed for such settings all contribute to poor access to geographically proximate care. Asthma interventions will be more effective when adapted to the ethnic, social, and economic characteristics of specific populations (De Oliveria et al., 1999).

INTERACTIONS AMONG COMMUNITY-LEVEL INFLUENCES AND THEIR MEDIATORS

A critical characteristic of community-level analysis has no doubt become apparent and has perhaps frustrated the reader. This is the tremendous complexity of interactions among community-level influences and the factors that mediate their effects on individuals.

As an example of complexity among mediators of community-level influences on asthma, consider the effects of violence. In the same Boston pediatric cohort discussed above, parental reports of keeping children indoors because of fear of neighborhood violence were related to increased risk of wheeze and physicians' diagnosis of asthma before the age of two years (Wright et al., 1998b). Reasonable hypotheses for this association include (1) increased exposure to indoor allergens; (2) increased sedentary lifestyle, which may be linked to obesity in children; (3) diminished stress-buffering factors such as social networks; and (4) influence on perceived control. Notably, recent studies have linked obesity to asthma (Camargo et al., 1999; Stenius-Aarniala et al., 2000) and suggested that obesity has increased among families living in poverty in the United States (Gortmaker et al., 1996). Parents who are worried about their children's safety in their neighborhood because of crime may keep their children indoors and otherwise restrict their social behavior, and thus their ability to develop support networks may be compromised (Sampson, 1992; see also Chapter 6). Psychopathology (e.g., posttraumatic stress disorder [PTSD], depression) influenced by life stress and chronic exposure to violence may also prevent a child from forming relationships that are necessary to promote normal social development. Fear of crime fosters a distrust of others and can contribute to social isolation (Krause, 1992), thereby limiting the formation of social networks that are especially important to health and well-being in high-risk urban populations faced with the cumulative effects of many other ecological stressors (e.g., poverty, low education, poor housing).

This complexity reflects the very nature of community-level influences. This no doubt challenges research in the field and may place community-level influences outside some kinds of knowing, but it is important that scholarship approach this complexity as something to be studied, not something to be controlled for.

LESSONS LEARNED FROM COMMUNITY
APPROACHES TO ASTHMA INTERVENTION

This section focuses on research in low-income, predominantly African-American neighborhoods in St. Louis, Missouri. After reviewing the identification of problems that underlie the disproportionate asthma burden in this group, we discuss two community- and peer-based approaches to intervention, the Neighborhood Asthma Coalition (NAC) and the Asthma Coach.

As in other cities described earlier, increases in hospitalizations for asthma among St. Louis children had been most pronounced among low-income African-American children (Bertolis et al., 1994). In particular, a study of five St. Louis children who had died from asthma in 1987 showed that they were African American and from low socioeconomic backgrounds (Birkhead et al., 1989). Common causes underlying these five cases included lack of prescribed corticosteroids in two decedents with known severe asthma and markedly subtherapeutic or zero serum theophylline levels at the time of death in all four of the cases in which measurements could be made. A similar pattern characterized fourteen pediatric asthma deaths in Brooklyn, New York (Rao et al., 1991). Review of these and similar cases suggests that most asthma deaths reflect a "slow-onset late-arrival" pathway marked by symptoms worsening over at least several hours but usually several or many days, disregard or passive acceptance of asthma and its symptoms, and delayed seeking of acute care (Strunk, 1993). The findings discussed in the section on access to health care above (Haire-Joshu et al., 1993) indicate that low-income groups tend to see asthma as an acute, periodic disease that can be treated with over-the-counter medication and tend to delay treatment for symptom exacerbation.

Problems also existed in receipt of regular asthma care. The guidelines of the National Asthma Education Program recommend regular outpatient care three times a year. Review of records for the first 103 subjects enrolled in the Neighborhood Asthma Coalition found that, during the year prior to enrollment, fewer than 4% had had three or more regular visits for asthma, and 77% had not seen a physician for asthma care other than in an emergency department (Matsumoto et al., 1994).

Profound Real-World Barriers to Basic Asthma Management

Among African-American children with asthma in the NAC, 10% had no insurance and 66% were covered by Medicaid, but economics was only part of the problem in low levels of regular asthma care. Audits of charts of community providers revealed a number of other problems for those in study neighborhoods: (1) episodic care promoted by not making appointments for regular follow-up visits, (2) no place for patients to call when acute symptoms occurred, (3) no plan of action for response to symptoms if medications did not stop symptoms or prevent progression, (4) rescue medication not prescribed and therefore not available at home, (5) prescription of medications that were not state-of-the-art (e.g., many patients who have had previous hospitalization or multiple emergency department visits were simply prescribed oral albuterol), and (6) no regular education provided about asthma. Further assessment included discussions with pediatricians serving the neighborhoods in order to develop an understanding of their perspectives on asthma care in their neighborhoods. We found a high level of motivation by practitioners, but also areas of discouragement, for example, having experienced high rates of "no-shows" among those given regular follow-up appointments. Our observations and discussions suggested a reciprocal relationship among the lack of patient understanding of the importance of regular care, poor attendance at such care, reluctance to offer such care, and continued lack of understanding of its importance because it was not offered or promoted (Sussman, 1992).

Rationale for Community- and Peer-Based Approaches to Asthma Education

A number of factors suggest the pertinence of community approaches to the problems detailed above. First, lack of understanding or appreciation of regular asthma care and progressive asthma management point to the role of peers and informal channels in communicating key messages, especially to low-income groups who may be alienated from more "mainstream" channels of communication (Mitchell et al., 1981; Blendon et al., 1989; Braithwaite and Lythcott, 1989). African Americans are relatively isolated from formal channels of information, such as physicians and other professionals, and thus may be more influenced by informal networks of friends and family. Information may be effectively exchanged within such networks (Rogers and Kincaid, 1981). African Americans appear to use their extended kin network for social support more than do whites (Dressler, 1985). Unfortunately, this probably contributes to the isolation of African Americans from formal health education and media and to their reduced use of formal and professional health services (Birkel and Repucci, 1983). However, a community organization's emphasis on implementing campaigns through peers may recruit such informal networks into supporting program goals. As informal networks are key sources of social support, reaching them brings this additional force to bear on program targets.

A second reason for emphasizing peer and community interventions is based on well-established findings in psychology that peers are especially effective in modeling changes in attitudes and behavior about which learners may be fearful or anxious (Meichenbaum, 1971; Kazdin, 1974). In the study of asthma deaths in the neighborhoods described above (Birkhead et al., 1989), families of decedents appeared not to have grasped the seriousness of their children's asthma. Consequently, the family, friends, and neighbors of children with asthma constitute a key target group for asthma education.

Community Organization

A community organization program, the NAC, was developed to engage not only children with asthma but also their parents, friends, and neighbors to encourage regular asthma care, daily management, and a broad understanding of the burdens posed by asthma and support for its care. Community organization usually entails participation of target audiences in planning and promoting programs and allows people to develop programs that meet their particular needs. This participation encourages them to assist and support one another's efforts and gain further assistance and support from formal and informal social structures and organizations. Such approaches may hold special promise for African Americans (Braithwaite and Lythcott, 1989; Fisher et al., 1992) and other underserved groups.

The NAC used a community organization approach (Rothman, 1968; Bracht, 1990; Minkler, 1990) to recruit members from four low-income, predominantly African-American neighborhoods of St. Louis into program governance, planning, and implementation. Detailed descriptions of the NAC and some of its distinctive program features have been reported (Fisher et al., 1992, 1994) along with demonstration that a community approach to asthma care can engage the intended audiences in program planning and implementation, be implemented within the settings of underserved, low-income and/or minority groups, and reach those it is designed to help (Fisher et al., 1996). In the following section the general characteristics and several illustrative aspects of the program are described.

Key Messages for a Neighborhood Program

The observations that low-income parents of children with asthma and adults with asthma tended to see asthma as an acute, periodic disease that could be treated with over-the-counter medication and that they also tended to delay treatment for symptom exacerbation led us to identify several key concepts for the NAC education activities: (1) take asthma seriously, (2) take asthma medicine for asthma symptoms, (3) when symptoms persist or worsen, follow an asthma action plan developed with your doctor, and (4) when symptoms continue or worsen, get help. As well as being pertinent to the needs identified, these messages are appropriate for a community program because they are simple and can be understood and passed on by neighborhood residents working in a wide variety of settings and activities.

Activities and Promotions as Channels for Education

Wellness councils and staff recognized that, on their own, didactic multisession asthma management classes were unlikely to attract audiences.

Combining this with the recognition of the relative simplicity of the key curricular messages noted above, a decision was made to focus the program on community-based activities and events that would be attractive and not presuppose extended commitment to repeated attendance. Accordingly, promotional events and activities have included (1) Back-to-School Parties with an "Ask the Doc" session and a talk on self-management; (2) Asthma Skate-Outs supported by a local businessman who donated roller skating passes for 100 participants; (3) a Halloween party; (4) a Teens on the Move conference (general health promotion and values clarification) supported by fourteen local businesses, including a local supermarket chain whose stores predominate in St. Louis African-American neighborhoods; (5) birthday celebrations for children in the program; (6) an annual NAC Calendar distributed to all participants by mail; (7) wellness councils developing a plan and recruiting the mayor of St. Louis to declare the month of March Asthma Awareness Month; (8) coverage on four TV and three radio talk shows and ten articles in print (9) presentations by parents in the NAC Speakers Bureau in numerous community settings, including presentations by staff and/or parents at thirteen schools; (10) participation by 108 churches in an asthma awareness prayer program or hosting presentations on asthma; (11) local radio station sponsorship of events (health fairs); and (12) distribution of flyers and leaflets by community groups and in shopping malls.

Concurrent with its wide range of activities and promotions, the NAC included asthma management classes for parents and children based on *Open Airways*. Initially, attendance was very low, often limited to three to five parents, even though ten to thirty parents were recruited for several classes. However, as the NAC gained popularity through the other activities and promotional events, interest in the more didactic presentations increased. In addition to presentations at health centers, churches, and community centers, the asthma management curriculum was taught through the neighborhood summer asthma camp, described below. On reflection, the mix of promotions, activities, and classes constitutes a versatile range of educational strategies consistent with a proactive approach (Prochaska et al., 1997) that stresses a range of activities with levels of commitment and educational complexity appropriate for individuals at different stages of readiness to improve asthma management (Abrams et al., 1986).

Engagement of the Audience

The NAC was implemented in four neighborhoods, each with a wellness council as part of a broader "Wellness Initiative" of the Grace Hill agency, our collaborator in this and several other health promotion programs. Evaluation was based on surveys from a cohort of parents of children who received emergency care for asthma and lived in either program neighborhoods or comparison neighborhoods. The parents were recruited merely with the agreement that they complete quarterly surveys (for each of which they were paid $10). This would provide an assessment of the extent the program could reach and engage them. Despite having agreed to do nothing but complete phone surveys, parents of 14% of the children in the program neighborhoods participated in at least one committee meeting involved in program planning and implementation, and parents of 17% assisted in actual implementation of program activities. In addition, twenty-two neighborhood residents were trained to help run summer asthma camps, described below, assisting in group educational activities. Despite the many stressors noted above, low-income parents can make active contributions to programs.

Beyond those who participated in program planning and implementation, the program reached a number of parents and children through their participation in activities and classes. Over the first two years of its implementation, 64% of children (and/or their parents or family members) in the evaluation cohort from program neighborhoods participated in at least one program activity. Consistent with the discussion above regarding the importance of health promotion activities that do not require commitment to extended attendance, participation was highest at low-demand events, such as holiday parties and skate-outs, which were promoted as enjoyable occasions, not educational activities. Forty-seven percent of children and/or parents from the program neighborhoods attended at least one such activity. Next most popular were the more traditional educational programs such as camp and the asthma management courses, with 39% attending at least one such session.

Peer Coaches in Reaching the Underserved

In addition to peer understanding of key concepts of asthma care, more general peer support appears important. Pilot data from the NAC directly suggested that social support for parents is important in asthma management and morbidity. Parents' social isolation was categorized according to responses to questions regarding how many family members and how many friends they could talk to about personal problems or call on for a favor. Children of socially isolated parents (those below the median on support from family and from friends) were reported to have more frequent days and nights with asthma symptoms, more days of activity limitation, poorer asthma management practices, and more emergency department visits compared to those of nonisolated parents or caregivers (Fisher et al., 1993). This relationship between parents social isolation and children's symptoms led investigators to recognize that neighborhood activities and naturally occurring informal networks might not reach some parents and their children. More generally, the linkage of social support to disease management (House et al., 1988), the burden and isolation many parents of asthmatic children experience (e.g., Schwam, 1987), and the need for stabilizing and supportive resources in the lives of mortality-prone asthmatic children (Strunk et al., 1985; Strunk, 1987) all indicate the importance of providing some direct support to parents and their children.

Initial plans to provide parents and their children support for asthma management included "Asthma Advocates," volunteer neighborhood residents who would take a strong role in assisting parents and children. In a review by the wellness councils and staff, this model appeared unfeasible. Given their own substantial burdens, neighborhood residents would not have the time as volunteers to master asthma knowledge and then assume the responsibility for ongoing support and monitoring of cases. Further, in its interest in channeling resources to neighborhood residents, Grace Hill maintains a policy of emphasizing paying jobs for substantial and skilled effort. Thus, a job line for CASS workers (named by the wellness councils for "change asthma with social support") entailed general assistance in program development and individualized contacts with parents and children, emphasizing promotion of attendance at programs, general support, assistance with overcoming barriers to asthma care, and basic asthma education stressing the core messages ("take asthma seriously," "when symptoms continue or worsen, get help") along with trigger management, medication adherence, and attendance at regular follow-up care. One CASS worker was assigned to each neighborhood and, in working with each neighborhood's wellness council, spent a considerable amount of time developing and implementing NAC activities as well as maintaining contacts with parents and children.

Initial evaluation of the CASS workers indicated they had been successful in being viewed as supportive, friendly, and nonauthoritarian. To do this, interviews were conducted with both parents and the CASS workers themselves. Responses indicated CASS workers provided a range of instrumental, informational, and emotional support, including specific tips on asthma management (Sylvia et al., 1993). In forced-choice questions, both the parents and the CASS workers themselves saw the CASS workers more as friends and equals than as doctors or authorities and as providing encouragement rather than checking up on people (Sykes et al., 1993; Sylvia et al., 1993).

Evaluation of the NAC indicated the CASS workers contributed to the benefits of the program. Contacts with CASS workers and attendance at educational programs were each statistically significant predictors of reductions in emergency care, after control for child's age and parent's education (Fisher, 1997a). Consequently, a separate study has focused on the impact of such a peer worker, now called the "Asthma Coach". This project examines the contribution of the peer coach to the promotion of coordinated preventive care and provision of individual support for the parents of ninety-three low-income African-American children (ages 2–8), all of whom were enrolled in Medicaid and had been hospitalized at St. Louis Children's Hospital for asthma.

Within several days of their child's discharge, parents are recruited to participate in surveys to evaluate the coach program. As with the NAC, enrollment entails no commitment to participate with a coach if randomized to receive one. Thus, the ability of the coach to engage the parent is a fairly unbiased estimate of this approach to reaching a group that often has been difficult to engage in educational programs.

After randomization the coach attempts to contact the parent and arrange an extended phone interview or home visit, following an idealized outline of home visits, phone contacts, and curriculum guides, but using flexibility in their implementation. One dimension of flexibility is the readiness of the parent to participate. When first contacted, many parents decline, indicating that, after hospitalization, their child is fine and does not need any more help. The coach's response is crucial. Rather than categorizing the parent as refusing treatment and closing the case or, perhaps, making several more calls within one to two weeks to try to persuade the parent to "enter treatment," the coach maintains a friendly, nondemanding tone and tells the parent that she will call back in a month or so to see how things are going. Amid the variability in sources and availability of care for low-income groups, the simple reliability of the coaches in following up a month later may be an especially critical step in establishing productive rapport with parents. The coach continues with nondemanding regular contacts. After several contacts, most parents express interest in becoming involved. The coach then proceeds with a sequence of home visits (and/or contacts in neighborhood settings such as a library or restaurant) and phone contacts. Seven key behaviors are addressed: (1) using the Asthma Action Plan that had been given to the parent as the child left the hospital, (2) using regular medicine, (3) giving rescue medicines as prescribed on the Asthma Action Plan, (4) attending regular follow-up care every four months, (5) establishing a partnership with the primary care physician, (6) keeping the child away from second-hand smoke, and (7) avoiding contact with cockroach allergen. After completing the curriculum parents are weaned to monthly phone contacts, but the curriculum is restarted in the event of the child's rehospitalization. Each case is given two years' access to a coach. The rationale for this approach rests on proactive approaches to health promotion that are tailored to fit the individual's readiness to change (Prochaska et al., 1997) and on research on nondirective social support that shows advantages, outside of acute or emergent situations, of support that cooperates with and accepts current feelings and choices rather than directing or seeking to control the recipient (Fisher, 1997a; Fisher et al., 1997b).

The coaches have been successful in reaching the audience of low-income, Medicaid-enrolled parents who, as noted, often are hard to engage in health promotion activities. In a preliminary audit before completion of the study, coaches were able to establish working relationships, defined as at least one substantive phone or face-to-face contact, with 27.2% of parents within the initial seven days. This figure rose to 44.5% in thirty days, 70.6 % in sixty days, and 85.8 % in ninety days. These contacts were also maintained. In the ninety days preceding the audit coaches had at least one substantive contact with 80.4% of the parents assigned. Thus, Asthma Coaches are able to reach and engage this important group. Although the study is incomplete, the coaches' notes indicate appreciable progress in the seven key behaviors, ranging from 45% making progress with using regular asthma medicines to 77% making progress with exposure to cockroach allergen (Tarr et al., 2000).

But What Does It Have to Do with Asthma?

Reflecting this chapter's emphasis on the complex and diverse relationships among community-level factors and the pathways of their impacts, both the NAC and the Asthma Coach programs have addressed topics that might seem to have little pertinence to asthma management. Reflecting research on exposure to violence and asthma, community events by the NAC included a safe Halloween party and promotion focused on enjoying the holiday but minimizing the risks of trick-or-treating. It also included programs for teens on conflict resolution and avoidance of violence. Reflecting the diverse stressors that may undermine asthma management, the Asthma Coaches have worked with parents not only on key asthma management practices but also on a number of stressors in their lives, including problems with landlords or welfare benefits, domestic disputes and violence, and seeking employment.

SUMMARY

Populations in communities that experience environmental inequities may also be characterized by high levels of poverty, low social capital, lack of opportunity and employment, high violence and crime rates, lack of perceived control, and hopelessness. It is unlikely that the health problems of these disadvantaged populations can be solved without understanding the potential role of such social determinants of health. For example, improvements in living conditions and life opportunities may be more effective as interventions aimed at encouraging disadvantaged populations to attend to health education and make behavioral changes (McKinlay, 1975).

Community-based participatory research, which focuses on physical as well as social environmental inequities through active involvement of community members, organizational representatives, civic institutions, neighborhood health centers, and researchers at all stages of both research and intervention processes, offers an invaluable tool for community empowerment. It may have long-lasting effects on building social capital, influencing policy, and thus affecting public health (Herbert, 1996; Israel et al., 1998). Such research may also point to unique interventions to decrease the morbidity associated with chronic illnesses such as asthma.

REFERENCES

Abrams D, Elder J, Lasater T, Artz L (1986). Social learning principles for organizational health promotion: An integrated approach. *Health and Industry: A Behavioral Medicine Perspective.* M. D. C. T. J. Coates. New York, Wiley.

Acierno R, Kilpatrick D, Rsesnick H, Saund C (1996). Violent assault, posttraumatic stress disorder, and depression: Risk factors for cigarette use among adult women. *Behav Modif* 20: 363–384.

Addington W and Weiss K. (1999). Targeting asthma in Chicago: Community stories. *Chest* 116: 198S.

Adler N, Boyce T, Chesney M, Chen C, Folkman S, Kahn R, Syme S (1994). Socioeconomic status and health: The challenge of the gradient. *Am Psychol* 49: 15–24.

U.S. Environmental Protection Agency (1998). National air quality and emissions trends report, 1996. EPA-454/R-97-013. Research Triangle Park, N.C.: U.S. EPA.

Anda R, Williamson D, Escobedo L, Mast E, Giovino G, Remington P (1990). Depression and the dynamics of smoking: A national perspective. *JAMA* 264: 1541–1545.

Anderson H, Baily P, Cooper J, Palmer J, West S (1983). Morbidity and school absence caused by asthma and wheezing illness. *Arch Dis Child* 37: 180–186.

Anderson RM, Funnell MM, Arnold MS, Barr PA, Edwards GJ, Fitzgerald JT

(2000). Assessing the cultural relevance of an education program for urban African Americans with diabetes. *Diabetes Educator* 26(2): 280–289.

Apter A, Reisine S, Affleck G, Barrows E, ZuWallack R (1998). Adherence with twice-daily dosing of inhaled steroids. Socioeconomic and health-belief differences. *Am J Respir Crit Care Med* 157: 1810–1817.

Attar B, Guerra N, Tolan P (1994). Neighborhood disadvantage, stressful life events and adjustment in urban elementary-school children. *J Clin Child Psychol* 23: 391–440.

Bandura B (1977). Self-efficacy: Towards a unifying theory of behavioral change. *Psychol Bull* 84: 191–215.

Beckham J, Roodman A, Shipley R, Hetzberg M, Cunha G, Kudler H, et al. (1995). Smoking in Vietnam combat veterans with posttraumatic stress disorder. *J Trauma Stress* 8: 461–472.

Bertolis P, Strunk R, Arfken C, Goodman G, Knutson A, Bloomberg G (1994). A nine year study of hopsitalizations for asthma in children in St. Louis. *J Allergy Clin Immunol* 93(1): 293.

Birkel R and Repucci N (1983). Social networks, information-seeking, and utilization of services. *Am J Community Psychol* 11: 183–203.

Birkhead G, Attaway N, Strunk R, Townsend M, Teutsch S (1989). Investigation of a cluster of deaths of adolescents from asthma: Evidence implicating inadequate treatment and poor patient adherence with medications. *J Allergy Clin Immunol* 84(4): 484–491.

Blendon R, Aiken L, Freeman H, et al. (1989). Access to medical care for black and white Americans: A matter of continuing concern. *JAMA* 261: 278–281.

Boney-McCoy S and Finkelhor D (1995). Psychosocial sequelae of violent victimization in a national youth sample. *J Consult Clin Psychol* 63: 726–736.

Bor W, Najman J, Anderson M, Morrison J, Williams G (1993). Socioeconomic disadvantage and child morbidity: An Australian longitudinal study. *Soc Sci Med* 9: 27–30.

Bracht N, ed. (1990). *Health Promotion at the Community Level.* Newbury Park, Calif: Sage.

Braithwaite R and Lythcott N (1989). Community empowerment as a strategy for health promotion for black and other minority populations. *JAMA* 261(2): 282–283.

Brunner E (1997). Socioeconomic determinants of health: Stress and biology of inequality. *BMJ* 314: 1472–1476.

Breslau N, Davis G, Andreski P, Petersen E (1991). Traumatic events and posttraumatic stress disorder in an urban population of young adults. *Arch Gen Psychiatry* 48: 216–222.

Busse W, Kiecolt-Glaser J, Coe C, Martin R, Weiss S, Parker S (1994). Stress and asthma: NHLBI Workshop Summary. *Am J Respir Crit Care Med* 151: 249–252.

Camargo CG, Field A, Colditz G, Speizer F (1999). Body mass index and asthma in children age 9–14. *Am J Respir Crit Care Med* 159: A150.

Carr W, Zeitel L, Weiss K (1992). Variations in asthma hospitalizations and deaths in New York City. *Am J Public Health* 82: 59–65.

Castro F, Maddahian E, Newcomb M, Bentler P (1987). A multivariate model of the determinants of cigarette smoking among adolescents. *J Health Soc Behav* 28: 273–289.

Chen E, Matthew K, Boyce TW (2002). Socioeconomic differences in children's health: how and why do these relationships change with age. *Psychol Bull* 128(2): 295–329.

Cockroft D, O'Brrne P, Swystun V, Bhagat R (1995). Regular use of inhaled albuterol and the allergen-induced late asthmatic response. *J Allergy Clin Immunol* 96: 44–49.

Cohen S and Lichtenstein E (1990a). Partner behaviors that support quitting smoking. *J Consult Clin Psychol* 58: 304–309.

Cohen S and Lichtenstein E (1990b). Perceived stress, quitting smoking, and smoking relapse. *Health Psychol* 9: 466–478.

Crain E, Kercsmar C, Weiss K, Mitchell H, Lynn H (1998). Reported difficulties in access to quality care for children with asthma in the inner city. *Arch Pediatr Adolesc Med* 152: 333–339.

Crain E, Weiss K, Bijur P, Hersh M, Westbrook L, Stein R (1994). An estimate of the prevalence of asthma and wheezing among inner-city children. *Pediatrics* 94: 356–362.

Cunningham J, Dockery D, Speizer F (1996). Race, asthma and persistent wheeze in Philadelphia schoolchildren. *Am J Public Health* 86: 1406–1409.

Curry S, Wagner E, et al. (1993). Assessment of community-level influences on individual's attitudes about cigarette smoking, alcohol use, and consumption of dietary fat. *Am J Prev Med* 9: 78–84.

De Oliveria M, Faresin S, Bruno V, de Bittencourt A, Fernades A (1999). Evaluation of an educational programme for socially deprived asthma patients. *Eur Respir J* 14: 908–914.

Dekker C, Dales R, Bartlett S, et al. (1991). Childhood asthma and the indoor environment. *Chest* 100: 922–926.

Diaz T, Sturm T, Matte T, Bindra M, Lawler K, Findley S, Maylahn C (2000). Medication use among children with asthma in East Harlem. *Pediatrics* 105: 1188–1193.

Diez-Roux A, Nieto J, Muntaner C, Tyroler H, Comstock G, Shahar E, Cooper L, Watson R, Szklo M (1997). Neighborhood environments and coronary heart disease: A multilevel analyses. *Am J Epidemiol* 146: 48–63.

Dohrenwend B and Dohrenwend B (1969). *Social Status and Psychological Disorder*. New York: Wiley.

Donahue J, Weiss S, Livingston J, Goetsch M, Greineder D, Platt R (1997). Inhaled steroids and the risk of hospitalization for asthma. *JAMA* 277: 887–891.

Dressler W (1985). Extended family relationships, social support and mental health in a southern black community. *J Health Soc Behav* 26: 39–48.

Dressler W (1991). *Stress and Adaptation in the Context of Culture: Depression in a Southern Black Community*. Albany, NY: State University of New York Press.

DuRant R, Getts A, Cadenhead C, Emans S, Woods E (1995). Exposure to violence and victimization and depression, hopelessness, and purpose in life among adolescents living in and around public housing. *Develop Behav Pediatr* 16: 233–237.

Ernest P, Demissie K, Joseph L, Locher U, Becklake M (1995). Socioeconomic status and indicators of asthma in children. *Am J Respir Crit Care Med* 152: 570–575.

Evans G (2001). Environmental stress and health. In Baum A, Revenson T, Singer J, eds.: *Handbook of Health Psychology*. Mahwah, NJ: Lawrence Erlbaum Associates, pp. 365–385.

Feigelman W and Gorman B (1989). Toward explaining the higher incidence of cigarette smoking among black Americans. *J Psychoactive Drugs* 21: 299–305.

Fingerhut L and Warner M (1997). Injury chartbook. In: *Health, United States, 1996–1997*. Hyattsville, Md: National Center for Health Statistics.

Fisher E, Auslander W, Sussman L, Owens N, Jackson-Thompson J (1992). Community orgainzation and health promotion in minority neighborhoods. *Ethn Dis* 2(Summer): 252–272.

Fisher E, Brownson R, Luke D, Summer W, Heath A (in press). Cigarette Smoking. In Raczynshi J, Bradley L, Leviton L, eds.: *Health Behavior Handbook*. Washington, DC: American Psychological Association.

Fisher E, Sussman L, Shannon W, Arfken C, Sykes R, Strunk R (1997a). *Neighborhood Asthma Coalition Impacts among Low Income, African American Children*. San Francisco: The American Thoracic Society.

Fisher EJ (1997). Two approaches to social support in smoking cessation: Commodity Model and Nondirective Support. *Addict Behav* 22(6): 819–833.

Fisher EJ, La Greca A, Greco P, Arfken C, Schneiderman N (1997b). Directive and nondirective support in diabetes management. *Int J Behav Med* 4(2): 131–144.

Fisher EJ, Strunk R, Sussman L, Arfken C, Sykes R, Munro J, Haywood S, Harrison D, Bascom S (1996). Acceptability and feasibility of a community approach to asthma management: The Neighborhood Asthma Coalition (NAC). *J Asthma* 33(6): 367–383.

Fisher EJ, Sussman L, Arfken C, Harrison D, Munro J, Sykes R, Sylvia S, Strunk R (1994). Targeting high risk groups: Neighborhood orgazination for pediatric asthma management in the Neighborhood Asthma Coalition. *Chest* 106(4): 248S–259S.

Fisher EJ, Sylvia S, Sussman L, et al. (1993). Social isolation of caretakers of African American children with asthma is associated with poor asthma management. *Am Rev Resp Dis* 147: A982.

Fleming A, Sterling-Scott R, Carabello G, Imari-Williams I, Allmond B, Foster R, Kennedy F, Shoemaker W (1992). Injury and violence in Los Angeles: Impact on access to health care and surgical education. *Arch Surg* 127: 671–676.

Fong R (1995). Violence as a barrier to compliance for the hypertensive African-American. *J Natl Med Assoc* 87: 203–207.

Ford J, Findley S, Mc Lean D, Nachman S, Trowers R (1998). Fatal asthma in perspective: relation between individual and community risk factors. In Sheffer A, ed.: *Fatal Asthma*. New York: Marcel Dekker, pp. 45–51.

Ford J, McLean D, Richardson L, Findley S, Copeland L, Felton C (1996). Identifying barriers to asthma management in Harlem. *Am Rev Respir Crit Care Med* 153: A419.

Gortmaker S, Must A, Sobol A, Peterson K, Colditz G, Dietz W (1996). Television viewing as a cause of increasing obesity among children in the United States, 1986–1990. *Arch Pediatr Adolesc Med* 150: 356–362.

Gottlieb G, Beiser A, O'Connor G (1995). Poverty, race and medication use are correlates of asthma hospitalization rates: A small area analysis in Boston. *Chest* 108: 28–35.

Guendelman S and Schwalbe J (1986). Medical care utilization by Hispanic children: How does it differ from black and white peers? *Med Care* 24: 925–940.

Haan M, Kaplan G, Camacho T (1987). Poverty and health: Prospective evidence from the Alameda County Study. *Am J Epidemiol* 125: 989–998.

Haan M, Kaplan N, Syme S (1989). Socioeconomic status and health: Old observations and new thoughts. In Bunker J, Gomby D, Kehrer B, eds.: *Pathways in Health*. Menlo Park, Calif: Henry J. Kaiser Family Foundation, pp. 76–135.

Haire-Joshu D, Fisher EJ, Munro J, Wedner H (1993). A comparison of patient attitudes toward asthma self-management among acute and preventive care settings. *J Asthma* 30(5): 359–371.

Heinrich J, Richter K, Magnussen H, Wichmann H (1998). Is the prevalence of atopic diseased in East and West Germany already converging? *Eur J Epidemiol* 14: 239–245.

Herbert C (1996). Community-based research as a tool for empowerment: The Haida Gwaii Diabetes Project example. *Can J Public Health* 87: 109–112.

Herman A (1988). Political violence, health, and health services in South Africa. *Am J Public Health* 8: 767–768.

Heurtin-Roberts S and Reisin E (1992). The relation of culturally influenced lay models of hypertension to compliance with treatment. *Am J Hypertens* 5(11): 787–792.

Hirsch T (1999). Indoor allergen exposure in West and East Germany: A cause for different prevalences of asthma and atopy? *Rev Environ Health* 14: 159–168.

Holden G (1991). The relationship of self-efficacy appraisals to subsequent health related outcomes: A meta-analysis. *Soc Work Health Care I* 16: 53–93.

House J, Landis K, Umberson D (1988). Social relationships and health. *Science* 241: 540–544.

Huang J and Johnson J (1998). Does small area income inequality influence the hospitalization of children? A disease-specific analysis. New York Academy of Sciences, Bethesda, MD.

Isaacs M (1992). *Violence: The Impact of Community Violence on African American Children and Families.* Arlington, Va: National Center for Education in Maternal and Child Health.

Israel B, Schulz A, Parker E, Becker A (1998). Review of community-based research: Assessing partnership approaches to improve public health. *Annu Rev Public Health* 19: 173–202.

Jatulis D, Meng Y, Eashoff R, et al. (1998). Preventive pharmacologic therapy among asthmatics: Five years after publication of guidelines. *Ann Allergy Asthma Immunol* 81: 82–88.

Jones C, Qureshi S, Rona R, Chinn S (1996). Exercise-induced bronchoconstriction by ethnicity and presence of asthma in British nine year olds. *Thorax* 51: 1134–1136.

Kaplan B and Mascie-Taylor C (1985). Biosocial factors in the epidemiology of childhood asthma in a British national sample. *J Epidemiol Community Health* 39: 152–156.

Kaplan B and Mascie-Taylor C (1988). Asthma and wheezy bronchitis in adolescents: Biosocial correlates. *J. Asthma* 25: 125–129.

Karvaonen S and Rimpela A (1996). Socio-regional context as a determinant of adolescents' health in Finland. *Soc Sci Med* 43: 1467–1474.

Kaufman J and Kaufman S (2001). Assessment of structured socioeconomic effects on health. *Epidemiology* 12: 157–167.

Kawachi I, Kennedy B, Wilkinson R (1999). Crime: Social disorganization and relative deprivation. *Soc Sci Med* 48: 719–731.

Kawachi I and Kennedy BP (1999). Income inequality and health: Pathways and mechanisms. *Health Serv Res* 34(1 pt 2): 215–227.

Kazdin A (1974). Covert modelling, model similarity, and reduction of avoidance behavior. *Behav Res Ther* 5: 325–340.

Kennedy B, Kawachi I, Prothrow-Smith D (1996). Income distribution and mortality: Test of the Robin Hoos Index in the United States. *BMJ* 312: 1004–1007.

Kennedy B, Kawachi I, Prothrow-Smith D, Lochner K, Gupta V (1998). Social capital, income inequality, and firearm violent crime. *Soc Sci Med* 47: 7–17.

Kirkman-Liff B and Modragon D (1991). Language of interview: Relevance for research of Southwest Hispanics. *Am J Public Health* 81: 1399–1404.

Kleinschmidt I, Hills M, Elliott P (1997). Smoking behavior can be predicated by neighborhood deprivation measures. *J Epidemiol Community Health* 87: 1113–1118.

Krause N (1992). Stress and isolation form close ties in later life. *J Gerontol* 46: S183–S194.

Kumanyika SK (1998). Obesity in African Americans: Biobehavioral consequences of culture. *Ethn Dis* 8(1): 93–6.

La Veist T (1993). Segregation, poverty, and empowerment: Health consequence for African Americans. *Milbank Q* 71: 41–64.

Lang D and Polansky M (1994). Patterns of asthma mortality in Philadelphia from 1969 to 1991. *N Engl J Med* 331: 1542–1546.

Ledogar RJ, Penchaszadeh A, Garden CC, Iglesias G (2000). Asthma and Latino cultures: Different prevalence reported among groups sharing the same environment. *Am J Public Health* 90(6): 929–935.

Lewis S, Richards D, Bynner J, Butler N, Britton J (1995). Prospective study of risk factors for early and persistent wheezing in childhood. *Eur Respir J* 8: 349–356.

Littlejohns P and Macdonald L (1993). The relationship between severe asthma and social class. *Respir Med* 87: 139–143.

Lochner K, Kawachi I, Kennedy B (1999). Social capital: A guide to its measurement. *Health Place* 5: 259–270.

Marder D, Targonsky P, Orris P, Persky V, Addington W (1992). Effect of racial and socioeconomic factors. *Chest* 101(suppl): 79S–83S.

Martinez F, Cline M, Burrows B (1992). Increased incidence of asthma in children of smoking mothers. *Pediatrics* 89: 21–26.

Martinez P and Richters J (1993). The NIMH Community Violence Project II. Children's distress symptoms associated with violence exposure. *Psychiatry* 56: 22–35.

Matsumoto D, Arfken C, Fisher EJ, Jaffe D, Strunk R (1994). Lack of association between greater number of regular follow-up visits for asthma and decreased emergency department (ED) visits for acute asthma in low income African American children. Paper presented at the 1994 American Academy of Allergy and Immunology meeting, Anaheim, CA.

McElmurry B, Buseh A, Dublin M (1999). Health education program to control asthma in multiethnic, low-income urban communities: The Chicago Health Corps Asthma Program. *Chest* 116: 198S–199S.

McKinlay J (1975). The help-seeking behavior of the poor. In Kosa J, Antonovsky A, Zola I, eds.: *Poverty and Health: A Sociological Analysis.* Cambridge, Mass: Harvard University Press, pp. 224–273.

McLean D, Hatfield-Timajchy K, Wingo P, Floyd R (1993). Psychosocial measurement: implications for the study of preterm delivery in black women. *Psychosocial Measurement* 9(Suppl 6): 39–81.

Meichenbaum D (1971). Examination of model characteristics in avoidance behavior. *J Per Soc Psychol* 17: 298–307.

Mielck A, Reitmeir P, Wjst M (1996). Severity of childhood asthma by socioeconomic status. *Int J Epidemiol* 25: 388–393.

Miller J (2000). The effects of race/ethnicity and income on early childhood asthma prevalence and health care use. *Am J Public Health* 86: 1406–1409.

Minkler M (1990). People need people: Social support and health. In Swencionis REO, ed.: *The Healing Brain: A Scientific Reader*. New York: Guilford Press, pp. 88–99.

Mitchell E (1991). Racial inequalities in childhood asthma. *Soc Sci Med* 32: 831–836.

Mitchell E, Stewart A, Pattermore P, Asher M, Harrison A, Rea H. (1989). Socioeconomic status in childhood asthma. *Int J Epidemiol* 18: 888–890.

Mitchell R, Barbarin O, Hurley D (1981). Problem solving, resource utilization, and community involvement in a black and white community. *Am J Community Psychol* 9: 233–246.

Mitchell R and Dawson B (1973). Educational and social characteristics of children with asthma. *Arch Dis Child* 48: 467–471.

Moudgil H and Honeybourne D (1998). Differences in asthma management between white European and Indian Subcontinent ethnic groups living in socioeconomically deprived areas in the Birmingham (UK) consultation. *Thorax* 53: 490–494.

Moudgil H, Marshall T, Honeybourne D (2000). Asthma education and qualtiy of life in the community: A randomised controlled study to evaluate the impact on white European and Indian subcontinent ethnic groups from socioeconomically deprived areas in Birmingham, UK. *Thorax* 55: 177–183.

Nelson D, Johnson C, Divine G, Strauchman C, Joseph C, Ownby D (1997). Ethnic differences in the prevalence of asthma in middle class children. *Ann Allergy Asthma Immunol* 78: 21–26.

National Institutes of Health (1991). Expert Panel Report I: Guidelines for the Diagnosis and management of Asthma. Washington, DC: National Institutes of Health, National Heart, Lung and Blood Institute.

National Institutes of Health (1997). Expert Panel Report II: Guidelines for the Diagnosis and Management of Asthma. Washington, DC: National Institutes of Health, National Heart Lung and Blood Institute.

Pachter LM and Weller SC (1993). Acculturation and compliance with medical therapy. *J Dev Behav Pediatr* 14(3): 163–168.

Partridge M (2000). In what way may race, ethnicity or culture influence asthma outcomes? *Thorax* 55: 175–176.

Pearce N, Beasley R, Burgess C, Crane J (1998). *Asthma Epidemiology: Principles and Methods*. New York: Oxford University Press.

Perrin J, Homer C, Berwick D, Woolf A, Freeman J, Wennberg J (1989). Variations in rates of hospitalization of children in three urban communities. *N Engl J Med* 320: 1183–1187.

Petermen C (1982). Learned helplessness and health psychology. *Health Psychol* 1: 153–168.

Pickett K and Pearl M (2001). Multi-level analyses of neighborhood socioeconomic context and health outcomes: A critical review. *J Epidemiol Community Health* 55: 111–122.

Pierson WE and Koenig JQ (1992). Respiratory effects of air pollution on allergic disease. *J Allergy Clin Immunol* 90(4 pt 1): 557–566.

Platts-Mills T, Ward GJ, Sporik R, et al. (1991). Epidemiology of the relationship between exposure to indoor allergens and asthma. *Int Arch Allergy Appl Immunol* 94: 339–345.

Prochaska JO, Redding CA, Evers KE (1997). The transtheoretical model and stages of change. In: K Glanz, FM Lewis and BK Rimer, eds. *Health Behavior and Health Education*, 2nd ed. San Francisco, CA: Jossey-Bass Inc., pp. 60–84.

Rabkin J and Struening E (1976). Life events, stress and illness. *Science* 194: 1013–1020.

Rao M, Kravath R, Abadco D, Arden J, Steiner P (1991). Childhood asthma mortality: The Brooklyn experience and a brief review. *J Assoc Acad Minor Phys.* 2(3): 127–130.

Reijneveld S (1998). The impact of individual and area characteristics on urban socioeconomic differences in health and smoking. *Int J Epidemiol* 27: 33–40.

Richards W (1989). Hospitalization of children with status asthmaticus: A review. *Pediatrics* 84: 11–118.

Roberts E (1997). Neighborhood social environments and the distribution of low birth weight in Chicago. *Am J Public Health* 87: 597–603.

Roberts S (1998). Community-level socioeconomic status effects on adult health. *J Health Soc Behav* 39: 18–37.

Robicsek R, Ribbeck B, Walker L (1993). The cost of violence: The economy of health care delivery for non-accidental trauma in an urban southeastern community. *NC Med J* 54: 578–582.

Rogers E and Kincaid D (1981). *Communication Networks: Toward a New Paradigm for Research.* New York: Free Press.

Romano R, Bloom J, Syme S (1991). Smoking, social support, and hassles in an urban African-American community. *Am J Public Health* 81: 1415–1422.

Rothman J (1968). Three models of community organization practice. In *Social Work Practice.* New York: Columbia University Press.

Salmond C, Crampton P, Hales S, Lewis S, Pearce N (1999). Asthma prevalence and deprivation: A small area analysis. *J Epidemiol Community Health* 53: 476–480.

Sampson R (1992). Family management and child development: Insight from social disorganization theory. In: WS Laufer, F Adler, and J McCord, eds. *Facts, Frameworks, and Forecasts: Advances in Criminological Theory.* pp. 63–93.

Sampson R, Raudenbush S, Earls F (1997). Neighborhoods and violent crime: A multilevel study of collective efficacy. *Science* 277: 918–924.

Schenker M, Samet J, Speizer F (1983). Risk factors for childhood respiratoy disease. *Am Rev Respir Dis* 128: 1038–1043.

Schwam J (1987). Assisting the parent of a child with asthma. *J Asthma* 24(1): 45–54.

Shagena M, Sandler H, Perrin E (1988). Concepts of illness and perception of control in healthy children and in children with chronic illnesses. *J Dev Behav Pediatr* 9: 252–256.

SIDRIA (Italian Studies on Respiratory Disorders in Childhood and the Environment) Collaborative Group (1997). Asthma and respiratory symptoms in 6–7 year old Italian children: gender, latitude, urban location, and socioeconomic factors. *Eur Resp J* 10: 1780–1786.

Sly R and O'Donnell R (1992). Association of asthma mortality with medical specialist density. *Ann Allergy* 68: 340–344.

Stein M, Wallston K, Nicassio P, Castner N (1988). Correlates of a clinical classification schema for the Arthritis Helplessness Index. *Arthritis Rheum* 31: 876–881.

Stenius-Aarniala B, Pousse T, Kvarnstrom J, Gronlund E, Ylikahri M, Mustajoki P (2000). Immediate and long term effects of weight reduction in obese people with asthma: Randomised controlled study. *BMJ* 320: 827–832.

Strunk R (1987). Asthma deaths in childhood: Identification of patients at risk and intervention. *J Allergy Clin Immunol* 80(3): 472–477.

Strunk R (1993). Dealth due to asthma: New insights into sudden unexpected deaths, but the focus remains on prevention (editorial) *Am Rev Respir Dis* 148: 550–552.

Strunk R, Mrazek D, Fuhrmann G, LaBrecque J (1985). Physiologic and psychological characteristics associated with deaths due to asthma in childhood: A case-controlled study. *JAMA* 254: 1193–1198.

Sussman L (1992). Hard-to-reach and resistant populations: Misguided concepts in health-related interventions and research. Paper presented at the 1992 annual meeting of the American Anthropological Association, San Francisco.

Sykes R, Arfken C, Sylvia S, Munro J, Sussman L, Bascom D, Harrison D, Owens N, Strunk R, Fisher E (1993). Neighborhood peer workers: Perceptions, problems, and promises. Paper presented at the 1993 Eighth National Conference on Chronic Disease Prevention and Control., Kansas City.

Sylvia S, Sykes R, Owens N, Munro J, Sussman L, Strunk R, Fisher EJ (1993). Role characteristics of neighborhood residents trained to support asthma management. Paper presented at the 1993 Society of Behavioral Medicine meeting, San Francisco.

Tarr K, Highstein G, Sykes R, Musick J, Strunk R, Fisher E (2000). Asthma coaches reach underserved Medicaid enrollees through nondirective support and practice strategies. Paper presented at 2000 meeting of the Society of Behavioral Medicine, Nashville, TN.

Taylor S, Repetti R, Seeman T (1997). Health Psychology: What is an unhealthy environment and how does it get under the skin? *Annu Rev Psychol* 48: 411–447.

Wagener D, Williams D, Wilson P (1993). Equity and environmental health: Data collection and interpretation issues. *Toxicol Ind Health* 9: 775–795.

Watson J, Cowen P, Lewis R (1996). The relationship between asthma admission rates, routes of admission, and socioeconomic deprivation. *Eur Respir J* 9: 2083–2087.

Weiss K, Gergen P, Crain E (1992). Inner-city asthma: The epidemiology of an emerging U.S. public health concern. *Chest* 101: 362S–367S.

Weiss K, Gergen P, Wagener D (1993). Breathing better or wheezing worse? The changing epidemiology of asthma morbidity and mortality. *Annu Rev Public Health* 14: 491–513.

Weiss S, Tager I, Speizer F, et al. (1980). Persistent wheeze: Its relation to respiratory illness, cigarette smoking and level of pulmonary functioning in a population sample of children. *Am Rev Respir Dis* 122: 687–703.

Weitzman M, Gortmaker S, Sobol A (1990). Racial, social, and environmental risks of childhood asthma. *Am J Dis Child* 144: 1189–1194.

Wilkinson RG (1996). *Unhealthy Societies. The Afflictions of Inequality.* London: Routledge.

Williams DR (1990). Socioeconomic differentials in health: A review and redirection. *Cos Psychol Q* 53: 81–99.

Williams DR (1998). African-American health: The role of the social environment. *J Urban Health* 75: 300–321.

Williams M, Baker D, Honig E, Lee T, Nowlan A (1998). Inadequate literacy is a barrier to asthma knowledge and self care. *Chest* 114: 1008–1015.

Wilson WJ (1987). *The Truly Disadvantaged: The Inner-City, the Underclass, and Public Policy.* Chicago: University of Chicago Press.

Wise P and Eisenberg L (1989). What do regional variations in the rates of hospitalization of children really mean? (editorial) *N Engl J Med* 320: 1209–1211.

Wright R, Hanrahan J, Tager I, Speizer F (1997). Effect of the exposure to violence on the occurrence and severity of childhood asthma in an inner-city population. *Am J Respir Crit Care Med* 155: A972.

Wright R, Rodriguez M, Cohen S (1998a). Review of psychosocial stress and asthma: An integrated biopsychosocial approach. *Thorax* 53: 1066–1074.

Wright R, Speizer F, Tager I, Hanrahan J (1998b). Children's distress and violence exposure: Relation to respiratory symptoms, asthma and behavior. *Am J Respir Crit Care Med* 157: A41.

Wright R and Steinbach S (2001). Violence: An unrecognized environmental exposure that may contribute to greater asthma morbidity in high risk inner-city populations. *Environmental Health Perspectives* 109:1085–1089.

Wright R and Weiss S (2000). Epidemiology of allergic disease. In Holgate S, Church M, Lichtenstein L, eds.: *Allergy,* 2nd ed. London: Harcourt.

Yach D (1988). The impact of political violence on health and health services in Capetown, South Africa, 1986: Methodological problems and preliminary results. *Am J Public Health* 78: 772–776.

Zapata B, Rebolledo A, Atalah E, King M (1992). The influence of social and political violence on the risk of pregnancy complications. *Am J Public Health* 82: 685–690.

III

THE CONTOURS OF NEIGHBORHOOD EFFECTS ON HEALTH

12
Residential Segregation and Health

Dolores Acevedo-Garcia
Kimberly A. Lochner

The evidence showing that neighborhood characteristics influence health continues to grow. However, neighborhoods exist in a larger context, and research on their role in health needs to relate neighborhood characteristics to city-wide processes. Residential segregation is a key variable in explaining the socioeconomic organization of metropolitan areas. Residential segregation "sorts" population groups into various neighborhood contexts and shapes the living environment at the neighborhood level. Integrating research on neighborhoods and health with that on segregation and health may help elucidate mechanisms at the level of the larger sociogeographic context as well as the neighborhood, which in turn may have implications for social and public health policy.

RACIAL RESIDENTIAL SEGREGATION

General Definition

Segregation refers to the differentiation of two or more population groups among subunits of a given social space. Population groups can be divided along racial/ethnic, social class, sex, or age lines. The social space can be a geographic social space such as a metropolitan area or a school district or an economic social space such as a labor market. Because this book is concerned with the relationship of neighborhood living conditions to health outcomes, we focus on residential segregation. We acknowledge, however, that other forms of segregation, such as racial segregation in hospital care (Smith, 1998), may also influence health.

Patterns of residential segregation are well documented in other developed and developing countries, such as South Africa (Christopher,

1994), Great Britain (Daley, 1998; Phillips, 1998) and Singapore (van Grunsven, 1992), but the relationship of residential segregation by race/ethnicity to health outcomes has been examined only in the United States and South Africa. Our focus is on the U.S. studies because the South African literature has examined residential segregation in combination with other facets of the apartheid system (Nightingale et al., 1990; Turton and Chalmers, 1990; Lubanga, 1993; Yach and Tollman, 1993; Heggenhougen, 1995; Kaufman, 1998; Sarkin, 1999).

Race/Ethnicity or Class

In the United States substantial evidence exists that race/ethnicity is the stronger force composed to social class driving residential segregation. Racial and ethnic segregation sorts individuals of comparable socioeconomic status into vastly different neighborhood environments. In 1990, for example, the probability that a poor person would live in a high-poverty neighborhood (i.e., a neighborhood where the poverty rate was at least 40%) was only 6.3% for whites but 22.1% for Hispanics and 33.5% for African Americans (Jargowsky, 1997). Although levels of racial segregation remain much higher than are levels of economic segregation,[1] segregation by class has been increasing, especially for African Americans and Hispanics (Jargowsky, 1996; Darden and Bagaka, 1997).

Additionally, in the United States racial residential segregation varies by demographic group. African Americans are considerably more segregated from the white population than are other racial/ethnic minorities (Massey and Denton, 1993). Prejudice and overall discrimination in housing and mortgage markets have shaped African-American segregation (Yinger, 1995). Hispanic and Asian segregation is considerably less pronounced than is black segregation (Massey and Denton, 1989), even though recent immigrants often settle in "ethnic enclaves" to ease their adjustment to U.S. society (Fernandez Kelly and Schauffler, 1996).

Discrimination versus Preferences

Segregation may originate from discrimination such as racial/ethnic prejudice. However, segregation may also result from choices or preferences, that is, members of various population groups may choose to live separate from other groups. Whether U.S. racial/ethnic residential segregation is driven by discrimination in either public or private housing markets or by choice has been the subject of considerable debate (Galster, 1988, 1989, 1996; Clark, 1989, 1991). However, because of the evidence of persistent racial discrimination in housing and mortgage markets (Yinger,

1995), most U.S. studies on segregation and health have hypothesized that residential segregation is a result of institutional racism (Collins and Williams, 1999; LaVeist, 1989, 1993; Polednak, 1991, 1993, 1996; Williams, 1997, 1998).

Dimensions of Residential Segregation

Segregation refers to the composition and spatial distribution of the population of a metropolitan area among neighborhoods. Residential segregation is a multidimensional construct consisting of five distinct geographic patterns: unevenness, isolation, clustering, centralization, and concentration (Massey and Denton, 1988; Massey et al., 1996). Because residential segregation refers to the separation of groups, usually blacks from whites, we refer to the dimensions in terms of black–white segregation. However, the dimensions apply equally to other race/ethnic groups as well as economic segregation, that is, poor from nonpoor. We briefly describe each of the five dimensions below. Fuller descriptions of each dimension, suggested indexes for measurement, and formulas are presented in the Appendix.

Unevenness refers to the distribution of blacks and whites across neighborhoods in an urban area, specifically the degree to which each neighborhood has the same proportion of blacks to whites as does the urban area overall. Isolation refers to the average probability of contact at the neighborhood level between blacks and whites. Clustering refers to ghettoization, that is, the degree to which black neighborhoods are contiguous to one another as opposed to dispersed across the metropolitan area. Centralization refers to the degree to which black neighborhoods are located near the metropolitan area's central city as opposed to its suburbs. The dimension of centralization is relevant in the U.S. context, in particular, because segregated minorities are concentrated in central cities, which are typically the oldest, most dilapidated, and most socioeconomically deprived part of the metropolitan area.[2] Concentration refers to the population density experienced by the segregated group across the metropolitan area relative to the density experienced by other groups (Massey and Denton, 1988).

Because of the multidimensional conceptualization of segregation, a group can be segregated on more than one dimension simultaneously. For example, blacks living in metropolitan areas with high levels of isolation might also experience high levels of clustering and concentration. Such patterns are referred to as hypersegregation. Although a high level of segregation on any one dimension can have deleterious social and economic consequences for the segregated group, as high levels of segregation accumulate across dimensions, the negative effects of segregation increase. In the United States not only do blacks, compared to Hispanics and Asians, experience higher levels of segregation on any single dimension, they also experience hypersegregation (Massey and Denton, 1989).

Residential Segregation, Concentration of Poverty, and Neighborhood Conditions

Residential segregation has long been studied as one of the crucial influences on the socioeconomic well-being of African Americans. The degree to which residential segregation by race/ethnicity, residential segregation by class, and economic conditions (e.g., income distribution) at the metropolitan area level explain poverty concentration among neighborhoods is the subject of a substantial body of research (Wilson, 1987, 1996; Massey and Denton, 1993; Jargowsky, 1997). Massey and Denton (1993) hypothesized that at the metropolitan area level, for a given poverty rate, residential segregation (i.e., unevenness) acts to concentrate poverty among neighborhoods.

In the sociological literature (see Appendix) the term *poverty concentration* usually refers to the distribution of poverty across neighborhoods. That is, like segregation, poverty concentration is an attribute of the entire metropolitan area (Massey and Denton, 1993; Jargowsky, 1997). However, the term is also often used to describe a high poverty rate at the neighborhood level (Wilson, 1996). Although the two meanings of the term are related and are often confused in both the sociological and the health literature on segregation, they are not interchangeable. Particular neighborhoods may have a high poverty rate whether or not they belong to a metropolitan area characterized by poverty concentration. In this chapter poverty concentration refers to the first meaning, that is, it is a metropolitan area attribute.

William Julius Wilson (1987, 1996) has argued that high poverty in African-American inner-city neighborhoods creates a uniquely disadvantaged social environment. Neighborhoods with high poverty are characterized by dilapidated and substandard housing, high unemployment rates, and low average wages. Exposure to such neighborhood conditions has been linked to high rates of teenage pregnancy as well as higher risks of joblessness and criminality among African-American men (Massey and Shibuya, 1995). The potentially deleterious consequences of racial residential segregation are not limited to central cities or to the urban poor. African Americans living in the suburbs are segregated in areas with lower income levels and higher crime rates (Alba et al., 1994; Logan and Alba, 1995).

SEGREGATION AND HEALTH

Empirical Evidence

The effects of segregation on health have been examined primarily in relation to the health status of U.S. blacks. Yankauer (1950) first demonstrated a relationship between the residential segregation of African Americans and infant mortality rates in urban areas. (For further discussion of studies relating residential segregation and infant health, see Chapter 10.) In recent years increasing interest has arisen in the health consequences of residential segregation in the United States.

We searched Medline for the years 1966 to June 2000 using *segregation* as a keyword and Sociofile for the years 1974 to February 2000 using *residential segregation* as a keyword. We included studies with the word *segregation* in the title or abstract, in which segregation referred to residential segregation. Because the majority of studies had mortality as an outcome, we chose only those studies. We also included studies of homicide if this was the main outcome of interest—and not part of a battery of crime outcomes. We also reviewed the references from these studies to identify studies published before 1966. We identified fifteen studies matching our criteria. Among these studies fourteen examined the association of racial (black) residential segregation and one examined economic residential segregation (Waitzman and Smith, 1998). The fourteen studies that focused on African-American segregation and mortality are presented in Table 12-1.

The studies presented in Table 12-1 demonstrate that black mortality rates are higher in urban areas with high levels of segregation. However, it is difficult to summarize the size of the effect of residential segregation on black mortality across these fourteen studies because, as the table shows, the outcome variables, samples of geographic areas, and years vary considerably. The few studies that examined the effect of racial residential segregation on white mortality rates had inconsistent findings (LaVeist, 1993; Fang et al., 1998; Collins and Williams, 1999).

Pathways between Segregation and Health

In general and in agreement with the sociological evidence, it is hypothesized that segregation affects health through concentrated poverty, the quality of the neighborhood environment, and the individual socioeconomic attainment of minorities (LaVeist, 1996; Williams, 1996, 1997). For example, Collins and Williams (1999), Guest and colleagues (1998), and Shihadeh and Flynn (1996) examined socioeconomic disadvantage (e.g., poverty, low education, unemployment) as the pathway through which

TABLE 12–1. Studies of Racial[1] Residential Segregation in Relation to Mortality

Study	Segregation Measure	Year	Geographic Area	Mechanisms[2]	Findings
Collins and Williams, 1999[3]	Isolation index	1990	107 U.S. cities with populations of least 100,000 and 10% black	Socioeconomic deprivation: % below poverty line, % persons not employed in managerial/professional positions	Black social isolation directly related to the black male and female all cause ($\beta = .30$, $p < .01$) and cancer ($\beta = .23$–.36, $p < .05$) mortality rate after adjustment for socioeconomic deprivation indicators[4]
Fang et al., 1998	Black pop. $\geq 75\%$; white pop. $\geq 75\%$	1990	177 ZIP codes in NYC	Primarily white areas confer "communal advantages"; primarily black areas experience poor physical environments and social unrest (mechanisms outlined in discussion but not tested)	% blacks in area unrelated to the black mortality rate (25–64 years) and inversely related to the black mortality rate (≥ 65 years); adjusted for socioeconomic indicators
Guest et al., 1998[3]	Isolation index	1990	40 black areas; 51 non-black areas, e.g. contiguous census tracts, in Chicago	Neighborhood socioeconomic conditions. % adults (≥ 25 years) with < high school degree % unemployed	Modest direct association between black isolation and the Black infant and working-age mortality rate, but statistically non significant. Effects appear to be mediated by % unemployed in area
Hart et al., 1998	Dissimilarity index	1990	114 U.S. MA	Segregation mediates negative relationship between degree of metropolitan governance	Dissimilarity was positively associated with black male mortlity; $\beta = 7.07$ ($p = .0002$)

		Year	Study population	Outcome	Findings
				(central city elasticity score) and black mortality	for black males; $\beta = 0.86$ (p = 0.41) for black females)[5]; central city elasticity was not significant after controlling for dissimilarity; model adjusted for MSA education, geographic location and poverty.
Polednak, 1996	Dissimilarity index	1990	38 and 92 U.S. MA	Poverty concentration and quality of life	In 38 MA, segregation was unrelated to the black IMR; in 92 MA, segregation directly related to the black IMR, but with adjustment for poverty and unmarried mother rate, the association with segregation did not hold
Shihadeh and Flynn, 1996[3]	Isolation index	1990	151 U.S. cities with populations of at least 100,000 and 5,000 blacks in	Economic factors: % black (16–64 years) employed; % blacks below poverty; % blacks renting vs. owning home. Cultural factors: % black teens (16–19 years) unemployed, not in school, no high school degree, not in armed forces; % black female headed HH. Political factors: black empowerment (ratio of % black city councilors to % city black voting age pop.)	Black isolation was directly related to the black homicide rate ($\beta = 0.31$, $p < .05$).[4] The effect is mediated, in part (approx. 25%), by socioeconomic, cultural, and political variables

(*continued*)

TABLE 12–1. Studies of Racial[1] Residential Segregation in Relation to Mortality (Continued)

Study	Segregation Measure	Year	Geographic Area	Mechanisms[2]	Findings
Bird, 1995	Dissimilarity index (based on MSA)	1990	34 U.S. states	Education (% > high school, % bachelor's degree); % black; % below poverty	Segregation was directly associated with the black IMR, adjusting for other state-level structural variables (β = .38, p < .05).[4]
LaVeist, 1993[3]	Dissimilarity index	1980	176 U.S. cities with a population of at least 50,000 and 10% black	% black below poverty; black political power (ratio of % black city councilors to % city black voting age pop)	Segregation was directly associated with the black IMR, adjusted for black poverty and political power (β = .065, p < .05).[5] Black political power was related to the black IMR, but the effect was not strong enough to significantly reduce the black–white disparity in IMR.
Peterson and Krivo, 1993	Dissimilarity index	1980	125 U.S. cities with a population of at least 100,000 and a black population of at least 50,000	Black social isolation; black socioeconomic deprivation	Segregation was directly related to the black homicide rate, adjusted for indicators of black socioeconomic status (β = .70, p < .01)[4]
Polednak, 1993; 1991	Dissimilarity index	1980	38 U.S. MA with populations at least 1 million	Quality of residential environment; quality and availability of health care	Segregation was directly related to the black–white ratio of the age-standardized mortality rate. Segregation was directly related to the black–white difference in

Potter, 1991	Isolation index	1980	27 MA	Black socioeconomic status	the IMR as well as the black IMR, adjusted for the black–white difference in poverty rate. Black isolation was directly associated with the white–black male life expectancy differential ($\beta = .54$, $p < .05$),[4] which was driven by the association between black isolation and the homicide differential.
LaVeist, 1989	Dissimilarity index	1980	176 U.S. cities with populations of at least 50,000 and 10% black	Socioenvironmental conditions	Segregation was directly associated with the black IMR ($\beta = .13$)[4] adjusted for socioeconomic factors and geographic region.
Massey et al., 1987	Racial compositional and pop. change (1970–1980)	1980	359 census tracts in Philadelphia	Neighborhood quality and environment	Black death rates were highest in established black census tracts and those with declining White population.
Yankauer, 1950	% nonwhite live births in area	1940	NYC health areas	Socioeconomic and physical environment of neighborhoods	The nonwhite and white IMR increased as the proportion of nonwhite births increased.

[1] Refers exclusively to the residential segregation of blacks from whites or nonblacks.

[2] Includes mechanisms that were explicitly tested or discussed.

[3] Examined mechanisms in model.

[4] Beta coefficients are standardized to distribution of variables used in study.

[5] Unstandardized coefficient.

MA, metropolitan area.

segregation affects mortality. All of these studies found that socioeconomic factors mediated part, but not all, of the association between segregation and mortality. However, these studies did not include distributional measures at the metropolitan area level (e.g., poverty concentration) nor socioeconomic indicators at the neighborhood or individual level. Rather they used aggregate indicators for the metropolitan area (e.g., poverty rate). Therefore, these studies did not directly test the role of poverty concentration nor possible pathways at the neighborhood or individual level.

Dimensions of Segregation

Although residential segregation is a multidimensional construct subsuming five distinct spatial patterns, health research has largely overlooked the complexity of residential segregation. In general, studies have used only one dimension of segregation, unevenness, measured by the dissimilarity index, yet most studies lack a conceptual justification for focusing on this segregation dimension. That is, why would segregation represented by spatial unevenness be the most appropriate dimension of segregation for the health outcome of interest? Among the studies that examined a dimension of segregation other than unevenness, two of the three that focused on segregation measured by isolation provided a strong theoretical justification for their choice of this dimension (Shihadeh and Flynn, 1996; Collins and Williams, 1999). Additionally, they addressed the issue of hypersegregation, defined as the conjunction of high dissimilarity and isolation.

The use of segregation in an unspecified manner impedes our understanding of why segregation is related to health. The reliance on one dimension of segregation, unevenness, has implications for the conceptualization and testing of specific pathways. For example, although the most widely discussed pathways pertain to disadvantaged neighborhood environments, unevenness is associated with only a few housing quality, neighborhood quality, and socioeconomic status indicators, while isolation is related to many more such indicators and concentration is most clearly linked to indicators of lower socioeconomic status for African Americans (Denton, 1994).

Several recent health studies have used population composition at the neighborhood level as a proxy for segregation (Fang et al., 1998). However, neighborhood population composition is not the same as either metropolitan area-wide segregation or neighborhood segregation. This is not merely a technical point. Not distinguishing between population composition and segregation is also a conceptual problem. As Jargowsky has argued, it is necessary to link within-neighborhood factors to a larger distribution of neighborhoods and to ask what metropolitan-area factors shape this larger distribution (Jargowsky, 1997). Neighborhood population composition is a within-neighborhood factor that is linked to the spatial distribution of the population across the metropolitan area. Residential segregation by race and by class contributes to the shape of this distribution. Studies of neighborhoods and health may incorporate neighborhood population composition as a neighborhood-level factor but should acknowledge that population composition is distinct from residential segregation.

In summary, the studies in Table 12–1 demonstrate that racial residential segregation in urban areas has a significant effect on both black infant and adult mortality rates, after adjusting for other socioeconomic and demographic characteristics of the area. However, existing studies have not fully used the multidimensional nature of segregation. Explanations of why and how residential segregation influences health, the testing of specific pathways, and the development of multilevel models remain underdeveloped.

NEW DIRECTIONS

The studies in Table 12–1 represent an important step in understanding the role that residential segregation plays in influencing health disparities. However, several areas need to be addressed in future studies if we are to fully understand the health consequences of segregation.

The Conceptualization and Operationalization of Segregation

An important conceptual and methodological issue for segregation and health research is to determine which dimensions of residential segregation are most relevant and to identify potential pathways to particular health outcomes. Earlier research on segregation and socioeconomic outcomes (Denton, 1994) and segregation and crime (Shihadeh and Flynn, 1996) has indicated the importance of recognizing that

1. Segregation has different dimensions
2. Each dimension is conceptually associated with distinct pathways to the outcome of interest
3. Each dimension is empirically correlated differently with the outcome of interest.

Future studies should choose a measure or measures of segregation and provide a justification for using that measure(s) by identifying the specific mechanisms linking it to the health outcome of interest. To date only a few studies on segregation and health have begun to address the relationship of various segregation dimensions to specific health outcomes and to provide a conceptual framework for doing so (Collins and Williams, 1999; Acevedo-Garcia, 2000; Acevedo-Garcia, 2001).

The Specification of Pathways Linking Segregation to Health

Segregation may be one of the structural factors at the metropolitan area level that contributes to the observed differences in neighborhood socioeconomic status and neighborhood quality and amenities. Various reviews of U.S. segregation and health research (Williams, 1996; Acevedo-Garcia, 2000) have concluded that the majority of studies in this area have conceptualized an indirect effect of residential segregation on health outcomes, primarily through neighborhood poverty. This can be summarized as a mediational model (Baron and Kenny, 1986), as shown in Figure 12–1. That is, segregation has an effect on social conditions at the neighborhood level, such as neighborhood poverty, which in turn influences health outcomes (pathway a). To the extent that segregation is hypothesized to have an effect on multiple mediator variables, segregation may have a residual statistical effect on the health outcome of interest (pathway c). This residual effect should not be confused with a conceptually grounded direct effect of segregation on health.

As mentioned earlier, studies often conflate metropolitan-area poverty concentration with neighborhood-level poverty. Future studies should explicitly address the role of racial/ethnic residential segregation

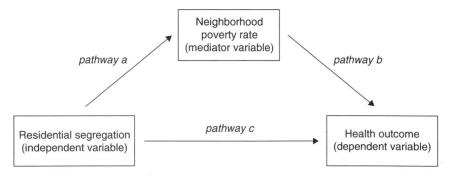

FIGURE 12–1. Mediational model.

in determining poverty concentration at the metropolitan-area level and, in turn, neighborhood socioeconomic characteristics thought to influence health outcomes. In addition, future studies should test the effect of segregation independently of poverty concentration.

Level of Analysis

In general, research on segregation and health has focused on ecological analyses at the metropolitan-area level. This has been due mainly to data availability. Nonetheless, ecologic studies prevent us from determining whether the health effects of segregation occur to those blacks living in predominantly black neighborhoods or to blacks living in predominantly white neighborhoods and from assessing the relationship between segregation and neighborhood living conditions. In order to untangle the complex processes by which segregation may influence health, we need data at different levels, including segregation and economic variables at the metropolitan-area level, neighborhood-level variables, and individual-level variables (see Chapter 3).

Class Segregation

U.S. research on segregation and health has focused on residential segregation by race/ethnicity. Only one study matching our criteria from Table 12–1 examined economic segregation (Waitzman and Smith, 1998). Future research should address the relationship of racial/ethnic segregation, economic segregation, and metropolitan-area economic variables (e.g., income distribution) to health outcomes.

Other Racial/Ethnic Groups

Because of the saliency of race in the United States and the large health disparities between African Americans and whites, the health literature has focused on black–white segregation. However, the variation in levels of residential segregation among U.S. minority groups suggests that future studies should compare the effect of segregation on health for African Americans, Hispanics, and Asians.

Protective Effects of Segregation

Most of the literature on residential segregation has examined the detrimental effects of segregation on socioeconomic, crime, and health outcomes for African Americans.[3] Although it is essential to continue exploring the adverse health consequences of segregation, future research should also examine the possibility that segregation may have positive effects. Future studies may focus on certain racial or ethnic groups for whom spatial concentration may (in combination with the quality of resources) be beneficial, for example, some U.S. immigrant groups (Fernandez Kelly and Schauffler, 1996). Additionally, some dimensions of residential segregation may be favorable for certain health outcomes. For example, studies have shown that discrimination adversely affects psychological distress and well-being for African Americans (Williams and Harris-Reid, 1999). Isolation could lead to better mental health for racial or ethnic minorities living in predominantly black neighborhoods because those living outside those areas may experience hostility and discrimination.

CONCLUSION

Both theoretically and empirically, research on neighborhood effects needs to relate neighborhood characteristics to broader social processes such as class segregation, racial/ethnic segregation, and residential mobility (Jargowsky, 1997; Sampson and Morenoff, 1997). For example, is the level of class segregation at the metropolitan-area level positively related to mortality/disease rates and individual-level outcomes at the neighborhood level, after controlling for the level of neighborhood deprivation? So far, U.S. research on segregation and health has not addressed this type of question. Multilevel studies that assume that neighborhoods do not occur in isolation but are influenced by their metropolitan area may enrich the research on neighborhoods and health.

NOTES

1. Economic segregation refers to segregation by income. However, in this chapter, economic segregation will be used interchangeably with the term class segregation.

2. In the United States, centralization may serve as an indicator of disadvantaged neighborhood conditions. However, in other societies the geographic concentration of poverty may have a different pattern. For example, in Latin American developing societies the urban periphery is generally more deprived than the central city (Lloyd-Sherlock, 1997).

3. Only a few studies (Fang et al., 1998) have suggested that residential segregation may also have positive or protective effects. However, this evidence is fragmentary.

REFERENCES

Acevedo-Garcia D (2000). Residential segregation and the epidemiology of infectious diseases. *Soc Sci Med* 51: 1143–1161.

Acevedo-Garcia D (2001). Zip code level risk factors for tuberculosis: Neighborhood environment and residential segregation, New Jersey, 1985–1992. *Am J Public Health* 91: 734–741.

Alba R, Logan JR, Bellair PE (1994). Living with crime: The implications of racial/ethnic differences in suburban location. *Social Forces* 73: 394–434.

Baron RM and Kenny DA (1986). The moderator–mediator variable distinction in social psychological research: Conceptual, Strategic and statistical considerations. *J Pers Soc Psychol* 51: 1173–1182.

Christopher AJ (1994). Segregation levels in the late apartheid city: 1985–1991. *J Econ Soc Geog* 85: 15–24.

Clark W (1989). Residential segregation in American cities: Common ground and differences in interpretation. *Population Research and Policy Review* 8: 193–197.

Clark W (1991). Residential preferences and neighborhood racial segregation: A test of the Schelling segregation model. *Demography* 28: 1–19.

Collins C and Williams DR (1999). Segregation and mortality: The deadly effects of racism. *Sociological Forum* 14: 495–523.

Daley PO (1998). Black Africans in Great Britain: Spatial concentration and segregation. *Urban Studies* 35: 703–724.

Darden J and Bagaka J (1997). Residential segregation and the concentration of low- and high-income households in the 45 largest U.S. metropolitan areas. *J Dev Societies* 13: 171–194.

Denton N (1994). Are African Americans still hypersegregated? In Bullard RD, Grigsby JE, Lee C, Feagin JR, eds.: *Residential Apartheid: The American Legacy*, vol. 2, CAAS Urban Policy Series. Los Angeles: CAAS Publications, pp. 49–81.

Fang J, Madhavan S, Bosworth W, Alderman MH (1998). Residential segregation and mortality in New York City. *Soc Sci Med* 47: 469–476.

Fernandez Kelly MP and Schauffer R (1996). Divided fates: Immigrant children and the new assimilation. In Portes A, ed.: *The New Second Generation*. New York: Russell Sage Foundation, pp. 30–53.

Galster G (1988). Residential segregation in American cities: A contrary review. *Population Research and Policy Review* 7: 93–112.

Galster G (1989). Residential segregation in American cities: A further response to Clark. *Population Research and Policy Review* 8: 181–192.

Galster G (1996). Racial discrimination and segregation. In Galster GC, ed.: *Reality and Research: Social Science and U.S. Urban Policy since 1960*. Washington, DC: Urban Institute Press, pp. 181–203.

Guest AM, Almgren G, Hussey JM (1998). The ecology of race and socioeconomic distress: Infant and working-age mortality in Chicago. *Demography* 35: 23–34.

Heggenhougen HK (1995). The epidemiology of functional apartheid and human rights abuses (editorial). *Soc Sci Med* 40: 281–284.

Jargowsky PA (1996). Take the money and run: Economic segregation in U.S. metropolitan areas. *American Sociological Review* 61: 984–998.

Jargowsky PA (1997). *Poverty and Place: Ghettos, Barrios, and the American City*. New York: Russell Sage Foundation.

Kaufman CE (1998). Contraceptive use in South Africa under apartheid. *Demography* 35: 421–434.

LaVeist TA (1989). Linking residential segregation to the infant mortality race disparity in U.S. cities. *Sociol Soc Res* 73: 90–94.

LaVeist TA (1993). Segregation, poverty, and empowerment: Health consequences for African Americans. *Milbank Q* 71: 41–64.

LaVeist TA (1996). Why we should continue to study race . . . but do a better job: An essay on race, racism and health. *Ethn Dis* 6: 21–29.

Lloyd-Sherlock P (1997). The recent appearance of favelas in Sao Paulo City: An old problem in a new setting. *Bull Latin Am Res* 16: 289–305.

Logan JR and Alba RD (1995). Who lives in affluent suburbs? Racial differences in eleven metropolitan regions. *Sociological Focus* 28: 353–364.

Lubanga N (1993). The legacy of apartheid in a changing South Africa. *Nursing & Health Care* 14: 512–519.

Massey D and Shibuya K (1995). Unraveling the tangle of pathology: The effect of spatially concentrated joblessness on the well-being of African Americans. *Soc Sci Res* 24: 352–366.

Massey D, White M, Phua V (1996). The dimensions of segregation revisited. *Sociological Methods and Research* 25: 172–206.

Massey DS and Denton NA (1988). The dimensions of residential segregation. *Soc Forces* 67: 281–315.

Massey DS and Denton NA (1989). Hypersegregation in U.S. metropolitan areas: Black and Hispanic segregation along five dimensions. *Demography* 26: 373–391.

Massey DS and Denton NA (1993). *American Apartheid: Segregation and the Making of the Underclass*. Cambridge, Mass: Harvard University Press.

Nightingale EO, Hannibal K, Geiger HJ, Hartmann L, Lawrence R, Spurlock J (1990). Apartheid medicine: Health and human rights in South Africa. *JAMA* 264: 2097–2102.

Phillips D (1998). Black minority ethnic concentration, segregation and dispersal in Britain. *Urban Studies* 35: 681–702.

Polednak AP (1991). Black–white differences in infant mortality in 38 standard metropolitan statistical areas. *Am J Public Health* 81: 1480–1482.

Polednak AP (1993). Poverty, residential segregation, and black/white mortality ratios in urban areas. *J Health Care Poor Underserved* 4: 363–373.

Polednak AP (1996). Segregation, discrimination and mortality in U.S. blacks. *Ethn Dis* 6: 99–108.

Sampson RJ and Morenoff JD (1997). Ecological perspectives on the neighborhood context of urban poverty: Past and present. In Brooks-Gunn J, Duncan GJ, Aber JL, eds.: *Neighborhood Poverty*, vol. 2. New York: Russell Sage Foundation, pp. 1–22.

Sarkin J (1999). Health and human rights in post-apartheid South Africa. *S Afr Med J* 89: 1259–1263.

Shihadeh ES and Flynn N (1996). Segregation and crime: The effect of black isolation on the rates of black urban violence. *Social Forces* 74: 1325–1352.

Smith DB (1998). The racial segregation of hospital care revisited: Medicare discharge patterns and their implications. *Am J Public Health* 88: 461–463.

Turton RW and Chalmers BE (1990). Apartheid, stress and illness: The demographic context of distress reported by South African Africans. *Soc Sci Med* 31: 1191–1200.

van Grunsven L (1992). Integration versus segregation: Ethnic minorities and urban politics in Singapore. *J Econ Soc Geog* 83: 196–215.

Waitzman NJ and Smith KR (1998). Separate but lethal: The effects of economic segregation on mortality in metropolitan America. *Milbank Q* 76: 341–373.

Williams D (1997). Race and health: Basic questions, emerging directions. *Ann Epidemiol* 7: 322–333.

Williams DR (1996). Racism and health: A research agenda (editorial). *Ethn Dis* 6: 1–8.

Williams DR (1998). African-American health: The role of the social environment. *J Urban Health* 75: 300–321.

Williams DR and Harris-Reid M (1999). Race and mental health: Emerging patterns and promising approaches. In Horwitz AV and Scheid TL, eds.: *A Handbook for the Study of Mental Health.* Cambridge: Cambridge University Press, pp. 295–314.

Wilson WJ (1987). *The Truly Disadvantaged: The Inner City, the Underclass, and Public Policy.* Chicago: University of Chicago Press.

Wilson WJ (1996). *When Work Disappears: The World of the New Urban Poor.* New York: Knopf.

Yach D and Tollman SM (1993). Public health initiatives in South Africa in the 1940s and 1950s: Lessons for a post-apartheid era. *Am J Public Health* 83: 1043–1050.

Yankauer A (1950). The relationship of fetal and infant mortality to residential segregation. *Am Sociol Rev* 15: 644–648.

Yinger J (1995). *Closed Doors, Opportunities Lost: The Continuing Costs of Housing Discrimination.* New York: Russell Sage Foundation.

Appendix: Residential Segregation, Poverty Concentration, and Related Concepts in Sociological Literature

Concept Name	Concept Definition (Measure)	Source
Metropolitan Area Economy		
Metropolitan area mean income	Average household income	Jargowsky, 1997
Metropolitan area income inequality	Coefficient of variation of the household distribution of income, i.e. standard deviation of household income, divided by mean household income	Jargowsky, 1997
Geographic Concentration of Poverty		
MA poverty rate	% of total number of MA persons that are poor (below federal poverty line)	Massey and Denton, 1993
High poverty neighborhood	Neighborhood where poverty rate ≥40%	Jargowsky, 1997
Neighborhood poverty rate (NPR)	% of MA total population that resides in high-poverty neighborhoods	Jargowsky, 1997
Concentration of poverty (affluence)	% of MA poor (affluent) population that resides in high poverty (affluence) neighborhoods	Jargowsky, 1997; Waitzman and Smith, 1998
Poverty concentration	Exposure to poverty across neighborhoods (based on isolation index)	Massey and Denton, 1993

For a given MA (j) and a racial/ethnic group (m), the index of exposure to poverty (EP_{jm}), is given by

$$EP^{jm} = \sum_{i=1}^{N} \frac{x_i^{jm}}{X^{jm}} \frac{e_i^j}{t_i^j}$$

where x_i^{jm}, t_i^j, and X^{jm} are the number of members of the group m in census tract i, the total population of census tract i, and the number of members of the minority group m for the entire MA j; e_{ji} is the number of persons living in poverty; N is the total number of census tracts in MA j. For example, $EP^{jm} = 0.15$ indicates that in MA j, the typical member of group m lives in a census tract where 15% of the population lives in poverty.

Residential Segregation by Race/Ethnicity

Dissimilarity

The dissimilarity index (D), which may be interpreted as the proportion of the minority racial/ethnic group of interest (m) that would need to move across subunits in order to achieve an even distribution, is given by

$$D^{jm} = \sum_{i=1}^{N} \frac{t_i |x_i - X|}{2TX(1 - X)}$$

where t_i and x_i are the total population and minority proportion of areal subunit (i.e., census tract) i, and T and X are the population size and minority proportion of the whole geographic area, i.e., MA (j), which is subdivided into N areal subunits. Ranges from 0, no residential segregation, to 1, complete residential segregation.

Massey and Denton, 1988

Isolation

The isolation index (P), which measures the extent to which a member of a racial/ethnic group (m) is likely to be in contact with members of this same group (as opposed to members of other groups), is given by

$$P^{jm} = \sum_{i=1}^{N} \frac{x_i^{jm}}{X^{jm}} \frac{x_i^{jm}}{t_i^i}$$

Massey and Denton, 1988

(continued)

Appendix: Residential Segregation, Poverty Concentration, and Related Concepts in Sociological Literature (Continued)

Concept Name	Concept Definition (Measure)	Source
	where x, X, and t are defined as above; e.g., $P^{jm} = 0.6$ indicates that in MA j, the average member of group m, lives in a census tract where the probability that (s)he will have contact with another member of group m is 0.6. Ranges from the overall proportion minority in the entire MA, no residential segregation, to 1, complete residential segregation.	Massey and Denton, 1988
Concentration	Concentration refers to the relative space occupied by a minority group in a geographic area. If a group occupies a small share of the total area, it is said to be residentially concentrated. A simple concentration index (C) can be derived from an application of the dissimilarity index defined above, $$C^{jm} = \frac{1}{2} \sum_{i=1}^{N} \left| \frac{x_i}{X} - \frac{a_i}{A} \right|$$ where x_i and X_i are defined as before; a_i equals the land area of subunit i, and A is the total land area of the geographic area (i.e., MA) j. This index may be interpreted as the share of minority members that would have to move across subunits in order to achieve a uniform density of minority members over all units. Ranges from 0, no residential segregation, to 1, complete residential segregation. Massey and Denton (1988) have proposed two more complex indexes of concentration, the absolute concentration index, ACO, and the relative concentration index, RCO.	

Centralization

Centralization refers to nearness to the center of the urban area, which in the largest and oldest US MAs is often characterized by dilapidated housing and socioeconomic deprivation. The absolute centralization index is given by

$$ACE = \sum_{i=1}^{N} C_{i-1} A_i \sum_{i=1}^{N} C_i A_{i-1}$$

where the N areal subunits are ordered by increasing distance from the central business district, C is the cumulative proportion of X in subunit i, and A is the cumulative proportion of land area through subunit i. Ranges from 1 to -1. Positive values indicate tendency of group X to live close to the center of the MA; negative values indicate tendency to live in the outlying areas; 0 denotes a uniform distribution throughout the MA.

Massey and Denton, 1988

Clustering

Clustering is the extent to which areal subunits inhabited by minority members adjoin one another, or cluster, in space. The preferred measure of this dimension is the index of spatial proximity (SP) given by the average of intergroup proximities (P_{xx}, P_{yy})

$$SP = \frac{XP_{xx} + YP_{yy}}{TP_{tt}}$$

where T, X, and Y are the population size, minority proportion, and majority proportion of the whole geographic area. To illustrate, the measure of spatial

Massey and Denton, 1988

(continued)

Appendix: Residential Segregation, Poverty Concentration, and Related Concepts in Sociological Literature (Continued)

Concept Name	Concept Definition (Measure)	Source
	proximity for group X, i.e., the average proximity between members of group X, is given by $$P_{xx} = \sum_{i=1}^{N} \sum_{j=1}^{N} \frac{x_i x_j c_{ij}}{X^2}$$ where c_{ij} represents a distance function between areas i and j, and x and X are defined as before. SP equals 1 when there is no differential clustering between X and Y, and is greater than 1 when members of each group live closer to one another than to each other.	
Residential Segregation by Class		
Neighborhood sorting index (NSI) and neighborhood distribution of income	$$NSI = \frac{\sigma_N}{\sigma_H}$$ where σ_N is the standard deviation of the neighborhood income distribution and σ_H is the standard deviation of the household income distribution. The neighborhood distribution of income is the distribution of households by the mean household income of the neighborhood in which they live—each neighborhood is weighted by the number of households it contains. The household distribution of income is the distribution of households by their own income. If there were no income	Jargowsky, 1997

	segregation, all neighborhoods would have the same mean income and σ_N, and thus NSI would be zero. At the other extreme, if there were perfect income segregation, all households would live in neighborhoods where the mean income approximated their own. In this case, σ_N would approach σ_H, and thus NSI would approach 1.$$NSI^2 = \frac{\sigma_N^2}{\sigma_H^2}$$$NSI^2$ is the proportion of the total variance in household income among, rather than within, neighborhoods	
Dissimilarity of the poor (affluent)[1]	Proportion of poor (affluent) families that would have to move in order to achieve an even socioeconomic distribution throughout the metropolitan area. See dissimilarity index above. Thresholds: poor—below federal poverty line; affluent—≥$75,000 (top 12% of the 1989 family income distribution).	Waitzman and Smith, 1998
Isolation of the poor (affluent)[1]	Exposure to poverty (affluence) across neighborhoods (defined by Massey and Denton (1993) as poverty concentration). See isolation index above. Thresholds: poor—below federal poverty line; affluent—≥$75,000 (top 12% of the 1989 family income distribution).	Waitzman and Smith, 1998

[1]The dissimilarity and the isolation index are not independent of the mean and variance of the income distribution. For this reason, Jargowsky has proposed the use of NSI and NSI^2 (Jargowsky, 1997).

Sources: Jargowsky, PA (1997). *Poverty and Place: Ghettos, Barrios, and the American City.* Russell Sage Foundation, New York. Massey, DS and Denton NA (1988). The Dimensions of Residential Segregation. *Social Forces* 67: 281–315. Massey, DS and Denton NA (1993). *American Apartheid: Segregation and the Making of the Underclass.* Harvard University Press, Cambridge, Mass. Waitzman, NJ and Smith KR (1998). Separate but lethal: The effects of economic segregation on mortality in metropolitan America. *Milbank Quarterly* 76: 341–373.

13

Neighborhoods and Networks: The Construction of Safe Places and Bridges

Lisa F. Berkman
Cheryl Clark

The idea that the environment, both natural and built, shapes patterns of social relationships is not new. Work in the 1950s illustrated the effects of housing on friendship formations and patterns of network interaction (Festinger et al., 1950). As others in this volume have noted, community-based studies that focus on patterns of formal and informal affiliation have a long and prominent history in sociology (Dubois, 1899; Wirth, 1938; Fischer, 1982; Sampson, 1988). As societies have become increasingly urbanized, however, and as people have become increasingly geographically mobile and new forms of communication have developed, serious questions have arisen about the extent to which networks are shaped by geographic location, specifically neighborhoods. These questions spill over into a larger issue regarding conceptions of the constitution of communities in general and the gains in well-being that may accrue from geographically "local" communities versus non–spatially based communities.

Early neighborhood studies implicitly identified themselves as community studies, embracing most central domains of networks. In recent decades rigorous efforts have been made to distinguish social networks and more formal affiliations from geography, or "place," and neighborhoods from communities. Drawing these distinctions has both advantages and disadvantages. The main advantage is that distinguishing between networks and communities allows us to test specific hypotheses related to the influence of neighborhoods on social ties, and vice versa. The distinction presses us to be explicit about our assumptions. We can then examine the structure of social relationships without assuming that they are bounded by geography or other things (e.g., kinship). The disadvantage is that disaggregating has led to less work on the relationship between the physical and the social environments in terms of, for instance, how neighborhoods and housing might shape network structure and influence function. For example, a great deal of the work on social networks has focused on how social status or similarities in background with regard to religion, occupation, race and ethnicity, age, and gender shape network structure and patterns of support (Laumann, 1973; Fischer et al., 1977, 1982). While this work is embedded in urban sociology, little of it examines neighborhoods or the built environment in relation to social networks. More recent work has focused on the fact that affluent people often associate with other affluent people and poor people with poor people, and has little orientation to the influence of place in determining these interactions. Though there are important exceptions (Massey and Denton, 1993; Wilson, 1996), much of the earlier and less formal work on social networks and family was oriented toward the influence of new towns, new housing, or the destruction of stable neighborhoods on social ties and support (Young and Willmott, 1957; Gans, 1962; Liebow, 1967). Our aim in this chapter is to review selected evidence about the effect of neighborhoods on social networks with regard to some specific groups. However, we also hope to clarify the difference between neighborhood and community. Our intent is to identify the extent to which a strong sense of community is maintained by social ties within neighborhoods.

Social networks form a web of associations that serve a myriad of functions, including the provision of support and access to material resources. They also serve to shape norms of behavior, they provide opportunities for social engagement and participation, and they have the capacity to produce social capital (Berkman and Glass, 2000). Social network analysis started when social scientists could not explain the patterning of behavior on the basis of kinship or geographic location alone (Barnes, 1954; Bott, 1957). When social scientists focused on actual social exchanges, however, they often found that individuals were embedded in a web of social relations that were functional although they did not fit the social scientists' preconceived notions of community. As Wellman (1988) and others have noted, a network approach permits us to test empirically whether relations are spatially clustered in the form of neighborhoods (or, for that matter, kinship). Because the functions of social networks are thought to have an important influence on a broad array of health outcomes for perhaps a broad array of reasons, it is important to identify the conditions that determine these networks. One of the ways in which neighborhoods may influence health is by shaping such social networks.

Definitions of neighborhood are not easy to come by. Neighborhood boundaries are commonly measured in empirical studies using proxy indicators such as census tracts or electoral wards. Macintyre identifies four dimensions of neighborhoods that help in defining them: services and amenities, the social environment, the physical environment, and reputation. In reality, most definitions of neighborhood build on bureaucratic boundaries in quantitative research. Spatial areas labeled and treated as coherent neighborhoods have come to be regarded as a natural phenomenon (Wellman and Leighton, 1979). In qualitative and ethnographic studies, definitions of neighborhoods are often based on either bureaucratically defined areas or smaller areas bounded by what individuals themselves define as their neighborhood.

Definitions of community often entail elements of both networks and geography. Wellman (1979), for instance, describes three elements of community: networks of interpersonal ties providing support and sociability, residence in a common locality, and solidarity sentiments and activities (Hillery, 1955; Wellman and Leighton, 1979). Because the study of communities has been firmly rooted in the study of neighborhoods, consideration of the role of community, or at least a clear understanding of the distinction between community and a geographically defined entity, is central to the chapter.

In looking at the interface among neighborhoods, networks, and communities, rather than focus on national samples or samples of predominately white middle- or working-class communities, we will highlight work in two populations, gay and lesbian and African-American urban populations. These populations give us "windows" into the interface among social ties, community, and neighborhood, and they are particularly important from a public health standpoint. Interest in them rests on the idea that men and women in minority groups may face particular challenges in maintaining social ties both with one another and to other groups that assure their health and well-being in physical, mental, and social terms. In order to illustrate the issues linking neighborhoods, networks, and communities in these groups, we have selected several studies that are particularly insightful.

A final overlay to the chapter is an examination of the relationship between community, social ties, and geography. In a seminal paper on communities, Wellman and Leighton (1979) identified three competing arguments by which we can evaluate the link between community and neighborhoods or networks. The first of these is that communities are "lost" in the fray of modern urban life, which entails substantial social disorganization stemming from large-scale social transformation of bureaucratic institutions. Investigators who find support for this argument often see individuals in urban settings as isolated and lacking strong ties capable of providing solidarity and assistance. The second argument identifies the community as "saved," by which investigators mean that neighborhood-based communities have persisted in modern industrial societies and continue to serve as important sources of support and sociability (Wellman and Leighton, 1979). According to this perspective, city dwellers continue to be involved in a single neighborhood that provides a great deal of support across a number of domains, although they may simultaneously belong to nongeographically bound networks as well. The third argument is that neighborhood-based communities have been weakened, yet primary ties have remained stable and flourish in urban areas; they are just not organized within neighborhoods but rather across them. These dispersed networks are effective because of modern technological developments relating to transportation and communication. This view is based on the idea that social relations are "liberated" from geography. As we evaluate the role of neighborhoods in influencing social ties and a sense of community, we will do so through the lens of community as lost, saved, or liberated.

SAFE PLACES: GAY AND LESBIAN TIES IN THE CITY

One of the major advantages of the city according to many urban sociologists is the increased opportunities in urban areas to promote and sustain multiple and diverse subcultures. Urban social life provides a number of subcultures with means capable of integrating their members into intimate social worlds. Through the 1960s and 1970s a number of investigators suggested that such subcultures and communities could exist in "social worlds" that were not necessarily based on geographic places or neighborhoods. Fisher suggested that these worlds introduced functional alternatives to communities organized by physical space or geographic proximity alone. Indeed, a great deal of the research on social networks and urbanization has described the broadening geographical space in which urban networks effectively operate (Fischer, 1982; Wellman, 1997). As mentioned earlier in this chapter, this work counters observations based on neighborhood interactions alone that "community is lost" with a more balanced interpretation that such communities exist in both geographic as well as virtual space.

Hence, it is of some importance to examine the ways in which gay and lesbian communities in urban areas grow and develop and the ways in which they are geographically bounded or exist in non–space-dependent "social worlds." Although there is some literature on rural gay and lesbian communities (Kramer, 1995; Bell and Valentine, 1995), the majority of work describes gay male neighborhoods in urban areas. There is a large literature describing gay communities in European and North American cities—London's Soho (Binnie, 1995), Manchester's "Gay Village" (Corton, 1993; Whittle, 1994), Park Slope, Brooklyn (Rothenberg, 1995), San Francisco (Castells, 1983). The titles of some of these works, "Get Thee to a Big City (Weston, 1995), "How Far Will You Go" (Kelley, Pebody, et al., 1996) "Invented Identities" (Cant, 1997), speak to the central role cities play in the lives of many gay men and lesbian women who migrate to cities or to specific neighborhoods in cities to create nurturing communities. In research on the geography of sexuality, Valentine (1995; Binnie and Valentine, 1999) insightfully describes past work in this area, focusing largely on the geography of this work and noting the need to understand and balance these findings with the extent to which such communities, although still urban, exist without being spatially bounded. The move from spatial landscape to virtual spaces based on forms of communication in which face-to-face contact is not always essential parallels the growth of informal networks in other communities.

The advantages of neighborhood-based gay and lesbian communities are clear. As Valentine (1993) describes, heterosexuals meet friends in everyday environments: work, school, restaurants, and daily activities. How gay men and lesbians meet, create social networks, and socialize is a much more complex and challenging experience. Geographic, or physical, space makes an enormous difference in building gay and lesbian networks. Valentine notes that of 645 friends identified by 40 lesbians, fully 85% of them met in gay environments as opposed to heterosexual environments. Homes of friends, gay spaces, support groups, and gay pubs, clubs, and discos accounted for more than three-quarters of contacts. Because gay men and lesbians often must separate their private lives from their public lives to conceal their sexuality, personal communities become an essential way to prevent isolation and find support, material and psychosocial resources, and companionship. Safe places become those neighborhoods, houses, social events, support or political groups, and societies where it is safe to express one's identity without fear of disclosure or reprisal. Some evidence indicates that such spaces produce networks that are densely interconnected. Valentine, for instance, found that the lesbian social networks of the women she interviewed were more tightly woven than were those in other studies of urban networks (Wellman, 1979; Fischer, 1982). This may be an artifact of her recruitment method of snowball sampling (ensuring that contacts knew at least a few others), but future work in this area should certainly extend these analyses to other samples. In any case, gay neighborhoods (specifically in terms of areas within cities) have not only provided safe places but have had a wider impact on the social, cultural, and political life of urban areas, contributing to the gentrification of many neighborhoods, generating political power in terms of a "gay vote," and adding to the business and cultural life of the city.

Safe places are not exclusively bound by residential neighborhoods, however. Increasingly, geographers working in this area point to the development of communities oriented in time and space dedicated to gay, or more commonly lesbian, social activities for a specified period of time. Discos, bars, and community centers dedicated to gay and lesbian activities for certain time periods are important examples. Further along the continuum of place-bound communities are ordinary places that have specific significance to gay men and lesbians or women and therefore serve as gathering and meeting places that serve to create both real and imagined communities. Finally, investigators address the growing importance of nonspatial types of communities built on Internet ties, hotlines and crises services, and support groups, all of which exist in terms of network ties but not geographical spaces.

Gay and lesbian networks and communities appear to be based on both geographic (i.e., neighborhood) criteria as well as other nonspatially based institutional criteria (participation in voluntary associations such as social, political, and sports-based activities). While we have not discussed gender-based differences in community constructions, some authors have pointed out that often gay male communities are based on residential proximity, whereas lesbian communities, because of economic circumstances as well as other social and behavioral characteristics, may be less geographically bound (Valentine, 1995). Both provide important opportunities, are resources, and seem to serve and aid the development and maintenance of social networks.

If we were to describe gay and lesbian communities across a number of urban areas as "lost," "saved," or "liberated" based on the predominantly ethnographic data we have, we would most definitely describe them as "liberated." The historical development of these communities has not paralleled the stages of development of many other communities (for instance, those based on ethnic homogeneity) that we often view as starting from preindustrial states of tightly knit homogeneous networks that were then challenged by rapid urbanization and forced to change. Nonetheless, they currently function quite similarly to many other urban communities. Residentially based neighborhood communities exist, yet primary ties exist across neighborhoods and not just within them. Modern technological developments relating both to communication and transportation serve to keep geographically dispersed networks effective.

Gay men and lesbians often seem to belong to neighborhood networks as well as nongeographically bound networks supporting the "liberated-communities" perspective.

Bridges: Racial Segregation and Social Ties

> The student must clearly recognize that a complete study must not confine itself to the group, but specially notice the environment; the physical environment of the city, sections and houses, the far mightier social environment—the surrounding world of custom, wish, whim, and thought which envelopes this group and powerfully influences its social development.
>
> —W. E. B. DuBois (1899)

Theoretical Bridges: Racial Segregation and Social Isolation

The study of African-American inner-city neighborhoods provides an opportunity to review and integrate major social network theories in explaining the institutional and interpersonal mechanisms that historically and currently bind poverty and divestment in human capital to geographic locales. In the spirit of the sociologist W. E. B. DuBois, community-level theories and concepts from the field of social network analysis may be used to explain the maintenance of poverty and stunted opportunities in African-American inner cities. Namely, the phenomenon of "social isolation," or the absence of ties to individuals and institutions that provide social and economic opportunities, has been proposed as a major mechanism by which poverty is perpetuated among African-American inner-city residents (Wilson, 1996). Social isolation has been produced by a series of public policies, institutional practices related to housing and economic development, and private behaviors that have led to increasingly racially segregated neighborhoods in a number of American cities over the last several decades (Massey and Denton, 1993). Many of these neighborhoods have now become what Massey and Denton refer to as "hypersegregated," a phenomenon that leads to ever-increasing social isolation for neighborhood residents. Several other chapters in this volume describe in greater detail such neighborhoods and the causes and consequences of residence in them. In this chapter we focus on the extent to which neighborhood characteristics influence the networks of urban African Americans.

Social isolation among economically disadvantaged African Americans living in inner cities has become synonymous with the work of sociologist William Julius Wilson, who studied the consequences of race-based social and economic exclusion in *When Work Disappears*. Wilson writes that inner-city African Americans living in highly segregated neighborhoods find themselves "out of contact or sustained interaction with institutions, families, and individuals that represent mainstream society" (Wilson, 1996, p. 64). This sort of social isolation deprives inner-city residents not only of "conventional role models . . . but also of social resources . . . provided by mainstream social networks that facilitate social and economic advancement in modern industrial society" (p. 66).

Social Bridges: The Importance of Weak Ties

The social isolation that Wilson describes draws heavily on social network theory. Specifically, the structural and interpersonal forces that lead to racial segregation may exclude inner-city African Americans from participating in "weak ties," as described in the classic work of Granovetter (1973). Such weak ties are characterized not by intimacy, but by a lack of closeness and density among ties. These ties are considered essential for the diffusion of information across communities and critical, as Granovetter has shown, for access to new information and contacts for jobs. Employment at many socioeconomic levels is heavily influenced by weak ties (Granovetter, 1983). While most of the work on weak ties has been oriented toward employment opportunities, there is growing research on diffusion of many kinds of information and behaviors, even on the direct transmission of infectious diseases. It is easy to imagine how such ties that bridge networks could be such effective links. Apart from the media, bridging networks are likely to play a major role in information diffusion, and some recent work suggests that a small number of "hubs," or networks with multiple weak ties branching out to other networks, may play a particularly important role in this process.

The existence of effective weak ties in poor inner-city neighborhoods is closely related to whether we construe these neighborhoods as communities that are "lost," "saved," or "liberated." Briefly, to review, "lost" communities are those in which local neighborhood ties have been destroyed and either no longer exist or have lost their functionality. "Saved" communities posit the existence and effective functioning of local networks, and the "liberated" community is one in which effective networks exist at both a local level and in an unbounded, nonspatially defined manner. The communities defined by both Wilson (1996)and Massey and Denton (1993) come closest to matching the definition of a lost community. Although ethnographers have described the many close and strong bonds that exist among African Americans living in inner cities, the apparent lack of weak ties that results from hypersegregation may, in fact, prevent those communities from being strong and cohesive. Whether we see these communities as "liberated" rests in large part on the evidence concerning whether they have weak ties that serve not only to bind networks within neighborhoods but also to link inner city African Americans to networks that cross and transcend neighborhood boundaries.

What, then, is the evidence that weak ties exist and function to provide support and resources in African-American inner-city communities? Interestingly enough, little research exists in this area, especially quantitative work. However, a study of three African-American communities in California allows an exploration of local features that illustrate "saved" and "liberated" communities as well as cultural features that promote resiliency in those that may be considered "lost."

The study was done by Oliver (1988) using classical social network analysis to examine the ties of African Americans in three African-American neighborhoods in Los Angeles. The three neighborhoods, however, were very different from one another and served to provide rich and nuanced perspectives on ties in large urban areas. The first community was Watts. It fit most closely the representation of Wilson's inner city. Residents of Watts had low-paying jobs, and the community featured high unemployment, high population density, and poor housing and lacked the fundamental services and institutions needed by residents. The second community was Crenshaw-Baldwin Hills. While also an inner-city neighborhood, it was more economically heterogeneous than was Watts and included a solid African-American middle class and excellent housing stock. In Oliver's description it was "institutionally complete" in that it contained services and institutions needed for the social functioning of its residents (Breton, 1964). The third neighborhood was Carson, a working-class and middle-class suburb, not adjacent to any other African-American community in Los Angeles. It was unique in being among the most integrated cities in California, having 33% African Americans, 31% whites, and 22% Hispanics.

In an analysis of ties that provide different types of support, African-American residents of Crenshaw-Baldwin Hills reported receiving more of all types of support. They also reported giving more support, especially emotional support ($p < .05$) than did residents in either Watts or Carson. Residents of Watts received the least support. While more than 50% of the dominant relationships that provided support across all three neighborhoods were kin, respondents from Watts were more likely than were others to name neighbors and kin outside the household as major sources of support. They were less likely to name friends and slightly less likely to name coworkers and members of clubs or organizations to which they belonged as support providers.

When Oliver examined where members of the respondents' support networks lived, he found that 33% of those in Watts had supporters who lived in the neighborhood. Twenty percent of those living in Carson and Crenshaw-Baldwin Hills had network ties in the neighborhood. This difference was due in large part to the fact that people in Watts had many more kin and group members living in their neighborhood than did those living in the other communities. In Carson only 7% of kin (compared to 23% in Watts and 19% in Crenshaw-Baldwin Hills) lived in the neighborhood.

The best test of the variability of weak ties across these neighborhoods involved a test of network density and multistrandedness. Multistrandedness is the extent to which social ties cross several contexts and relationships. Most ties are single-stranded, that is, the relationship is with a kin, friend, or neighbor. Community residents in these three areas differed in the number of multistranded ties they had. Such ties were more common in Watts than in the other two communities (40% versus 32% and 30% for Crenshaw-Baldwin Hills and Carson, respectively).

This study is important in several respects. First, it illustrates the diversity of African-American neighborhoods, all in the larger metropolis of Los Angeles, that are often not differentiated. Second, the network structure, support, and resources vary by neighborhood. Only Watts, to a certain extent, fits the image of a tightly knit community filled with dense, multistranded networks often based on kin, church-based affiliations, and neighborhood-based ties. While in all three communities most residents reported the availability of a large number of ties across a number of types of relationships, Watts's residents maintained the most local ties and the fewest distal ties. The networks of Carson and Crenshaw-Baldwin Hills lend support to the idea that these communities are "liberated." Watts is somewhat lacking in weak ties that might serve as bridges to other nonlocal networks. Nonetheless, residents are hardly isolated in a network analytic sense, that is, without close ties to others. Thus, while residents of Watts maintain close ties, as assessed from these types of surveys, Watts remains a community institutionally "incomplete," lacking in neighborhood services that would help it thrive, including a public transportation system that would facilitate travel from Watts to other areas, and full local employment. While Watts may not fit the definition of a "lost" community, it clearly does not fit the "saved" or "liberated" community pattern, either. How can we classify Watts as socially isolated using Wilson's framework and simultaneously acknowledge the dense interconnectedness of Watts's social networks and its weak ties, which, although not as extensive as those in the other communities, are still evident?

In order to understand this phenomenon, it is helpful to turn to the ethnographic literature. These studies provide insights into the quality, functions, and resources that flow among close, tightly knit ties and among weaker, more extended ties. A large body of work produced between the 1960s and the early 1980s documents the importance of extended kin and close friends in protecting poor inner-city African Americans from the ravages of poverty and sustaining the values of family and friends. A review of the works *All our Kin* (Stack, 1974), *A Place on the Corner* (Anderson, 1976), and *Tally's Corner* (Liebow, 1967) provides countless examples of how strong bonds serve to buffer the stresses of economic hardship and discrimination. These networks often function effectively even in the face of extremely scarce resources. However, over the last two decades Massey and Denton (1993) have noted that because of increasing hypersegregation, ethnographers now portray a bleaker scenario. They point out Anderson's (1990) work describing inner-city life in the 1980s that shows a considerable breakdown in bonds, especially between older, formerly respected seniors and younger men and women. "Residents keep more to themselves now and no longer involve themselves in their neighbors' lives as they did as recently as ten years ago" (Anderson, 1990). Street-smart young people became more important role models than wise elders as inner-city youths abandoned values they saw as hopeless in helping them achieve success. Such a shift may also help explain the dramatic rise in single-parenthood among African Americans in inner cities during this period.

Anderson's description stands, however, in contrast to Newman's (1999) compelling stories of young men and women working at low-paying jobs in Harlem during the 1990s. While she selected those who were working, clearly a subsample of inner-city young men and women, Newman's stories document time and time again the extent to which connections served to help young men and women find jobs. Furthermore, most of the respondents in Newman's accounts appear to have had many ties with others—friends, family, and coworkers. Many fathers, although often unmarried, cared deeply about their children and were simply struggling to make ends meet in an economic situation in which this was all but impossible. What is notable in Newman's ethnography is that while networks were large and isolation was rare, commonly the connections were unable to provide the kinds of support and resources that were needed. Ties were rarely "vertical," that is, leading to upward mobility, needs for child care often went unmet, and financial resources were unavailable. Newman's subjects could identify friends and relatives who were middle class and better off, many of whom had moved out of the inner city, yet they were rarely able to count on them for help finding a job or for financial resources, except, perhaps, in the direst circumstances.

While far from conclusive, it would seem that one must differentiate between the existences of networks and their capacity to provide resources. With regard to the existence of connections, strong and, to a lesser extent, weak ties exist even in the most highly impoverished, racially segregated communities. However, such ties often are not able, for a number of reasons, to provide the support and resources (material, instrumental, financial, or emotional) that are needed to sustain stable families, effective community organizations, and economic advancement. The situation appears to be substantially different for more economically advantaged communities and more racially integrated poor communities. In neighborhoods in which there is a convergence of poverty and racially based exclusion from weak ties, a breakdown may emerge in the connections between people, and a limited number of network members may remain to provide psychosocial and material resources to one another. Thus, it is important that weak ties be investigted.

In his work on social capital, Alejandro Portes (1998) describes the negative effects of social capital in a number of communities ranging from Balinese entrepreneurs to many immigrant groups in the United States. Essentially, when success is fragile, community solidarity comes at great cost and threatens to undermine the entire network. Under conditions of strong social capital and tightly knit networks, successful members are obligated to support needier extended family and community ties. Such demands may undermine the tenuous grasp of newly successful members on resources and pull down the entire community. In order to avoid this scenario, Portes suggests that more successful middle-class members distance themselves from their poorer relations. Thus, as Newman suggests, poorer blacks, like many immigrant groups, may well have ties to more middle-class relatives or members of their older communities, but they may not be able to call on them for support, either material, informational, or emotional. Weak ties exist but cannot be called upon for support.

If one of the critical factors that limits upward mobility in African-American inner-city neighborhoods is the dearth of weak ties that bridge to the larger society, it may be possible to design institutional interventions to take the place of these ties and harness resilient features of neighborhoods without swamping more successful members of the community with too many demands. It is also possible that the weak ties in poor African-American communities do not contain bridges to new resources or possibilities. Weak ties are only as good as the information and resources that flow through them. If this is the case, investment in resources within neighborhoods is vital to their success. Over time, with investments both in resources and in strengthening the structure of social ties, the nature of social isolation may be transformed.

CONCLUSION

Our aim in this chapter has been to examine the role of neighborhoods in the structure and functioning of networks. We have also aimed to classify communities as lost, saved, or liberated based on the structure and function of networks and the extent to which these networks are geographically bounded. We chose to examine two very different communities, gay and lesbian communities in cities and inner-city African-American communities. We focused our attention on these communities because (1) we thought geography might play a particularly important role in shaping networks and support and (2) we thought any information we might glean from our analyses might be useful in promoting the health and well-being of these men and women because of the discrimination both groups often experience in their daily lives. Furthermore, few network analyses have been conducted in these communities, and we hoped the identification of unsolved issues might promote more work in these areas.

Our findings, although far from conclusive, suggest that men and women living in urban communities today normally have ties within their neighborhoods and across the city. Networks are both local and nonlocal. In this way gay men and lesbians and African Americans are much like other urban dwellers. Both groups, however, invest a great deal in nurturing local relationships and sharing a common space, perhaps more so than many other urban groups. While our review suggests that "liberated" communities may be the norm for many groups at the beginning of the twenty-first century, not all groups reap the advantages of connections. Impovershed African-American men and women living in hypersegregated neighborhoods where they are excluded from meaningful ties to the larger society are most vulnerable. Our efforts in the future would be well directed to helping all communities, but especially those that experience discrimination, to build on the strength of local connections balanced with constructing bridges across communities.

REFERENCES

Anderson E (1976). *A Place on the Corner.* Chicago: University of Chicago Press.
Anderson E (1991). *Street Wise: Race, Class, and Change in an Urban Community.* Chicago: University of Chicago Press.
Barnes JA (1954). Class and committees in a Norwegian island parish. *Human Relations* 7: 39–58.
Bell D and Valentine G (1995). Queer country: rural lesbian and gay lives. *Journal of Rural Studies* 11: 113–172.

Berkman LF and Glass T (2000). Social integration, social networks, social support and health. In Berkman LF and Kawachi I, eds.: *Social Epidemiology*. New York: Oxford University Press, pp. 137–173.

Binnie J (1995). Trading places: Consumption, sexuality and the production of queer space. In Bell D and Valentine G, eds.: *Mapping Desire: Geographies of Sexuality*. London: Routledge, pp. 82–199.

Binnie J and Valentine G (1999). Geographies of sexuality: A review of progress. *Prog Hum Geogr* 23(2): 175–187.

Bott E (1957). *Family and Social Network*. London: Tavistock.

Breton R (1964). Institutional completeness of ethnic communities and the personal relations of immigrants. *Am J Sociol* 70: 193–205.

Cant B (1997). *Invented Identities: Lesbians and Gays Talk about Migration*. London: Cassell.

Castells M (1983). *The City and the Grassroots*. Berkeley: University of California Press.

Corton S (1993). *Anal Street: Manchester's Gay Village—Dissection of a "Community."* Manchester: Department of Geography, University of Manchester.

Dubois, W. E. B. (1899). *The Philadelphia Negro*. Philadelphia: University of Pennsylvania Press.

Festinger L, Schacter S, et al. (1950). *Social Pressures in Informal Groups*. New York: Harper & Row.

Fischer CS (1982). *To Dwell among Friends: Personal Networks in Town and City*. Chicago: University of Chicago Press.

Fischer CS, Jackson RM, et al. (1977). *Networks and Places: Social Relations in the Urban Setting*. New York: Free Press.

Gans H (1962). *The Urban Villagers*. Glencoe, Ill: Free Press.

Granovetter M (1973). The strength of weak ties. *Am J Sociol* 78: 1360–1380.

Hillery J (1955). Definitions of community: Areas of agreement. *Rural Sociol* 20: 111–125.

Kelley P, Pebody R, et al. (1996). *How Far Will You Go? A Survey of London Gay Men's Migration and Mobility*. London: GMFA.

Kramer J (1995). Bachelor farmers and spinsters: Gay and lesbian identities and communities in rural North Dakota. In Bell D and Valentine G, eds.: *Mapping Desire: Geographies of Sexualities*. London: Routledge, pp. 200–213.

Laumann EO (1973). *Bonds of Pluralism*. New York: Wiley.

Liebow E (1967). *Talley's Corner: A Study of Negro Streetcorner Men*. Boston: Little Brown.

Massey D and Denton N (1993). *American Apartheid: Segregation and the Making of the Underclass*. Cambridge, Mass: Harvard University Press.

Newman KS (1999). *No Shame in My Game*. New York: Russell Sage Foundation.

Oliver M (1988). The urban black community as network: Towards a network perspective. *Sociol Quart* 24: 623–645.

Portes A (1998). Social capital: Its origin and applications in modern sociology. *Annual Review of Sociology* 24: 1–24.

Rothenberg T (1995). "And she told two friends": Lesbians creating urban social space. In Bell D and Valentine G, eds.: *Mapping Desire: Geographies of Sexualities*. London: Routledge, 165–181.

Sampson R (1988). Local friendship ties and community attachment in mass society: A multilevel systematic model. *Am Sociol Rev* 53: 766–779.

Stack C (1974). *All Our Kin: Strategies for Survival in a Black Community.* New York: Harper & Row.

Valentine G (1993). Desperately seeking Susan: A geography of lesbian friendships. *Area 25* 1–15.

Valentine G (1995). Out and about: Geographies of lesbian landscapes. *J Urban Regional Res* 19: 96–112.

Wellman B (1979). The community question: The intimate networks of East Yorker. *Am J Sociol* 84: 1201–1231.

Wellman B (1988). The community question re-evaluated. In Smith MP, ed.: *Power, Community and the City.* New Brunswick, NJ: Transaction Publishers, pp. 81–107.

Wellman B, Wong RYL, Tindall D, Nazer N (1997). A decade of network change: Turnover, persistence and stability in personal communities. *Social Networks* 19(1): 27–50.

Wellman B and Leighton B (1979). Networks, neighborhoods and communities. *Urban Affairs Quart* 14: 363–390.

Weston K (1995). Get thee to a big city: Sexual imaginary and the great gay migration. *GLQ: A Journal of Lesbian and Gay Studies* 2(3): 253–277.

Whittle S (1994). Consuming differences: The collaboration of the gay body with the cultural state. In Whittle S, ed.: *The Margins of the City: Gay Men's Urban Lives.* Aldershot: Ashgate Publishing, pp. 27–41.

Wilson W (1996). *When Work Disappears: The World of the Urban Poor.* New York: Vintage Books.

Wirth L (1938). Urbanism as a Way of Life. *Am J Sociol* 44(1): 1–24.

Young M and Willmott P (1986). *Family and Kinship in East London,* rev. ed. Harmondsworth: Penguin.

14

Neighborhoods, Aging, and Functional Limitations

Thomas A. Glass
Jennifer L. Balfour

Why Study Neighborhoods and Aging?

Thousands of years before the appearance of modern physicians, medicines, hospitals, schools of public health, or even written language and complex society, humans relied on local kinship-based forms of social organization as the primary survival resource. Evolutionary forces that selected humans for a long postreproductive life span suggest the possibility that the integration of older persons within the social fabric of the larger community is an essential (and potentially biologically programmed) human propensity and need (Davis and Daly, 1997). Evolutionary biologists argue that transmission of knowledge from grandparents to progeny (Lewis, 1999) and intergenerational food sharing (Hawkes et al., 1998, p. 1336) may have served as driving forces for extending human longevity.

One implication of these arguments is that humans are subject to evolutionary forces that have selected for the importance of geographically local forms of social organization. The residential neighborhood represents a modern analogue, to the ancient tribal landscapes in which humans evolved. This adds to the potential relevance of studying neighborhood influences on the health of older adults. The social and physical characteristics of neighborhoods may determine not only whether seniors remain living in the community, but the continuing presence of older persons within neighborhoods may have implications for all residents.

From a demographic point of view, significant social transformation will be required for societies to adjust to the inevitability of population aging. Dramatic increases in the percentage of persons over 65, along with continuing increases in life expectancy, will create substantial demographic, political, and cultural pressures on existing institutions. While infectious disease preoccupied public health at the beginning and end of the twentieth century, the dominant epidemics of the twenty-first century are likely to be dementia and functional disability—both chronic, progressively degenerative, complex diseases of late life. While numerous risk factors have been identified for physical disability (including comorbid conditions, inactivity, social isolation, lack of access to care, poverty, and several poor health habits), all of these factors have been explored almost exclusively at the individual level (Stuck et al., 1999). A similar statement can be made about cognitive function and physical health more broadly.

THE QUESTION OF DIFFERENTIAL VULNERABILITY

One important question is whether aging is accompanied by increasing vulnerability to the deleterious effects of *bad* neighborhoods or by increasing needs for compensatory services and resources. This is important for deciding whether the intersection of aging and neighborhood effects is of special significance. If older persons become increasingly vulnerable to the effects of their neighborhood environments, then they are an especially appealing group in which to study neighborhood effects. Evidence of increased vulnerability comes from several quarters. First, older adults have a longer duration of exposure to potentially unhealthy environments compared to younger adults (Elreedy et al., 1999). Second, the impact of exposure to poor environmental contexts may be more severe for older adults owing to increased biological and psychological vulnerability with age (Lawton, 1977; House and Robbins, 1983; Rodin, 1986). Changes in physical and cognitive capacity associated with normal aging or age-related diseases may reduce an individual's competence, exacerbate barriers to service use, and increase vulnerability to environmental stresses. For example, Carp (1986) showed increased sensitivity to physical barriers in the environment among older adults with mobility impairments. In their study of the presence of in-home environmental hazards, Gill and colleagues (1999) found a high prevalence of "significant environmental hazards" among community-dwelling seniors; unsafe conditions were no less common in the homes of disabled persons, who have less ability to cope safely with these hazards.

Changes in cognitive capacity may also pose barriers to services and may increase vulnerability to environmental stress. In an experimental study Lipman (1991) showed that older persons have more difficulty recognizing landmarks and organizing travel routes within their own neighborhoods. A subsequent study by Simon (1992) supports the view that changes in cognition and spatial organization lead to lower levels of service use and a diminished life-space diameter. These age-related changes are likely to make seniors more vulnerable to the effects of environmental change or deterioration. Older persons demonstrate increased rates of hearing impairment, cognitive impairment, and depression in response to noise and other environmental stresses (Roberts et al., 1997). Several studies have also shown that residential instability, which can be caused by neighborhood factors, is especially stressful for older persons (Schulz and Brenner, 1977; Colsher and Wallace, 1990; Armer, 1993).

A third reason that neighborhoods and home environments may be more critical for older persons compared to younger is the changing pattern of spatial use (Lawton et al., 1980; Carp, 1986; Ward et al., 1988; LaGory and Fitzpatrick, 1992). Whereas younger adults may be exposed to many contexts, including work, community, and recreation, older adults often experience their residential communities as the most salient environmental context (Lawton, 1977). As the spatial area of resource use diminishes with age, the resources available within the immediate community become increasingly important (Bourg, 1975; Cantor, 1975; Regnier, 1974, 1997). Finally, because the social networks of older persons often shrink because of the deaths of spouses, family, and friends and the relocation of children, older persons rely more heavily on access to community sources of integration, such as senior centers (Miner et al., 1993) and neighbors (Bohland and Davis, 1979). As reflected in a recent editorial in the *American Journal of Public Health* by Satariano (1997), there is a growing recognition that we must turn our attention to features of the social and physical environment to better understand how physical and mental disability is both promoted and prevented. In summary, the dominant public health crises of the next century will require us to go beyond people to examine the role of places.

Toward that end, the goals of this chapter are

- to selectively review existing literature on both outcomes and mechanisms,
- to provide a conceptual framework for understanding the role of neighborhoods in aging,
- to elucidate the primary domains of neighborhood influence and the associated mechanisms or pathways through which they operate,
- to highlight several important methodological challenges associated with this line of inquiry, and
- to propose new lines of research as well as several important public policy implications.

SELECTED REVIEW OF THE LITERATURE

Before proposing a conceptual and causal model to motivate future research, a brief and selective review of existing studies of neighborhood effects on the health and well-being of older persons will be presented.

Neighborhoods and Mortality

To date at least eight prospective contextual analyses of neighborhood effects on mortality have been done. For our purposes we consider only those studies that examine contextual effects on mortality in older persons. As will become apparent, contrary to the hypothesis of increasing vulnerability with old age, neighborhood effects on all-cause mortality appear to weaken late in life. Waitzman and Smith (1998) carried out a multilevel study of 10,101 adults in the 1971 to 1974 wave of the National Health and Nutritional Examination Survey (NHANES I). They examined whether persons in two age categories (25–54 and >54 years) living in federally designated poverty areas (based on U.S. Census figures) had elevated risk of mortality. Numerous individual-level covariates were considered, including household income, years of formal education, smoking, drinking, exercise, and marital status. While a significant contextual effect (net of individual characteristics) was found on all-cause mortality in the younger age group (*RR* of 1.78; 95% *CI* of 1.33–2.38), no significant excess risk of death was found for older subjects.

Anderson and colleagues (1997) linked data from the National Longitudinal Mortality Study to census tract information for 239,187 persons to assess eleven-year mortality risk among black and white men and women associated with median census tract income adjusted for individual family income. Again, while area effects on mortality were found for younger persons, among persons age 65 years or greater only individual family income was associated with mortality, and only for white men. Similar findings were observed in an analysis of black–white differences in mortality by census tract (LeClere et al., 1997).

In a seminal study Haan and colleagues (1987) found that residence in a poverty area was associated with nine-year risk of all-cause mortality after adjustment for age, sex, race, individual markers of socioeconomic status (SES), and baseline health. However, when mortality rates were examined stratified by age, sex, and racial group, mortality rate differentials were highest between the ages of 45 and 64. After age 65 mortality rates among poverty area residents were not higher than those of non–poverty-area residents.

There are several potential explanations for the observed deterioration of neighborhood influences on mortality at the end of the life course. The most obvious reason is selective mortality. In the poorest, most at-risk neighborhoods the force of mortality is likely to play itself out comparatively early in the life course. Those who survive past age 65 in high-risk neighborhoods are likely to be the "hearty" survivors who do not reflect general population patterns. A second reason for the insensitivity of mortality outcomes to contextual effects may have to do with the relative ubiquity of the outcome itself. That is, risk factors that are clearly observed for less-common outcomes are often more difficult to detect in populations in which the outcome of interest is highly prevalent. Studies of older persons often fail to find associations among risk factors that are firmly established in younger populations because of the shear frequency of mortal outcomes (Kaplan et al., 1999). High blood pressure and cholesterol are examples (Krumholz et al., 1994). Third, existing studies of area-based measures of SES and mortality have used inadequate measures. Robert (1996) has shown that when measures of wealth (rather than just income) are included, area differences in mortality can be seen until at least age 85. For a variety of reasons, mortality may not be the best outcome to use to study the impact of residential neighborhood on aging, or, perhaps, next-generation measures of neighborhood characteristics with improved reliability and sensitivity will paint a clearer picture of this complex association.

Neighborhood Effects on Disability and Physical Functioning

To date only a small number of studies have examined the influence of residential neighborhood on functioning and risk of disability among older persons. Studies of this kind are sorely needed (see the editorial by Satariano, 1997). In a recent review of longitudinal studies of risk factors for disability, Stuck and colleagues (1999) found the following risk factors for functional status decline (in alphabetical order): cognitive impairment, depression, disease burden (comorbidity), increased and decreased body mass index, lower extremity functional limitation, low frequency of social contacts, low level of physical activity, no alcohol use compared to moderate use, poor self-perceived health, smoking, and vision impairment. These authors noted that they could "not find a single study analyzing physical environment as a predictive factor" (p. 461). In short, research on the role of the physical or social environment in the etiology of functional decline is in its infancy. However, the widespread adoption of Verbrugge and Jette's model of the disablement process has been promising (Verbrugge and Jette, 1994). In their model environmental factors can increase the risk of disability directly or can exacerbate the negative impact of other individual-level risk factors.

The prevalence of disability varies across geographic area. A recent study used 1990 census data to examine the geographic distribution of disability among older adults in the United States (Lin, 2000). Using residents of the northeastern United States as the comparison group, white residents of the Deep South (excluding Florida) had a 50% increase in risk of disability, while black residents of any of the southern regions (Deep South, Florida, or southwest central) had a significant 10% increase in risk of disability. The associations remained after adjusting for age, sex, marital status, education, income, source of income, and rural area. It is unknown whether these regional patterns reflect neighborhood differences or patterns existing at higher levels of aggregation.

Characteristics of the area appear to be related to prevalence of disability. Two ecologic studies examined the relationship between census tract characteristics and prevalence of physical disability in selected U.S. counties. After adjusting for age and sex distributions, both studies found that census tract SES was inversely associated with disability prevalence in the general population (Satin and Monetti, 1985) and in the older population (Balfour, 1999). Other factors associated with increased prevalence of physical disability were higher residential instability and, once area SES was accounted for, lower density of housing units (Balfour, 1999).

Several studies by Robert and colleagues are particularly important in showing that comorbidity and health status may be sensitive to environmental context at older ages (Robert et al., 1996; Robert, 1998, 1999). These studies, using data from nationally representative studies, show that community socioeconomic context is associated with self-reported health and chronic disease independently of individual SES and that the effect of community SES on self-assessed health increased with age (Robert and Li, 2001). Two studies examined the association between neighborhood environment and functional status. Robert (1998) found that, after adjusting for individual SES, community SES was not associated with an index of functional disability. In contrast, Balfour and colleagues (under consideration) found a strong relationship between the socioeconomic deprivation of a census tract and the prevalence of disability in mobility and instrumental activities of daily living after adjustment for individual socioeconomic factors and health characteristics.

Studies that have used longitudinal data to examine this question are especially rare. One exception is the work of Balfour and colleagues, who examined the association between negative features of neighborhoods and the health of older adults using data from three studies (Balfour, 1999;

Balfour and Kaplan, 2002). Residence in a multiple-problem neighborhood was found to be associated with incident loss of physical function in all three studies. In these reports a substantial fraction of older adults perceived one or more serious problems in their neighborhoods. Residence in a multiple-problem neighborhood was associated with functional loss and depression independently of individual SES, health status, and health behaviors at baseline, with odds ratios ranging from 1.5 to 2.25. As might be expected, different patterns of effect were observed across neighborhood types: in the urban and dense suburban environment, physical barriers were found to be associated with loss of physical function (adjusted odds ratio $OR_{adj} = 2.28$, 95% $CI = 1.10–4.72$). In wealthy suburban areas resource inadequacy (rather than physical barriers) increased the risk of functional loss ($OR_{adj} = 1.51, 95\% CI = 0.87–2.61$). In small towns the presence of both physical barriers and lack of access to resources were associated with functional loss ($OR_{adj} = 1.87, 95\% CI = 0.82–4.28$). Both neighborhoods with many challenges and barriers as well as neighborhoods lacking services and social stimulation appear to be detrimental. However, these studies were limited by a lack of independent neighborhood assessment and the small number of neighborhood characteristics that were measured.

Neighborhood Effects on Nursing Home Admission

Few studies have sought to examine the effect of neighborhoods on risk of institutionalization. However, it is well recognized that characteristics of the social and physical environment are important determinants of who will require long-term care services (Wolinsky et al., 1992; Freedman, 1993; Freedman et al., 1994). The work of Wolinsky (1993) and Miller and colleagues (1999) has illustrated the complex ways in which residential mobility in late life can be explained in terms of the fit between the environment and the functional capacities of the individual. For both dementia patients and dementia-free controls, housing type is related to the probability of nursing home placement: living in a retirement home, supervised apartment, or assisted living facility increased the likelihood of subsequent institutionalization (Smith et al., 2000). Wolf (1978) showed that ecological features (percentage of residents who were foreign-born and number of available primary care providers) explained half the variance in long-term care use rates in thirty-nine catchment areas in Massachusetts. Finally, using data from the Longitudinal Study on Aging, Coward (1995) found that incontinent seniors residing in less-urbanized and thinly populated areas were more likely to enter a nursing home than were those living in other kinds of residential settings.

Neighborhood Effects on Mental Health

The study of neighborhood influences on mental health dates at least to sociological studies of the classic "Chicago School." For example, early work showed that high rates of mental disorder emerged in the most dilapidated and run-down areas of the city (Faris and Dunham, 1939, as cited in Krause, 1996). Theorists have long suggested that neighborhood deterioration may be especially important for older persons (Carp, 1967). To the extent that neighborhood conditions are stressful or supportive, neighborhoods might be expected to increase or decrease the risk of poor mental health. The evidence is somewhat limited. The best work done in this area is the paper by Roberts and colleagues (1997), who examined risk of major depressive episodes in older persons using data from the 1994 and 1995 cohorts of the Alameda County Study. Neighborhood problems were significant and independent predictors of the risk of a major depressive episode.

Because the study of environmental influences on health has to some extent been housed in the field of environmental psychology, a good deal of literature exists on neighborhood influences on mental health in late life. After surveying the psychological and urban planning literatures, Halpern (1995) concluded that the planned environment may influence the mental health of people of all ages through four channels: (1) stress, (2) social networks and support, (3) social labeling and symbolic effects, and (4) the planning process itself. However, few studies of neighborhoods and mental health use clinical diagnoses or recognized measures of psychological and emotional function. The majority of studies employ generalized measures of well-being, reported satisfaction, or presence/absence of positive and negative life conditions as outcomes. For example, fear of crime is used as an indicator of diminished mental health. While this work underscores the multidimensionality of well-being as a construct, it nevertheless indicates that a rigorous psychiatric epidemiology of neighborhoods is lacking.

Numerous studies exist of housing and neighborhood satisfaction, satisfaction with social network contacts, perceived security, activity participation, and mobility (see Lawton et al., 1975, for a review). Residential satisfaction is often treated as a proxy for general well-being (Carp and Christensen, 1986; Lawton, 1980). While the use of measures of neighborhood satisfaction as a mental health outcome is circular, these studies show that environmental satisfaction measures correlate well with neighborhood conditions measured both subjectively and objectively. The most consistent associations are found using multidimensional scales that are believed to measure neighborhood conditions including SES, safety, aesthetics, reputation, land use, terrain and density, social integration, and service quality. For example, Barresi (1983) studied a national sample of low- and middle-income elderly and found that environmental satisfaction and neighborhood sociability were key determinants of well-being in later life. The field would be strengthened by using standardized measures of mental health and well-being not based on residential or neighborhood satisfaction.

Studying older residents of eighteen small towns in Kansas, Windley and Scheidt (1982) used factor analysis to derive five neighborhood factors: satisfaction with dwelling features, environmental constriction, community satisfaction, community involvement, and community expectations of isolation and withdrawal. They found that perceived environmental constriction was negatively associated with activity and mental health, while community satisfaction and dwelling satisfaction were positively associated with activity and mental health. This finding anticipates a conceptual model that differentiates perceived environmental constriction and satisfaction.

CONCEPTUAL FRAMEWORK: LAWTON'S ECOLOGICAL MODEL OF AGING

Several general models of neighborhood effects on health have helped in the development of this chapter (Mayer and Jencks, 1989; Macintyre et al., 1993; especially Macintyre and Ellaway, 2000). The model presented below draws most heavily on the work of M. Powell Lawton (Lawton and Simon, 1968; Lawton, 1974, 1980, 1983, 1990a, 1990b; Lawton et al., 1973, 1976, 1980), whose impact on the study of ecological factors and aging has been immeasurable. In a series of influential papers Lawton and colleagues explicated their ecological model of aging (hereafter, EMA) (Lawton, 1980; Lawton, 1982; Lawton, 1990; Lawton and Nahemow, 1973; Lawton et al., 1976). The following discussion extends and modifies Lawton's model in the hopes that it might serve as a useful theoretical starting point for future research.

To briefly summarize the model, the EMA is concerned with person–environment fit. Individual behaviors are contingent on the dynamic interplay between the demands of the environment (called press) and the person's ability to deal with that demand (referred to as competence). Lawton makes clear that his model of environment involves "extra-individual" factors related to both physical and social features of the environment. Specific details about the nature of environmental press have not yet been developed. Behavioral competence is the "theoretical upper

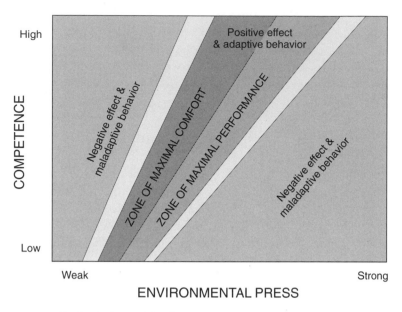

FIGURE 14–1. Ecological model of aging. Source: Adapted from Lawton and Nahemow (1973).

limits of capacity of the individual to function in the areas of biological health, sensation and perception, motor behavior and cognition" (Lawton, 1982, p. 38). Competencies are not directly measured but can be observed indirectly through assessment of multiple items across multiple domains. Much of Lawton's subsequent work sought to develop such measures; the well-known geriatric depression scale (GDS) and the morale scale are by-products.

The EMA is depicted in Figure 14–1 (taken from Lawton et al., 1973). As shown, environmental press can be positive, negative, or neutral. When competence and press are in balance, the resulting behavior is adaptive, resulting in positive well-being. If, however, either component is out of balance, maladaptive behavior results. An important feature of the model is that environments can be harmful both because they are overly demanding or because they demand too little. When competence far outstrips press, boredom and atrophy occur; when press exceeds competence, withdrawal and isolation occur. Both maladaptions can therefore lead to increased risk of disability and deterioration. This is an especially important insight for gerontology, the "use-it-or-lose-it" hypothesis. Environmental perspectives such as the EMA help to generate testable hypotheses about the conditions under which an individual might "use" or "lose."

The EMA is, however, not without limitations. It has been applied rather narrowly to examine residential satisfaction and general well-being but has rarely been used to study physical health. The model has proven to be difficult to operationalize in epidemiologic research. It is unclear how person–environment fit operates across time. Another limitation is the absence of a clear elaboration of pathways through which neighborhood characteristics lead to increased or deceased risk of adverse health. The model is also difficult to operationalize because the measurement of environmental press has not been adequately refined. For this reason the EMA has been narrowly applied to studies of nursing homes and retirement communities. Finally, the EMA underemphasizes the inverse of environmental press. Features of the environment that are conducive to functioning and to high levels of competence (or, in our terms, that *buoy* behavioral competence) may be as important as those features of the environment that exert demands. Several extensions and modifications of Lawton's model have been proposed by Wister (1989) and Brown (1995), although neither model addresses these issues sufficiently. In what follows, we attempt to address such limitations by extending the EMA, with special attention to several epidemiologic considerations: what are the etiologic pathways and how can sources of environmental press and buoy be classified.

Extension of the Ecological Model of Aging to Focus on Predictors of Disability

Our extension of the EMA is depicted in Figure 14–2 as a causal pathway (to be read temporally and causally from left to right). The model comprises five components, beginning with four specific dimensions of neighborhoods that are hypothesized to condition and shape the degree of person–environment fit (PEF) through the channels listed in the boxes. The resulting balance between personal competencies and environmental press/buoy is, in turn, hypothesized to alter the probability that adaptive or maladaptive behavioral responses will be chosen. These behavioral responses then lead to health and functional outcomes through four subpathways. Finally, a set of exacerbating factors can alter the causal process either by increasing the downward balance of PEF or by altering patterns of behavioral response. Next, each of these components is described in greater detail.

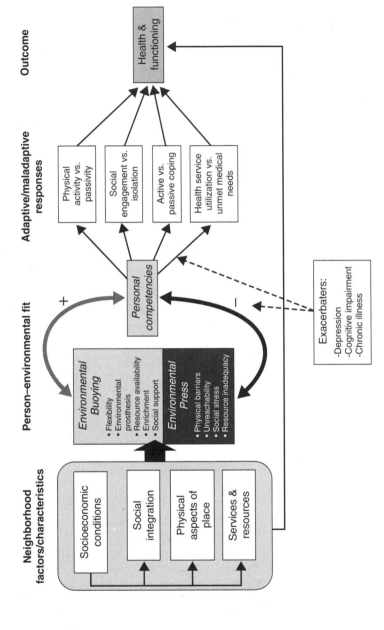

FIGURE 14–2. Causal model of neighborhood effects on aging (an extension of the EMA).

DOMAINS OF NEIGHBORHOOD INFLUENCE ON AGING

Borrowing from work that appears in this volume (see Chapters 1 and 2) and elsewhere (Macintyre et al., 1993), four dimensions of neighborhoods were selected to represent potentially independent sources of influence on the aging process. These four dimensions include socioeconomic conditions, social integration, physical aspects of place, and available services and resources. These are also neighborhood domains that are potentially modifiable and thus may constitute reasonable targets for intervention.

Socioeconomic Conditions

A substantial body of literature has documented the association between the socioeconomic character of places and the health and well-being of older adults (Chapman and Beaudet, 1983; Satin et al., 1985; Anderson et al., 1997; Diez-Roux et al., 1997; LeClere et al., 1998; Robert, 1998; Balfour and Kaplan, 2002; Robert et al., in press). Area poverty and deprivation have proven to be moderately robust risk factors, independent of the individuals who live in those areas. Indeed, in many studies socioeconomic factors are the only variables that are measured and examined. A goal in developing the model presented in this chapter is to begin to "unpack" this association by explicating pathways or channels through which socioeconomic conditions may operate. While socioeconomic factors may drive the availability of services and resources, the quality of the physical environment, and the levels of social integration, it is equally possible that these dimensions function independently of one another and from general socioeconomic characteristics.

The left-most portion of the model includes arrows that lead from socioeconomic conditions to the three other dimensions in recognition of the importance of the role of socioeconomic factors, along with the possibility that these factors may be partially independent. For example, many poor neighborhoods are tightly integrated socially (Portes, 2000). Examples exist of suburban neighborhoods where services and resources are quite meager. A major challenge for research on neighborhoods and health is to move beyond classifying neighborhoods solely on the basis of poverty and deprivation.

Neighborhood Social Integration

The study of how the social organization of neighborhoods affects residents is among the oldest and most deeply rooted subjects in social science. Macro-level theorists such as Durkheim (Durkheim, 1947, 1951) and Tonnies (1887/1963) treated entire nations as if they were *super-neighborhoods*. The so-called Chicago studies of neighborhood life in the 1930s and 1940s established a pragmatic brand of American sociology that was concerned with the problem of social integration at a smaller level (Faris et al., 1939). The Chicago Area Project is the latest incarnation of this tradition (Earls and Buka, 1997; Sampson, Raudenbush, Earls, 1997). The central insight that links these diverse studies is based on the work of Durkheim.

In his classic study *Suicide: A Study in Sociology* (1951) Durkheim noted the persistent pattern of suicide in certain areas and social groups over time. He argued that individuals are bonded to society by two forms of integration: attachment and regulation. Attachment is the extent to which an individual maintains ties with members of the society; regulation is the extent to which a society's values, beliefs, and norms control individual behavior (Turner, Beeghley, Powers, 1989). By studying these patterns of social integration, Durkheim was able to explain area-based variations in suicide rates. (To be precise, Durkheim identifies four forms of suicide: egoistic, altruistic, anomic, and fatalistic; only two are explained in terms of differential levels of social integration.) Thus, Catholic countries have lower suicide rates according to Durkheim's theory because the bonds that tie individuals to the group are tighter than in non-Catholic countries. The central insight that grows from the Durkheimian tradition is that places can be characterized according to varying degrees and types of social integration. The extent to which social organization is tight or loose determines the moral boundedness of persons who reside in that place. This, in turn, may affect the health and well-being of residents both directly and indirectly. Below, we highlight several features of social organization that have appeared in the literature. Three aspects of social integration are briefly discussed: social capital, fear and crime, and age concentration.

Social capital
The concept of social capital has been discussed elsewhere in this volume (see especially Chapters 1 and 6). To date, no studies have examined the effect of neighborhood social capital among older adults. However, the results of a study by Greenberg and colleagues (1997) suggests that higher levels of social capital are related to residents' levels of trust, residential stability, and willingness and ability to exercise control in their neighborhood. If social capital can be defined as a neighborhood high in trust, stability, and willingness and ability to exercise control in the neighborhood, many reasons exist to suppose a neighborhood high in social capital might be an environment low in environmental press and high in environmental buoying. The benefits of social capital for older persons may

accrue from the willingness of other residents to offer assistance to frail neighbors, from a greater feeling of security in such a neighborhood, or from increased opportunities for social activity and engagement with neighbors, as well as from the benefits of being in a community able to organize for what it needs.

Fear and crime

Older persons appear to be more fearful of neighborhood conditions in general than are young persons, although some interesting patterns emerge (Lebowitz, 1975). A study by Jeffords (1983) indicates that while older persons are more fearful of walking alone in their neighborhoods, they are actually less fearful alone in their homes than are younger adults. Age differences in reporting fear of crime diminish when the fear is warranted. In high-crime neighborhoods, older and younger adults report similarly high levels of fear (Baumer, 1985; Maxfield, 1984).

Evidence of an association between fear of crime and health outcomes is sparse. Fear of crime has been linked to psychological well-being in studies of older people residing in public housing (Lawton and Yaffe, 1980). Among a sample of low-income urban blacks aged 62 and older, fear of crime was associated with lower subjective well-being and limited mobility but was unrelated to self-reported health status (Bazargan, 1994). While the mechanisms through which crime and fear of crime might be related to health are unclear, Krause (1993) tested a plausible model and found that living in deteriorated neighborhoods tended to promote distrust of others and that older adults who were more distrustful of others tended to be more socially isolated. The negative health consequences of social isolation have been well documented (House et al., 1982, 1988; Berkman and Glass, 2000).

In addition to social capital and fear of crime, a general sense of neighborhood safety may be related to older adult health by influencing patterns of physical activity and exercise. Results from the Behavioral Risk Factor Surveillance System suggest that perceptions of neighborhood safety are strongly associated with level of physical activity (Anonymous, 1999). Differences in physical inactivity across levels of perceived neighborhood safety were especially pronounced among people aged 65 and older. Physical inactivity increased from 38.6% among older participants who rated their neighborhoods as "extremely safe" to 63.1% among older participants who rated their neighborhoods as "not at all safe."

Age concentration

On the one hand, a high older age concentration at the neighborhood level may be a marker for the presence of services or the availability of dense social support networks. This was the case in at least one qualitative study, in which the oldest members of a tightly knit neighborhood took care of one another on a daily basis (Rosel, 1983). Sherman (1985) studied patterns of service use and attitudes toward aging in more than 1,100 seniors in neighborhoods of high, moderate, and low older age concentration and found that living in areas with a high concentration of seniors was associated with increased knowledge of and access to services and persons (although older age concentration was not associated with attitudes toward the aged, as had been expected). On the other hand, some studies have suggested that high older age concentration is negatively associated with well-being (Usui and Keil, 1987). It is possible that having many neighbors who may need support is perceived by some as burdensome.

Physical Aspects of Neighborhoods

Studies of the impact of physical conditions on health and well-being in the elderly have tended to emphasize the physical deterioration of housing. For example, Krause (1996) showed declines in the self-assessed health of older adults residing in deteriorated neighborhoods compared to those living in neighborhoods that were better maintained. Neighborhood deterioration was measured by interviewer assessments of respondents dwellings, and of neighborhood homes, streets, sidewalks, and yards.

The physical conditions of neighborhoods may also affect health through differential exposure to environmental toxins. In a recent example data from the Normative Aging Study showed that older persons living in low-education neighborhoods had higher average tibia lead levels (a sensitive measure of the cumulative body burden of lead) compared with those living in a more-educated area (Elreedy et al., 1999). This association held only for men who themselves had lower levels of education.

The literature on aging shows a general pattern of increasing vulnerability with age to negative features of the environment. This is perhaps nowhere clearer than in studies of frail elders. Mild to moderate levels of physical disability leave seniors more vulnerable to adverse physical surroundings. Guralnik (1996) notes that "Physical disability is associated with restrictions that affect all aspects of daily life." This leads, among other things, to a constriction of life-space diameter (or the range of one's daily functional activities). In a study of participants in the Women's Health and Aging Study (WHAS), among the one-third most disabled women older than 65, 34% did not leave their neighborhood in a typical week, and 15% did not leave their home (Simonsick et al., 1995).

Several studies suggest that loud noise, such as from construction and machinery, reduces altruistic and helping behavior (Mathews and

Canon, 1975; Page, 1977; Cohen and Weinstein, 1981; Moser, 1988). Noise may also explain lower levels of social interaction on busy streets (Appleyard and Lintell, 1972; Korte et al., 1975). High noise levels may also be associated with increased levels of cardiovascular stress (Cohen et al., 1981). In their study of 3,000 elderly tenants of 153 planned housing environments, Lawton and colleagues (1980) found that quiet neighborhoods were associated with a more active lifestyle and greater well-being. While many of these studies did not focus on older residents, studies in general support the inference that a neighborhood with high noise levels may be more isolating and less supportive of its residents. These studies also demonstrate how poor physical conditions affect levels of social integration.

Services and Resources

Adults of all ages, including older adults, report that access to resources and services is a vital component of the ideal neighborhood. Two studies have examined age variation in features of neighborhoods perceived to be most important. Blake (1975) found that eleven features of the neighborhood factored into three dimensions: access to high-quality and varied goods and services (such as medical care, jobs, and stores); relationships with others; and access to sources of personal development such as outdoor recreation, entertainment, and clubs. Carp and Carp (1982) found that access to resources and services, including stores, restaurants, and public transportation, was among the top three features of an ideal neighborhood among adults aged 25 and older. In both studies adults of all ages seemed to share the same concept of a desirable living environment. While some differences were seen in how younger vs. older adults ranked these attributes in absolute terms, the relative rankings by age group were similar, leading to the conclusion that older and younger people share a recognition of community attributes necessary for the common good. In the study by Carp and Carp, there were some significant differences in neighborhood attributes valued by older and younger adults. For example, younger adults rated distance to schools, jobs, and the freeway as more important than did older people, while older people rated distance to a bus stop as more important. However, for other services, such as distance to food shopping, access to rapid transit, and good walking conditions, few age differences were found. Access to high-quality services, both necessary and recreational, was an important component of the ideal neighborhood for all adults.

Centrality of location (a proxy for access to services) measured as nearness to city center was positively associated with well-being, defined as active and autonomous use of time, space, and social networks (Carp,

1975). Conversely, inaccessibility to services and lack of human contact appeared to be reasons elders give for wanting to move out of a neighborhood (Brody, 1979). Summarizing the body of literature on service proximity, Lawton (1977) concluded: "From the fairly large body of material on resource-use by the elderly, the conclusion is that the shorter the distance between a subject and a resource, the greater the likelihood that he will use it" (page 278).

Proximity to resources and services may be more important to older persons with diminished physical competency, and frail older persons may be less likely to travel across town or to adjacent neighborhoods to shop for groceries. Among women aged 60 and older living alone, more than half reported a desire to have services located within walking distance or within their own block (Carp et al., 1982). Desired services included grocery stores, pharmacies, doctors' offices, banks, bus stops, places of worship, libraries, restaurants, beauty shops, a senior center, a nutrition program for the elderly, and a fire station. The emphasis on proximity is interesting in light of the potentially negative consequences of having services close by (such as increased traffic flow, noise, and presence of strangers). Nevertheless, the ideal neighborhood for women older than 60 living alone was one rich in services.

Few studies have examined receipt of services by older adults directly. In one exception Frongillo (1992) found that older persons who lived farther from services were more likely to go one or more days without eating. Talbot and Kaplan (1991) found that proximity to well-maintained parks and other green spaces was associated with significantly higher levels of life satisfaction among older residents.

PERSON–ENVIRONMENT FIT

In the proposed model depicted in Figure 14–2, Lawton's ideas on the importance of a balance between features of the environment and individual behavioral competence is retained. To this basic scheme an additional component has been added. In Figure 14–2, environment *buoys* competence as well as challenges it. In addition to the demand characteristics of neighborhoods, environmental factors may support and reinforce competence, may facilitate adaptation, and may offer what Kleemeier (1959) has called "environmental prosthesis." The addition of this component changes the dynamic balance at the heart of the Lawton model by recognizing the dual effect of the neighborhood environment. In what follows several of the general ways that neighborhoods both press and buoy are addressed.

The anatomy of environmental press has not been thoroughly elaborated. In the proposed model (and based on the literature reviewed above) four features of the neighborhood environment are hypothesized to exert press on residents. These include physical barriers, inaccessibility of services and amenities, social stress, and resource inadequacy. Along with these sources of press are features of neighborhoods that buoy (or up-regulate) the person–environment fit (PEF) balance. These include environmental flexibility, environmental prosthesis, resource availability, personal growth and enrichment through opportunities for meaningful social engagement, and social support.

A concrete example may be useful in illustrating these points. Consider an elderly person who wishes to shop for food, a basic instrumental activity of daily living. Food shopping is an especially useful example because it involves multiple domains of function (lower extremity, upper extremity, mobility, and cognition) and because it is a core self-care task that has implications for autonomy and functional independence. As our fictitious senior leaves the safety of her home, she must confront physical barriers and obstacles. How far is the food store? How wide and accommodating are the sidewalks? Do curbs and other changes in the landscape make walking difficult? What is the quality of the lighting? Are there traffic, noise, or distracting environmental features that impede her progress?

In addition to physical barriers, the environment may harbor social stressors. How comfortable does the shopper feel? What is the level of receptivity to the presence of an older person? How safe or threatening is the area? Are there drug deals or other social activities in progress that make her feel ill at ease? Conversely, the social conditions in a neighborhood may buoy the shopper's confidence. Perhaps strangers are friendly and offer to help. Do people on the street know the person and inquire as to her welfare? Does she encounter an environment that reinforces her resolve to get to the food store even if she is having a "bad day"?

Once she reaches the food store, what does she encounter? Perhaps the food she wished to buy is of poor quality, expensive, or absent. Neighborhoods have been shown to vary in the extent to which they offer residents fresh fruits and vegetables and other healthy foods (Sooman et al., 1993). If hers did not, she might have traveled farther, an adaptive strategy that would be likely for a person with high behavioral competence (absence of frailty or mobility dysfunction) but unavailable to someone who was impaired in some way. At the food store there may be opportunities to interact socially with individuals and the community. She may encounter a friendly employee or a bulletin board that offers opportunities for personal growth and enrichment such as upcoming cultural events or volunteer opportunities.

Consistent with Lawton's model, the level of competence of the subject with respect to balance, gait, and mobility must be taken into account. If our imaginary person has had a stroke, uses a cane, requires a wheelchair, or is otherwise limited, each of the above environmental challenges exacts a heavier toll. In short, the subject's behavior will be shaped by the balance of environmental challenge and support in the context of that person's level of functional competence. If some critical threshold (or "tipping point") is exceeded, she may choose to stay home or to turn to family or friends to do her shopping, or she may rely on more formal services such as meals-on-wheels. To the extent that her basic competence decreases because of infirmity, or age-related losses in functional reserve, the impact of the neighborhood may increase. With each additional loss of competence, the constraining or supportive features of her surroundings may make a larger and larger difference in her ability to function.

ADAPTIVE VERSUS MALADAPTIVE BEHAVIORAL RESPONSES

Another feature of the model depicted in Figure 14–2 is that four primary behavioral response options are specified. These responses may be adaptive or maladaptive. It is through these pathways that the balance of press, buoy, and competence get *into the body* to affect functioning and health. Each set of behavioral responses represents a different domain: physical, cognitive, psychological, and social. Each implies a specific pathway through which either deterioration in function or maintenance of function can occur. The choice of adaptive versus maladaptive behavioral responses is hypothesized to depend on the balance between the components of the PEF section that lies to the left.

Below we develop an example of how the model functions at this stage through the variation that can be seen in adaptive compared to maladaptive behavioral responses involving activity versus passivity. This refers to the degree to which multiple physiological and cognitive systems are activated. To return to our earlier example, an adaptive behavioral response would be maintenance of a high level of physical and cognitive activity associated with shopping, social engagement, and other daily tasks. In turn, this pattern of activity would result in greater musculoskeletal and cardiovascular fitness (Tager et al., 1998; Broughton and Taylor, 1991; Astrand, 1992; De Backer et al., 1981). All systems of the body appear to benefit from continuous activity at the physiological level. On the other hand, if environmental press exceeds the individual's level of competence, then the resulting behavioral response may be maladaptive. Our senior may stay home and limit the extent and range of her activity. This, in turn, would result in atrophy, sarcopenia, and, eventually, elevated risk of disability (Buchner and Wagner, 1992; Fiatarone and Evans, 1993; Tennstedt and McKinlay, 1994; Walston and Fried, 1999). In this way, the seminal idea of "use-it-or-lose-it" can be seen within the context of neighborhood environments that determine, in part, which of the two outcomes is likely to occur.

PROBLEMS IN THE STUDY OF NEIGHBORHOOD EFFECTS ON ELDERLY PERSONS

In the study of neighborhood effects on late life, the standard conceptual difficulties associated with measuring neighborhoods certainly apply and are well documented elsewhere in this book. Several additional issues should be raised. Interstate migration patterns have created new forms of social organization in Sunbelt retirement communities. It is not yet clear whether these new forms of social organization are qualitatively similar to or different from the neighborhoods from which many of these migrants came. A cultural geographer who studied Sun City, Arizona, found that this new retirement community differs in important ways from more traditional neighborhoods and is "characterized by increased emphasis on surveillance, security, simulations, consumerism, and fragmentation of identities, in both life courses and landscapes" (Laws, 1995). Retirement communities are increasingly populated by relatively homogeneous groups of seniors who are disproportionately affluent, nondisabled, and consumeristic about services and resources. In addition, those who migrate to retirement communities may reflect a relative lack of social integration into their neighborhoods of origin. For example, Silverstein and Zablotsky (1996) found that migration to retirement communities is more likely among elderly persons who live alone and among those whose children do not live nearby.

Another general issue is the limitations associated with the use of unidimensional measures of neighborhoods, which fail to capture the complexity described in the model above. Great care must be taken when considering the social consequences of poverty when poverty is all that is assessed. There is a tendency to assume that impoverished areas are necessarily socially disorganized or depleted of social capital. In his presidential address to the American Sociological Association, Portes called this "mythical reasoning" (Portes, 2000). A rich tradition in sociology has shown that poor urban areas can be tightly integrated, with extensive patterns of social network integration and resource sharing (Whyte, 1943; Stack, 1974). Nevertheless, persons living in impoverished areas appear to have social contacts that are limited or constrained in their scope and capacity to mobilize resources effectively (Fernandez-Kelly, 1995).

Migration and Drift

Among the most serious challenges in studying area-based effects in late life is the social patterning of residential migration. Systematic patterns of late-life migration can lead to misclassification of exposure, which severely limits a researcher's ability to detect associations. For example, a consistent finding of studies of elderly persons is that newly disabled seniors tend to relocate (often great distances) to be near adult children who are in the best position to provide care (Silverstein and Angelelli, 1998). However, if newly disabled persons are more likely to migrate out of the neighborhoods under study, any neighborhood effects on disability risk will be obscured. The severity of this problem may differ according to other factors, such as poverty. South (1997) observed that older adults who reside in poor neighborhoods are much less likely to move to a nonpoor neighborhood than are younger adults, regardless of health status.

Demographers have shown that the dominant pattern of migration for persons aged 60 and older is from metropolitan to nonmetropolitan areas (Longino, 1982), suggesting that the stresses of urban life trigger decisions to relocate. Many older persons move as their competence decreases (as would be predicted by our extension of the EMA). On the other hand, using data from the American Housing Survey, Clark (1990) found that economic factors appear to play an equally important role in predicting residential mobility in seniors. In summary, researchers must pay close attention to the potential role of migration and duration of exposure to ensure that important associations are not underappreciated or obscured.

Do Area Effects Carry Over to Suburban and Rural Areas?

The majority of research on neighborhood influences on aging has been undertaken in urban areas. With the exception of a small number of studies (including the studies by Balfour, 1999, mentioned earlier, and Windley et al., 1982), very little is known about whether associations found in urban areas can be found in suburban and rural communities. At least one study of elderly residents in four small towns in Kansas suggests that economic threats to small-town life are particularly stressful to older residents, who are often highly invested in those towns (Norris-Baker and Scheidt, 1994).

The Proximity Problem

In a recent letter to the editor of the *American Journal of Epidemiology* regarding Yen and Kaplan's (1999) study of neighborhood social environment and mortality, Hook (2000) commented on the reported association between proximity to presumably health-related services (such as pharmacies and doctors' offices) and health outcomes. He asked, "why does proximity (a presumed measure of access) to, say, a barbershop measure anything at all directly pertinent to health?" (p. 1132). Arguments based on proximity to potentially beneficial services are problematic. Given our highly mobile society, it is possible for people to go several neighborhoods away in search of better services. How do we distinguish between services and facilities that might reasonably be expected to directly affect health (such as clinics and emergency rooms), as opposed to those that may be related only tangentially to health (such as barbershops)? When the number of bars, grocery stores, and gun dealers in a neighborhood is measured, it is not obvious what exactly is being measuring or what these may be indirect proxies for. Hook's question is a fair one that invites researchers to think more clearly about what is being measured. However, this argument demonstrates the potential utility of the model presented above. According to that model, the extent to which proximity to valued services is related to activity level and access to resources will depend on the individual's competencies and the supportiveness of the neighborhood. From these arguments, proximity of services would be hypothesized to be more relevant for seniors with mobility impairment. This is why older populations may be an especially important group for the study of area-based health effects.

Conclusion and Policy Implications

The goal of this chapter has been to make a case for the importance of studying neighborhood effects on functional limitations in late life. We have selectively reviewed existing literature and proposed a theoretical model to guide future research on the health effects of neighborhoods on older persons. In conclusion, several public policy issues are relevant. The twenty-first century will bring profound and transformative changes in the population age structure of all nations, including those in the developing world. In the coming decades upwards of one-fifth to one-quarter of the U.S. population will be age 65 or older. Even without the potential benefits of the genetic revolution, we are quickly becoming an older society. The cutting edge of these changes can be seen in countries like Italy, where unprecedented low birthrates and longer life expectancy have combined to create a demographic and political climate that is new and volatile (Golini and Lori, 1990; Havlik, 1993), yet, systems of social welfare and health care (to say nothing of the design of neighborhoods) have failed to keep pace with these demographic changes. Riley has referred to this as "structural lag" (Riley and Riley, 1994). A major policy challenge for the coming decades will be whether developed nations will begin to address these problems.

Among the most significant aspects of structural lag is the failure adequately to consider the needs of an increasingly older population in the design of residential neighborhoods. The dominant model of urban landscape architecture has been suburban sprawl and deurbanization. Where urban redevelopment has occurred, the dominant pattern in many cities has been "gentrification" involving high concentrations of young, single, affluent professionals displacing previously established neighborhoods, often leading to the displacement of long-time older residents (Eckert, 1979; Henig, 1981). The "Sun City" model has evolved in the retirement ghettos of the South and Southwest. This postmodern model of a neighborhood appears to meet the needs of some, but not all, seniors. Given the inevitable increase in the age of retirement that likely will be induced by population aging, along with the clear desire of older persons to remain productive and socially engaged, a model of retirement as a permanent sun-drenched vacation will not be adequate in the coming century.

In the 1980s Pavan (1987) argued that the needs of an aging society would best be met by small towns of compact size and structure permitting concentration of services to shore up the mobility of an increasingly frail urban population. This prescription is in marked contrast to the suburban sprawl and urban decay that have characterized urban planning (or lack of planning) over the ensuing decades. It is increasingly clear that the forms of urban planning and architecture that are likely to be most conducive to the maintenance of independence in the elderly are the forms that are growing less, rather than more, common. These issues are exacerbated in the increasing population of elderly homeless persons (Boondas, 1985).

Structural lag implies that the design of living spaces will eventually need to catch up to the demographic reality. The prospects for more short-term intervention are difficult to evaluate. Few environmental interventions aimed at bolstering the functional capacities of seniors have been attempted. It is hoped that research in this area will lead to intervention efforts in the future. Evidence suggests that interventions that target features of places can have greater impact than can those that target individuals (Lawton, 1980; Lawton et al., 1980). A crucial challenge is finding strategies of urban and residential design that buoy efficacy and a sense of control. The loss of self-determination is a source of fear among many older adults and a primary reason for resisting resettlement to nursing homes. Studies indicate that the neighborhood and built environment can be designed to promote and support self-determination and independence among older residents living in the community, low-cost community, and nursing homes (Vallerand et al., 1989).

Substantial progress has been made in designing nursing homes and assisted living facilities (Regnier and Gelwicks, 1981; Regnier, 1996, 1997; Regnier and Overton, 1997). Structural lag has been the systematic consideration for the design of urban and suburban neighborhoods optimally configured for a growing older population. The literature cited above contributes to our understanding of the basic components of a well-designed neighborhood. For example, time use studies have shown that environments that are designed to stimulate social activity lead to increased social and physical activity levels even among frail elderly persons, compared to similar people in unenriched environments (Carp, 1978).

In addition to thinking about eradication of physical barriers (as with handrails and sidewalk ramps), environmental design should consider ways to facilitate social engagement as well as other pathways of environmental influence. Among the most important factors is public transportation. Driving cessation leads to lower levels of social engagement (Marottoli et al., 2000), which calls for additional attention to the public transportation infrastructure. Rates of nursing home admission are substantially lower in Europe (especially Scandanavia) due in part to substantial investments in public resources such as transportation, parks, public facilities, and community-based services (Hokenstad and Johansson, 1996). The design of urban spaces clearly plays a role as well. In this country both public policy and private development efforts have ignored the needs of older persons. Perhaps as the political clout of this growing segment of the population coalesces, factors will conspire to reverse this trend. In the meantime, additional research aimed at identifying the mechanisms and pathways through which neighborhood context affects aging will better prepare us for the coming decades.

REFERENCES

Anderson RT, Sorlie P, Backlund E, Johnson N, Kaplan GA (1997). Mortality effects of community socioeconomic status. *Epidemiology* 8: 42–47.

Anonymous (1999). From the Centers for Disease Control and Prevention. Neighborhood safety and the prevalence of physical inactivity-selected states, 1996. *J Am Med Assoc* 281: 1373.

Appleyard D, and Lintell M (1972). The environmental quality of city streets: The residents' viewpoint. *J Am Inst Planners* 38: 84–101.

Armer JM (1993). Elderly relocation to a congregate setting. *Issues in Mental Health Nursing* 14: 157–172.

Astrand PO (1992). Physical activity and fitness. *Am J Clin Nutr* 556: 1231S–1236S.

Balfour JL (1999). Neighborhood environment and Loss of Physical Function in Older People: Evidence from Three Studies of Aging in the California Bay Area. Doctoral thesis dissertation. University of California Berkeley, Department of Epidemiology.

Balfour JL, Glass TA, Frick KD, Bandeen-Roche K, Volpato F, Guralnik JM (under consideration). Aging and place: Neighborhood socioeconomic deprivation and disability among older women. *Am J Public Health*

Balfour JL, and Kaplan GA (2002). Neighborhood environment and loss of physical function in older adults: prospective evidence from the Alameda County Study. *Am J Epidemiol* 155: 507–515.

Barresi CM, Ferraro KF, Hobey LL (1983). Environmental satisfaction, sociability, and well-being among urban elderly. *Int J Aging Hum Dev* 18: 277–293.

Baumer TL (1985). Testing a general model of fear of crime: Data from a national sample. *J Res Crime and Delinquency* 22: 239–255.

Bazargan M (1994). The effects of health, environmental, and socio-psychological variables on fear of crime and its consequences among urban black elderly individuals. *Int J Aging Hum Dev* 38: 99–115.

Berkman LF, and Glass TA (2000). Social integration, social networks, social support, and health. In Berkman LF and Kawachi I, eds.: *Social Epidemiology*. New York: Oxford University Press, pp. 137–173.

Blake B, Weigl K, Perloff R (1975). Perceptions of the ideal community. *J Appl Psychol* 60: 612–615.

Bohland JR and Davis L (1979). Sources of residential satisfaction among the elderly. In Golant SM, eds.: *Location and Environment of Elderly Populations*. New York: Wiley, pp. 95–109.

Boondas J (1985). The despair of the homeless aged. *J Gerontol Nurs* 11: 8–13, 36.

Bourg C (1975). Elderly in a southern metropolitan area. *Gerontologist* 15: 15–22.

Brody EM (1979). Service-supported independent living in an urban setting: The Philadelphia Geriatric Center community housing for the elderly. In Byerts TO, eds.: *Environmental Context of Aging*. New York: Garland, pp. 121–128.

Broughton DL and Taylor RJ (1991). Review: Deterioration of glucose tolerance with age: the role of insulin resistance. *Age Ageing,* 20: 221–225.

Brown V (1995). The effects of poverty environments on elders' subjective well-being: A conceptual model. *Gerontologist* 35: 541–548.

Buchner DM and Wagner EH (1992). Preventing frail health. *Clinics Geriatric Med,* 8: 1–17.

Cantor MH (1975). Life space and the social support system of the inner-city elderly of New York. *Gerontologist* 15: 23–26.

Carp FM (1978). Effects of the living environment on activity and use of time. *Int J Aging Hum Dev* 9: 75–91.

Carp FM (1967). The impact of environment on old people. *Gerontologist* 7: 106–108.

Carp FM (1975). Lifestyle and location within the city. *Gerontologist* 15: 27–34.

Carp FM (1986). Neighborhood quality perception and measurement. In Newcomer RJ, Lawton MP, Byerts TO, eds.: *Housing an Aging Society: Issues, Alternatives and Policy*. New York: Van Nostrand Reinhold, pp. 127–140.

Carp FM and Carp A (1982). The ideal residential area. *Res Aging* 4: 411–439.

Carp FM and Christensen DL (1986). Technical environmental assessment predictors of residential satisfaction. A study of elderly women living alone. *Res Aging* 8: 269–287.

Chapman NJ and Beaudet M (1983). Environmental predictors of well-being for at-risk older adults in a mid-sized city. *J Gerontol* 38: 237–244.

Clark WA and Davies S (1990). Elderly mobility and mobility outcomes: Households in the later stage of the life course. *Res Aging* 12: 430–462.

Cohen S, Krantz DS, Evans GW, Stokols D (1981). Cardiovascular and behavioral effects of community noise. *Am Scientist* 69: 528–535.

Cohen S and Weinstein N (1981). Non-auditory effects of noise on behavior and health. *J. Soc Issues* 37: 36–70.

Colsher PL and Wallace RB (1990). Health and social antecedents of relocation in rural elderly persons. *J Gerontol* 45: S32–S38.

Coward RT, Horne C, Peek CW (1995). Predicting nursing home admissions among incontinent older adults: A comparison of residential differences across six years. *Gerontologist* 35: 732–743.

Davis JN and Daly M (1997). Evolutionary theory and the human family. *Q Rev Biol* 72: 407–435.

De Backer G, Kornitzer M, Sobolski J, Dramaix M, Degre S, de Marneffe M, Denolin H (1981). Physical activity and physical fitness levels of Belgian males aged 40–55 years. *Cardiology* 67: 110–128.

Diez-Roux AV, Nieto FJ, Muntaner C, Tyroler HA, Comstock GW, Shahar E, Cooper LS, Watson RL, Szklo M (1997). Neighborhood environments and coronary heart disease: a multilevel analysis. *Am J Epidemiol* 146: 48–63.

Durkheim E (1947). *The Division of Labor in Society.* New York: Free Press.

Durkheim E (1951). *Suicide: A Study in Sociology.* New York: Free Press.

Earls F and Buka S (1997). *Project on Human Development in Chicago Neighborhoods. A Technical Report Presented to the National Institute of Justice.* Washington, DC: U.S. Department of Justice.

Eckert JK (1979). Urban renewal and redevelopment: High risk for the marginally subsistent elderly. *Gerontologist* 19: 496–502.

Elreedy S, Krieger N, Ryan PB, Sparrow D, Weiss ST, Hu H (1999). Relations between individual and neighborhood-based measures of socioeconomic position and bone lead concentrations among community-exposed men: The Normative Aging Study. *Am J Epidemiol* 150: 129–141.

Faris R and Dunham HW (1939). *Mental Disorders in Urban Areas.* Chicago: University of Chicago Press.

Fernandez-Kelly P (1995). Social and cultural capital in the urban ghetto: Implications for the economic sociology of immigration. In Portes A, eds.: *The Economic Sociology of Immigration: Essays in Network, Ethnicity and Entrepreneurship.* New York: Russell Sage Foundation, pp. 213–247.

Fiatarone MA and Evans WJ (1993). The etiology and reversibility of muscle dysfunction in the aged. *J Gerontol* 48: 77–83.

Freedman VA (1993). Kin and nursing home lengths of stay: A backward recurrence time approach. *J Health Soc Behav* 34: 138–152.

Freedman VA, Berkman LF, Rapp SR, Ostfeld AM (1994). Family networks: Predictors of nursing home entry. *Am J Public Health* 84: 843–845.

Frongillo EA Jr, Rauschenbach BS, Roe DA, Williamson DF (1992). Characteristics related to elderly persons' not eating for 1 or more days: Implications for meal programs *Am J Public Health* 82: 600–602.

Gill TM, Williams CS, Robison JT, Tinetti ME (1999). A population-based study of environmental hazards in the homes of older persons. *Am J Public Health* 89: 553–556.

Golini A and Lori A (1990). Aging of the population: Demographic and social changes. *Aging (Milano)* 2: 319–336.

Greenberg M and Schneider D (1997). Neighborhood quality, environmental hazards, personality traits, and resident actions. *Risk Anal,* 17: 169–75.

Guralnik JM (1996). Disability as a public health outcome in the aging population. *Annu Rev Public Health* 17: 25–46.

Haan M, Kaplan GA, Camacho T (1987). Poverty and health. Prospective evidence from the Alameda County Study. *Am J Epidemiol* 125: 989–998.

Halpern D (1995). *Mental Health and the Built Environment: More than Bricks and Mortar?* London: Taylor & Francis.

Havlik R (1993). Proceedings of the 1991 International Symposium on Data on Aging. Vitality Workshop. *Vital Health Stat* 5: 55–58.

Hawkes K, O'Connell JF, Jones NGB, Alvarez H, Charnov EL (1998). Grandmothering, menopause, and the evolution of human life histories. *Proc Natl Acad Sci USA* 95: 1336–1339.

Henig JR (1981). Gentrification and displacement of the elderly: An empirical analysis. *Gerontologist* 21: 67–75.

Hokenstad MC and Johansson L (1996). Eldercare in Sweden: Issues in service provision and case management. *Journal of Case Management* 5: 137–141.

Hook EB (2000). Re: "Neighborhood social environment and risk of death: Multilevel evidence from the Alameda County study." *Am J Epidemiol* 151: 1132–1133.

House JS, Landis KR, Umberson D (1988). Social relationships and health. *Science* 241: 540–545.

House JS and Robbins C (1983). Age, psychosocial stress and health. In Riley M, Hess BB, Bond K, eds.: *Aging in Society: Selected Reviews of Recent Research.* Hillsdale, NJ: Lawrence Erlbaum Associates, pp. 175–197.

House JS, Robbins C, Metzner HL (1982). The association of social relationships and activities with mortality: Prospective evidence from the Tecumseh Community Health Study. *Am J Epidemiol* 116: 123–140.

Jeffords CR (1983). The situational relationship between age and the fear of crime. *Int J Aging Human Dev* 17: 103–111.

Kaplan GA, Haan MN, Wallace RB (1999). Understanding changing risk factor associations with increasing age in adults. *Annu Rev Public Health* 20: 89–108.

Kleemeier RW (1959). Behavior and the organization of the bodily and the external environment. In Birren JE, eds.: *Handbook of Aging and the Individual.* Chicago, Ill: University of Chicago Press, pp. 400–451.

Korte C, Ypma A, Toppen C (1975). Helpfulness in Dutch society as a function of urbanization and environmental input level. *J Pers Soc Psychol* 32: 996–1003.

Krause N (1996). Neighborhood deterioration and self-rated health in later life. *Psychol Aging* 11: 342–352.

Krause N (1993). Neighborhood deterioration and social isolation in later life. *Int J Aging Hum Dev* 36: 9–38.

Krumholz HM, Seeman TE, Merrill SS, Mendes de Leon CF, Vaccarino V, Silverman DI, Tsukahara R, Ostfeld AM, Berkman LF (1994). Lack of association between cholesterol and coronary heart disease mortality and morbidity and all-cause mortality in persons older than 70 years. *JAMA* 272: 1335–1340.

LaGory M and Fitzpatrick K (1992). The effects of environmental context on elderly depression. *Journal of Aging and Health* 4: 459–479.

Laws G (1995). Embodiment and emplacement: Identities, representation and landscape in Sun City retirement communities. *Int J Aging Hum Dev* 40: 253–280.

Lawton MP (1982). Competence, environmental press, and the adaptation of older people. In Lawton MP, Windley PG, Byerts TO, eds.: *Aging and the Environment: Theoretical Approaches.* New York: Springer, pp. 33–59.

Lawton MP (1980). *Environment and Aging.* Monterey, Calif: Brooks/Cole.

Lawton MP (1983). Environment and other determinants of well-being in older adults. *Gerontologist* 23: 349.

Lawton MP (1977). The impact of environment on aging and behavior. In Birren JE and Schaie WK, eds.: *Handbook of the Psychology of Aging.* New York: Van Nostrand Reinhold, pp. 276–301.

Lawton MP (1990). Residential environment and self-directedness among older people. *Am Psychol* 45: 638–640.

Lawton MP (1980). Residential quality and residential satisfaction among the elderly. *Research in Aging* 2: 309–328.

Lawton MP (1974). Social ecology and the health of older people. *Am J Public Health* 64: 257–260.

Lawton MP (1990). Vulnerability and socioenvironmental factors. In Harel Z, Ehrlich P, Hubbard R, eds.: *The Vulnerable Aged: People, Services and Policies.* New York: Springer, pp. 104–115.

Lawton MP, Brody EM, Saperstein AR (1990). Social, behavioral, and environmental issues. In Brody SJ and Pawlson LG, eds.: *Aging and Rehabilitation.* New York: Springer, pp. 133–149.

Lawton MP, Kleban MH, Carlson DA (1973). The inner-city resident: To move or not to move. *Gerontologist* 13: 443–448.

Lawton MP and Nahemow L (1973). Ecology and the aging process. In Eisdorfer C and Lawton MP, eds.: *The Psychology of Adult Development and Aging.* Washington, DC: American Psychological Association, pp. 464–488.

Lawton MP, Nahemow L, Teaff J (1975). Housing characteristics and the well-being of elderly tenants in federally assisted housing. *J Gerontol* 30: 601–607.

Lawton MP, Nahemow L, Tsong Min Y (1980). Neighborhood environment and the well-being of older tenants in planned housing. *Int J Aging Hum Dev* 11: 211–227.

Lawton MP, Patnaik B, Kleban MH (1976). The ecology of adaptation to a new environment. *Int J Aging Hum Dev* 7: 15–26.

Lawton MP and Simon B (1968). The ecology of social relationships in housing for the elderly. *Gerontologist* 8: 108–115.

Lawton MP and Yaffe S (1980). Victimization and fear of crime in elderly public housing tenants. *J Gerontol* 35: 768–779.

Lebowitz BD (1975). Age and fearfulness: Personal and situational factors. *J Gerontol* 30: 696–700.

LeClere FB, Rogers RG, Peters K (1997). Ethnicity and mortality in the United States: Individual and community correlates. *Social Forces* 76: 169–198.

LeClere FB, Rogers RG, Peters K (1998). Neighborhood social context and racial differences in women's heart disease mortality. *J Health Soc Behav* 39: 91–107.

Lewis K (1999). Human longevity: An evolutionary approach. *Mech Ageing Dev* 109: 43–51.

Lin G (2000). Regional assessment of elderly disability in the U.S. *Soc Sci Med* 50: 1015–1024.

Lipman PD (1991). Age and exposure differences in acquisition of route information. *Psychol Aging* 6: 128–133.

Longino CF Jr (1982). Changing aged nonmetropolitan migration patterns, 1955 to 1960 and 1965 to 1970. *J Gerontol* 37: 228–234.

Macintyre S and Ellaway A (2000). Ecological approaches: Rediscovering the role of the physical and social environment. In Berkman LF and Kawachi I, eds.: *Social Epidemiology.* New York: Oxford University Press, pp. 332–348.

Macintyre S, Maciver S, Sooman A (1993). Area, class and health: Should we be focusing on places or people? *Journal of Social Policy* 22: 213–234.

Marottoli RA, Mendes de Leon CF, Glass TA, Williams CS, Cooney LM, Berkman LF (2000). Consequences of driving cessation: Decreased out-of-home activity levels. *J Gerontol B Psychol Sci Soc Sci* 55: S334–S340.

Mathews KE and Canon LK (1975). Environmental noise level as a determinant of helping behavior. *J Pers Soc Psychol* 32: 571–577.

Maxfield MG (1984). The limits of vulnerability in explaining fear of crime: A comparative neighborhood analysis. *J Res Crime and Delinquency* 21: 233–250.

Mayer SE and Jencks C (1989). Growing up in poor neighborhoods: How much does it matter? *Science* 243: 1441–1445.

Miller ME, Longino CF Jr, Anderson RT, James MK, Worley AS (1999). Functional status, assistance, and the risk of a community-based move. *Gerontologist* 39: 187–200.

Miner S, Logan JR, Spitze G (1993). Predicting the frequency of senior center attendance. *Gerontologist* 33: 650–657.

Moser G (1988). Urban stress and helping behavior: Effects of environmental overload and noise on behavior. *Journal of Environmental Psychology* 8: 287–298.

Norris-Baker C and Scheidt RJ (1994). From "Our Town" to "Ghost Town"?: The changing context of home for rural elders. *Int J Aging Hum Dev* 38: 181–202.

Page RA (1977). Noise and helping behavior. *Environment and Behavior* 9: 311–334.

Pavan R (1987). The aging of man and society. *Archives of Gerontology and Geriatrics* 6: 3–9.

Portes A (2000). The hidden abode: Sociology as analysis of the unexpected, 1999 ASA Presidential address. *American Sociological Review* 65: 1–18.

Regnier V (1997). Design for assisted living. Familiar surroundings and activities are key for residents with dementia. *Contemporary Longterm Care* 20: 50–56.

Regnier V (1996). Long-term care design: strategies for planning the next generation of assisted living facilities. *Journal of Healthcare Design* 8: 47–51.

Regnier V and Gelwicks LE (1981). Preferred supportive services for middle to higher income retirement housing. *Gerontologist* 21: 54–58.

Regnier V and Overton J (1997). Factors affecting the growth of assisted living. *Balance* 1: 18–38.

Regnier VA (1974). Neighborhood settings and neighborhood use: Cognitive mapping as a method for identifying the macro-environment of older people. Conference Paper. The Gerontological Society of America, Portland, Oregon.

Regnier VA (1997). The physical environment and maintenance of competence. In Willis SL and Schaie WK, eds.: *Societal Mechanisms for Maintaining Competence in Old Age.* New York: Springer, pp. 232–274.

Riley MW and Riley JW Jr (1994). Age integration and the lives of older people. *Gerontologist* 34: 110–115.

Robert S and House JS (1996). SES differentials in health by age and alternative indicators of SES. *Journal of Aging and Health* 8: 359–388.

Robert SA (1998). Community-level socioeconomic status effects on adult health. *J Health Soc Behav* 39: 18–37.

Robert SA (1999). Neighborhood socioeconomic context and adult health. The mediating role of individual health behaviors and psychosocial factors. *Ann N Y Acad Sci* 896: 465–468.

Robert SA and Li LW (2001). Age variation in the relationship between community socioeconomic status and adult health. *Research in Aging* 32: 233–258.

Roberts RE, Kaplan GA, Shema SJ, Strawbridge WJ (1997). Does growing old increase the risk for depression? *Am J Psychiatry* 154: 1384–1390.

Rodin J (1986). Aging and health: Effects of the sense of control. *Science* 233: 1271–1276.

Rosel N (1983). The hub of a wheel: A neighborhood support network. *Int J Aging Hum Dev* 16: 193–200.

Sampson RJ, Raudenbush SW, Earls F (1997). Neighborhoods and violent crime: A multilevel study of collective efficacy. *Science* 277: 918–924.

Satariano WA (1997). The disabilities of aging—looking to the physical environment. *Am J Public Health* 87: 331–332.

Satin MS and Monetti CH (1985). Census tract predictors of physical, psychological, and social functioning for needs assessment. *Health Serv Res* 20: 341–358.

Schulz R and Brenner G (1977). Relocation of the aged: A review and theoretical analysis. *J Gerontol* 32: 323–333.

Sherman SR, Ward RA, LaGory M (1985). Socialization and aging group consciousness: The effect of neighborhood age concentration. *J Gerontol* 40: 102–109.

Silverstein M and Angelelli JJ (1998). Older parents' expectations of moving closer to their children. *J Gerontol B Psychol Sci Soc Sci* 53: S153–S163.

Silverstein M and Zablotsky DL (1996). Health and social precursors of later life retirement-community migration. *J Gerontol B Psychol Sci Soc Sci* 51: S150–S156.

Simon SL, Walsh DA, Regnier VA, Krauss IK (1992). Spatial cognition and neighborhood use: The relationship in older adults. *Psychol Aging* 7: 389–394.

Simonsick EM, Phillips CL, Skinner EA, Davis D, Kasper JD (1995). The daily lives of disabled older women. In Guralnik JM, Fried LP, Simonsick EM, Kasper JD, Laferty ME, eds.: *The Women's Health and Aging Study: Health and Social Characteristics of Older Women with Disability*. Bethesda, Md: National Institute on Aging, pp. 50–69.

Smith GE, Kokmen E, O'Brien PC (2000). Risk factors for nursing home placement in a population-based dementia cohort. *J Am Geriatr Soc* 48: 519–525.

Sooman A, Macintyre S, Anderson A (1993). Scotland's health—a more difficult challenge for some? The price and availability of healthy foods in socially contrasting localities in the west of Scotland. *Health Bull (Edinb)* 51: 276–284.

South SJ and Crowder KD (1997). Residential mobility between cities and suburbs: Race, suburbanization, and back-to-the-city moves. *Demographics* 34: 525–538.

Stack C (1974). *All Our Kin*. New York: Harper & Row.

Stuck AE, Walthert JM, Nikolaus T, Bula CJ, Hohmann C, Beck JC (1999). Risk factors for functional status decline in community-living elderly people: A systematic literature review. *Soc Sci Med* 48: 445–469.

Tager IB, Hollenberg M, Satariano WA (1998). Association between self-reported leisure-time physical activity and measures of cardiorespiratory fitness in an elderly population. *Am J Epidemiol* 147: 921–931.

Talbot JF and Kaplan R (1991). The benefits of nearby nature for elderly apartment residents. *Int J Aging Hum Dev* 33: 119–130.

Tennstedt SL and McKinlay JB (1994). Frailty and its consequences. *Soc Sci Med* 38: 863–865.

Tonnies F (1887/1963). *Community and Society.* New York: Harper & Row.

Turner JH, Beeghley L, Powers CH (1989). *The Emergence of Sociological Theory.* Chicago: Dorsey Press.

Usui WM, Keil TJ (1987). Life satisfaction and age concentration of the local area. *Psychol Aging* 2: 30–35.

Vallerand RJ, O'Connor BP, Blais MR (1989). Life satisfaction of elderly individuals in regular community housing, in low-cost community housing, and high and low self-determination nursing homes. *Int J Aging Hum Dev* 28: 277–283.

Verbrugge LM and Jette AM (1994). The disablement process. *Soc Sci Med* 38: 1–14.

Waitzman NJ and Smith KR (1998). Phantom of the area: Poverty-area residence and mortality in the United States. *Am J Public Health* 88: 973–976.

Walston J and Fried LP (1999). Frailty and the older man. *Med Clin North Am* 83: 1173–1194.

Ward R, LaGory M, Sherman S (1988). *The Environment and Aging.* Tuscaloosa: University of Alabama Press.

Whyte WF (1943). *Street Corner Society.* Chicago: University of Chicago Press.

Windley PG and Scheidt RJ (1982). An ecological model of mental health among small-town rural elderly. *J Gerontol* 37: 235–242.

Wister AV (1989). Environmental adaptation by persons in their later life. *Research on Aging* 11: 267–291.

Wolf RS (1978). A social systems model of nursing home use. *Health Serv Res* 13: 111–128.

Wolinsky FD, Callahan CM, Fitzgerald JF, Johnson RJ (1993). Changes in functional status and the risks of subsequent nursing home placement and death. *J Gerontol* 48: S94–S101.

Wolinsky FD, Callahan CM, Fitzgerald JF, Johnson RJ (1992). The risk of nursing home placement and subsequent death among older adults. *J Gerontol* 47: S173–S182.

Yen IH and Kaplan GA (1999). Neighborhood social environment and risk of death: Multilevel evidence from the Alameda County Study. *Am J Epidemiol* 149: 898–907.

15

Neighborhoods, Health Research, and Its Relevance to Public Policy

JODY HEYMANN
ARON FISCHER

In many areas of medical and public health research, identifying health risks leads directly to recommendations for change. Sometimes these recommendations involve encouraging individuals to change risk behavior. When smoking was shown to cause cancer, individuals were warned to stop smoking or never to start. When diet and physical activity was proven to reduce the risk of heart disease, people were encouraged to eat right and exercise. To be sure, public policies can make these individual actions easier. City-wide bans on smoking in public places, safe public space available for exercising, and healthy food offerings in company cafeterias are just a few examples of the many ways that collective policies can make healthy steps by individuals easier and more probable. However, while public policies may help individuals reduce personal risk factors, they are not necessary for individuals to act.

Other research findings, such as those that identify occupational or environmental health risks, do require collective responses. After a body of research revealed that even low levels of lead could harm the nervous systems of children, concerned families could do little on their own to shield themselves from the lead in gasoline fumes and in the paint of public buildings. In order to protect children from these exposures, the government limited the use of lead products in gasoline and schools. Similarly, since people cannot protect themselves from the hazardous actions of drunk drivers in other cars, stricter laws against drinking and driving were crucial to reduce that health risk. Even in cases such as these where the remedy is clear, enacting the necessary public policy changes can involve long and difficult political battles (Isaacs and Schroeder, 2001). Still, such cases are more straightforward than those discussed in this volume because research findings directly informed thinking on the nature of solutions.

Like other social or environmental research, research on neighborhoods and health requires a collective response to be useful; individuals living in injurious neighborhoods often lack the option to leave, even if they want to. Yet, addressing the health hazards of living in troubled neighborhoods is a uniquely difficult task because no targeted intervention of a traditional variety is likely to alleviate the health risks of these neighborhoods. Rather, these health risks will probably continue to exist as long as troubled neighborhoods themselves exist. Improving the nature of neighborhoods has proven a far more complex and intractable problem than placing fluoride in water or taking lead out of paint (Ferguson and Dickens, 1999).

WILL ANY OF THIS RESEARCH MAKE A DIFFERENCE IN PUBLIC POLICY AND PRACTICE?

The preceding chapters make a major contribution to our understanding of the health effects of neighborhoods. Bringing together for the first time a range of mature, cross-disciplinary research on the question, this book offers a comprehensive survey of the existing evidence about neighborhoods and health, defines the conceptual and methodological challenges future research must confront, and suggests a variety of promising new means to meet those research challenges. Despite the important further research that remains to be done, however, the evidence that neighborhoods have independent effects on health outcomes is already cumulatively very substantial. While the research agenda presented in this volume needs to be carried out, it is not premature to begin considering policy responses to the health risks of distressed neighborhoods. If we want existing as well as future research to do more than sit on shelves in journals and books, we need to step back and examine critically its salience to action.

Is it useful to have research that demonstrates the health effects of living in troubled neighborhoods? If the research does nothing more than highlight the undesirability of some neighborhoods, then the answer is no. Ordinary citizens have long sought to avoid living in areas with high crime rates, troubled schools, discrimination, concentrated poverty, and many of the other problems outlined in this volume. Indeed, one reason for the persistence of distressed neighborhoods may be that better-off residents leave as soon as they have the means to do so (Wilson, 1987; Mincy,

1994; Jargowsky, 1997), nor has the fact that living in some neighborhoods is bad for you gone unnoticed by academia. From popular literature to academic writing, the list of books that address troubled neighborhoods was extensive well before the health effects of neighborhoods were carefully studied. Before the twentieth century, fiction by Charles Dickens, mortality studies by Engels, satires on the health effects of socioeconomic disparities by Swift, and exposés about tenement conditions by Jacob Riis asserted the problems of concentrated poverty. Since then landmark works of policy and scholarship such as the Kerner Commission report (1968), *The Underclass* by Ken Auletta (1982), and *The Truly Disadvantaged* by William Julius Wilson have explored the impacts of neighborhoods.

If it has long been the case that people have known about the problems of distressed neighborhoods, then the barriers to improving these neighborhoods must be more than just lack of awareness. What has kept those who develop public policy and programs from successfully addressing these problems to date? At least five obstacles have stood in the way of markedly improving conditions in the hardest hit neighborhoods in many countries during the past century.

1. *Competing for resources.* Hard-hit neighborhoods are widespread. Efforts to improve the quality of life in these neighborhoods will be neither cheap nor easy in most countries. More than ten million Americans lived in U.S. Census tracts with poverty rates of 40% or more in 1990, and even in the midst of a booming economy in the year 2000, eight million Americans still lived in concentrated poverty (Jargowsky, 1997; Jargowsky, 2003). Meanwhile, demand for increased spending in other social areas, such as health care and education, remains high. In the political climate of recent years, social spending priorities must compete in many countries for a fiscal bidget that remains relatively constant or shrinks, because few governments raise taxes and others cut them (McFate et al., 1995). Budgets are further constrained by recent economic declines and increased demands for spending on security. For this reason, even when policy makers accept the principle that improving neighborhoods is a public responsibility, substantial debate always arises about whether resources could be better used for other projects.
2. *Addressing problems raised by competing values.* In addition to questions about competing uses of fiscal resources, efforts to improve neighborhoods have been hindered by questions about competing values. Some of the traditional policies to solve neighborhood problems conflict with widely held values. For example, if the most effective way to decrease crime is "zero tolerance" for small infractions, how does that policy affect on social relationships or justice?

3. *Reaching agreement on individual vs. public responsibility*. Regardless of research findings, popular debates have long focused on the extent to which poverty and the quality of neighborhoods in which the poor live are the responsibility of society and the extent to which they are the responsibility of individuals. Some political constituencies argue that poverty and poor neighborhoods are caused by individual failings rather than by social conditions. In a recent U.S. survey, slightly more than half of respondents believed that people are poor due more to their "not doing enough to help themselves" than due to "circumstances beyond their control," while substantial majorities listed "lack of motivation," "moral failings," "drug abuse," and "too many single-parent families" as major causes of poverty (National Public Radio/ Kaiser Center/Kennedy School, 2001). Such beliefs lead to the conclusion that poverty alleviation is the responsibility of individuals and religious institutions rather than of society as a whole. The belief in individual responsibility appears to be less prevalent in the United Kingdom, where most people consider social class to be a key determinant of individual well-being (Schlesinger and Lee, 1993; Evans, 1997). Nevertheless, the opinion of many policy makers and voters that troubled neighborhoods are the responsibility of residents and not of the larger society can be a major barrier to the enactment of public policies.

4. *Obtaining political support*. Together, these factors make it difficult to gather political support for efforts to address neighborhood problems. Notwithstanding arguments to the contrary made by some conservatives, the majority of Americans do believe the government should have a role in helping the disadvantaged (Heclo, 1994). Still, limits to public support remain a significant problem in the United States. In public opinion polls Americans consistently give less support to social welfare benefits than do Europeans (Bobo and Smith, 1994). The percentages are somewhat higher in Europe, but aid to the disadvantaged remains a subject of real debate.

   Thus, even when policy makers may have resolved in their own minds that improving hard-hit neighborhoods outweighs other priorities, questions remain as to whether public opinion will back the sort of large-scale effort that would be required. Currently, aid to poor nations and welfare for poor families each make up less than 1% of United States gross domestic product (U.S. Dept. of Commerce, 2000).

5. *Finding tested solutions*. Even after the majority agree that addressing the problems of neighborhoods is a social responsibility, is more important than other goals, and is worth a large investment of resources, proven means of improving neighborhoods would still be lacking. This

is true even when there is agreement about "root problems" in hard-hit neighborhoods. For example, if lack of educational opportunities for children and marketable skills for adults perpetuate neighborhood poverty, then we can try to improve schools and increase training opportunities for everyone in the hardest-hit communities (Durlauf, 1996), but no one has demonstrated a reliable and replicable system for improving the quality of the worst public schools. Furthermore, even when programs can successfully increase the educational opportunities available to some individuals, that does not mean they will stay in the neighborhood. If insufficient social capital is the problem, then we can try to foster community organizations and to increase political participation (Putnam, 2000), but no proven means of restoring a sense of community to fragmented neighborhoods exists.

WHICH BARRIERS RESEARCH CAN HELP TO BREAK DOWN

Will studying the relationship between neighborhoods and health help address any of these five barriers to effective action? The research presented and proposed in this book will help overcome some of them, but others will remain even after this research program is complete and disseminated. In order to overcome the final obstacles standing in the way of better policies to improve hard-hit neighborhoods, a new way of conceptualizing and prioritizing research will be needed.

New knowledge about the health consequences of poor neighborhoods may help with the first barrier described, the question of resource allocation. Resource allocation decisions inevitably involve debates about costs and benefits. If improving the quality of neighborhoods improves public health outcomes, it becomes easier to argue for the benefits society can anticipate from the measures to be taken: many economic benefits accrue from having a healthier population. It is unclear, however, whether the need to document these additional benefits is the missing inducement when it comes to increasing resources for neighborhoods. Those who would benefit most from neighborhood programs still lack the political and economic power that is so critical to having their interests met and protected.

Learning about the relationship between neighborhoods and health may provide information that helps with the second barrier—balancing competing values—but it is unlikely to provide final answers. Improving the public health will be added to fighting poverty and combating racial inequality as values served by policies to improve embattled neighborhoods, but dilemmas regarding competing values will remain. For example, if integrated neighborhoods improve health but monolingual immigrants prefer to live in neighborhoods where the language they speak predominates, what action should be taken, if any? If "zero tolerance" of any loitering or infraction is the most effective way to combat high crime rates that lead to poor health, but this policy results in serious consequences for some minor offenders, what should be done? How to balance competing values is not new to public health policy, but it is rarely resolved by research alone.

Research on neighborhoods and health may also help with the third barrier by tipping the debate between individual and social responsibility in the direction of social responsibility. As this book documents, the evidence is mounting that neighborhoods have a significant impact on health *independent* of individual characteristics. The ethical implications of these data are clear. Only the most naïve observer could argue that people live in bad neighborhoods purely by free choice. If social conditions rather than individual behavior cause the problem, then society must share some of the responsibility for solving it.

It remains to be seen whether knowing the health benefits of improving neighborhoods will weaken the fourth barrier: finding the political will to act. The effect of the research on political will is likely to vary from country to country. In countries like the United Kingdom and Canada, where a national health service already exists and where there is a generally shared belief that the government has a responsibility for caring for the health of all citizens, showing that neighborhood quality affects health may be seen as immediately relevant to policy makers' choices about how to improve the health of communities. In countries like the United States, where there is neither national health insurance nor universal acceptance that the government is responsible for caring for citizens' health, evidence that links the nature of neighborhoods with the health of individuals may have more of an uphill battle to fight in shaping political will and influencing policy decisions (Schlesinger and Lee, 1993; Jimenez, 1997). Those who do not think the government should be involved in providing medical care for those who cannot afford it may be unmoved by the more indirect arguments about the health benefits of improving neighborhoods.

Although current research on neighborhoods and health will not overcome all the political barriers to improving neighborhoods, on balance it is likely to improve the odds that initiatives designed to address neighborhood conditions will be taken seriously. Nevertheless, one barrier to improving neighborhoods exists that the evidence on neighborhoods and health will not even begin to break down, and that is how little we really know about *how* to improve the quality of neighborhoods.

Even if the causal relationship between neighborhoods and health is fully understood and that research is effectively disseminated, the practical question of which programs work and which do not will remain. Now, we know a little about improving neighborhoods, but we need to know much more.

PAST EFFORTS TO IMPROVE NEIGHBORHOODS

Initiatives focused on improving the conditions of hard-hit neighborhoods are not a recent innovation. On the contrary, such efforts occurred in different forms throughout the twentieth century. In the United States the settlement houses of the 1900s focused on meeting the health and service needs of families in poor neighborhoods (Halpern, 1996). In the New Deal Era of the 1930s, "slum clearance" became a major public policy debate, with dilemmas over the relative roles of public and private institutions that foreshadowed many of today's arguments about the role of government. The Great Society initiatives of the 1960s sought to defeat inner-city poverty with a variety of social programs, including the Community Action Program and community development corporations (O'Connor, 1999). The 1990s saw such projects as "comprehensive community initiatives" and empowerment zones designed to improve neighborhoods (Lehman and Smeeding, 1997).

While each of these efforts affected change, none provided a recipe for addressing the needs of troubled neighborhoods. For example, during the 1970s and 1980s neighborhood poverty became more common, not less (Rusk, 1999; Jargowsky, 1997). While some indicators associated with distressed neighborhoods, notably violent crime, declined in the 1990s, little evidence indicates that these figures represent general improvements in the conditions of poor neighborhoods. Instead, while some neighborhoods have improved, others have declined.

For some of the major issues facing troubled neighborhoods, no effective solutions have been found. Residential segregation is one example. The first steps are clear enough: ensure that there are no barriers to individuals moving into neighborhoods. Programs to do this already have a policy foundation, the Fair Housing Act of 1968, which made discrimination in selling houses or providing mortgages illegal. Efforts to improve enforcement of the act have made progress in establishing legal precedents against housing discrimination (Massey and Denton, 1993). However, explicit discrimination is no longer the primary cause of segregation, and the steps to address the less blatant causes are less clear. Devastating disparities in residential segregation continue, with African-

American families far more likely than other groups to live in neighborhoods of concentrated poverty (Orfield, 1997; Rusk, 1999).

Challenges to Conducting the Necessary Research

Compared to public health successes of the past, such as the advent of immunizations and the improvement of sanitary services, our understanding of how to solve neighborhood problems is limited. In fact, we know more about improving individuals' lives by moving them out of hard-hit neighborhoods than we do about healing neighborhoods themselves (Rosenbaum, 1995; Katz et al., 2001; Ludwig et al., 2001). This perhaps should not come as a surprise. The mechanisms by which neighborhoods affect public health and well-being are far more complex than are those of polio or water-borne bacteria. Moreover, the research necessary to learn what works and what does not in improving neighborhood conditions faces at least four substantial challenges.

1. *Randomization is a rare option.* The gold standard for most medical and public health trials is randomization, yet randomization at the neighborhood level is difficult to accomplish. Politically, it is hard to convince people that it is worth spending money on major neighborhood initiatives of uncertain value, and, ethically, the case is usually made for randomization when researchers do not know which arm of a study will prove to be better. If the evidence is strongly suggestive that the neighborhood that receives the intervention will be better off, how does one convince neighborhoods to be willing to be randomized and risk a substantial chance of receiving no help? If the evidence is not strongly suggestive, how does one obtain the support necessary to obtain the needed resources? Making the case that resources should be provided and participants should volunteer for uncertain risks and benefits is difficult enough in a clinical trial; it is far more difficult in the political sphere.

    Hancock and colleagues (1997) conducted a thorough review of the research literature that evaluates community action projects designed to reduce cancer and cardiovascular disease rates. They reviewed the studies they found according to standard scientific criteria, including sampling design, use of control procedures, quality of study instruments, and techniques used in data analysis. None of the articles they found met all of the criteria they agreed upon for rigorous science.

2. *Sorting out the influence of multiple factors is difficult.* When conditions in a given neighborhood are poor, often many interventions to improve the deleterious conditions will be tried simultaneously. State and local governments may change their public policies toward the individual neighborhood and nonprofit organizations may bring in special programs, all concurrent with a study that is being implemented. This presents large challenges to sorting out effects. If a neighborhood does improve, what led to that, and if conditions worsen, what was the cause?

Interventions are often attempted in hard-hit communities that have many initiatives occurring simultaneously. The multiplicity of initiatives makes sense, given the high need in the communities, yet it makes determining which one is effective, if any, difficult or impossible. Spergel and Curry's (1990) work on youth gangs and interventions aimed at decreasing their violence documents the number of organizations often involved with this single problem in a given community.

3. *Problems of sample size limit study power.* It is difficult to have a large enough sample size of neighborhoods in which an intervention is being tried to determine statistically whether an effect is significant. In other social or biomedical science studies, sample sizes of 100 individuals would be considered small, but to put together a sample size of 100 neighborhoods is an enormous and frequently impossible undertaking. This is particularly the case for purposeful interventions. (The chance is better of putting together this sample size to study the impact of policies that have de facto been implemented differentially across states for political reasons). In their discussion of how best to evaluate the effect of community interventions even on a common problem such as heart disease, Feldman and colleagues (1996) note how difficult it is to obtain a sample size large enough to document the health effects of community interventions while taking into account the other natural differences that occur in communities.

4. *Findings frequently may not be generalizable.* When a program to improve conditions appears to work well in one or several neighborhoods, the question of generalizability remains an important one. Programs that work well to fight discrimination in economically homogeneous neighborhoods may not succeed in economically heterogeneous neighborhoods. Projects that address income inequalities in communities with high levels of social capital and trust may be ineffective in communities with low levels of social capital and trust. Programs that are politically feasible in a strong economy may be impossible to sustain in recessions.

ADDRESSING THE CHALLENGES TO
SOLUTION-ORIENTED RESEARCH

It is important to note that health researchers are not alone in struggling with the difficulties of studying neighborhood interventions. In the policy conclusions to the Social Science Research Council's two-volume report on the influence of neighborhoods on child and adolescent development, Jeffrey Lehman and Timothy Smeeding write, "We still have breathtakingly little knowledge about the effects of public interventions. . . . There would seem to be great potential value in federal support for carefully structured programmatic experimentation, coupled with rigorous evaluation, in order to augment that knowledge" (Lehman and Smeeding, 1997, p. 269). Health researchers can take the same approach, working with communities to develop and rigorously test solutions to neighborhood health risks. Nationwide, anecdotal reports of localized programs that work are numerous. Using these scattered programs as the bases for experimental or comparative studies, researchers on neighborhoods and health may be able to take advantage of the diversity of American neighborhood interventions to achieve rigorous and useful results.

The best solution-oriented research to date has been conducted on moving people out of hard-hit neighborhoods. The most important examples of policy experiments relevant to neighborhoods are the housing programs that randomly assign participants to receive different benefits—the Gautreaux Assisted Housing Program in Chicago and the subsequent Moving to Opportunity housing voucher programs in various American cities (Rosenbaum, 1995; Katz et al., 2001; Ludwig et al., 2001). The quasi-experimental nature of the earlier program and the explicitly experimental design of the later, with participants randomly designated to one or more policy "treatments," allowed researchers to compare outcomes among people in comparable circumstances. These studies found that residents who received vouchers to move out of poor neighborhoods experienced statistically significant improvements in child outcomes.

As discussed above, research that evaluates policies aimed at entire neighborhoods rather than individuals faces many more obstacles. Nonetheless, the diversity of state and local approaches to neighborhood problems can be studied. When different localities take different approaches to solving neighborhood problems, rigorous comparison can help determine which solutions are effective. For example, one proposed strategy for reducing the negative effects of concentrated poverty has been the regional approach implemented in Minnesota, using tactics such as rezoning middle-class areas for affordable housing and sharing the property tax base among more and less affluent areas in order to reduce the political and social isolation of poor neighborhoods (Orfield, 1997). Comparative studies on the effects of zoning laws and property tax jurisdictions could shed light on the generalizability of this approach.

To be sure, confounding variables pose challenges to comparative policy studies, yet with the experiences of hundreds of affected neighborhoods to compare, important understanding regarding what will make a difference can be achieved. The methodologies discussed in this book and applied to understanding the problems now need to be applied to understanding the solutions.

CONCLUSION

Research on neighborhoods and health is providing a crucial balance to biomedical research. As essential as it us for us to understand the pathophysiological mechanisms of diseases, it is equally essential for us to understand the social and environmental factors that lead to illnesses.

Even so, the field examining neighborhoods and health is still at an early stage, and much remains to be done before this research fulfills its potential in improving population health. For the field to achieve its potential, researchers will need to think carefully about the remaining obstacles to moving from scientific understanding to policy and program changes that better health. They will find knowledge gaps they need to fill as well as practical challenges to turning that knowledge into policy (Heymann, 2000).

Undoubtedly, one of the greatest obstacles that remains is our limited understanding of how to improve conditions in hard-hit neighborhoods. Research designed to identify effective ways to improve neighborhoods will not be easy. Each approach carries its own array of difficulties to be resolved. Still, in the long run, unless we learn how to ameliorate troubled neighborhoods, knowledge of the need to improve them will be of little use. Critical challenges exist in conducting research to evaluate what will be an effective and generalizable way to address the problems neighborhoods face, but we will not be effective at reducing the health risks associated with neighborhoods unless we meet these challenges.

The research we know how to do best will not provide the answers we lack. The old story of the man looking for his keys under a lamppost on a dark street is relevant here. When asked if he lost his keys under the lamppost, he replied, "No, but that is where the light is." A critical key to meeting the health needs of individuals, their families, and their communities lies in improving the conditions they face in their neighborhoods, and an essential key to improving those conditions lies in learning how.

REFERENCES

Auletta K (1982). The Underclass. Woodstock, NY: Overlook Press.

Bobo L and Smith RA (1994). Anti-poverty policy, affirmative action, and racial attitudes. In Danziger SH, Sandefur GD, Weinberg DH, eds.: *Confronting Poverty: Prescriptions for Change.* New York: Russell Sage Foundation; Cambridge, Mass: Harvard University Press, pp. 365–395.

Danziger SH, Sandefur GD, Weinberg DH, eds. (1994). *Confronting Poverty: Prescriptions for Change.* New York: Russell Sage Foundations; Cambridge, Mass: Harvard University Press.

Durlauf S (1996). A theory of persistent income inequality. *J Econ Growth* 1: 75–93.

Evans G (1997). Political ideology and popular beliefs about class and opportunity: Evidence from a survey experiment. *Br J Sociol* 48(3): 450–470.

Feldman HA, McKinlay SM, Niknian M (1996). Batch sampling to improve power in a community trial: Experience from the Pawtucket Heart Health Program. *Evaluation Review* 20(3): 244–274.

Ferguson RF and Dickens WT, eds. (1999). *Urban Problems and Community Development.* Washington, DC: Brookings Institution.

Halpern R (1996). Neighborhood-based strategies to address poverty-related social problems: An historical perspective. In Kahn AJ and Kamerman SB, eds.: *Children and Their Families in Big Cities: Strategies for Service Reform.* New York: Cross National Studies Research Program, School of Social Work, Columbia University, pp. 30–86.

Hancock LH et al. (1997). Community action for health promotion: A review of methods and outcomes 1990–1995. *Am J Prev Med* 13(4): 229–239.

Heclo H (1994). Poverty politics. In Danziger SH, Sandefur GD, Weinberg DH, eds.: *Confronting Poverty: Prescriptions for Change.* New York: Russell Sage Foundation; Cambridge, Mass: Harvard University Press, pp. 396–437.

Heymann SJ (2000). Health and social policy. In Berkman L and Kawachi I, eds.: *Social Epidemiology.* New York: Oxford University Press, pp. 368–382.

Isaacs SL and Schroeder SA (2001). Where the public good prevailed. *Am Prospect* 12(10): 26–30.

Jargowsky PA (1997). *Poverty and Place: Ghettos, Barrios, and the American City.* New York: Russell Sage Foundation.

Jargowsky PA (2003). *Concentration of Poverty.* Washington DC: The Brookings Institution.

Jimenez MA (1997). Concepts of Health and national health care policy: A view from American history. *Social Serv Rev* 71(1): 34–50.

Katx L, Kling J, Liebman J (2001). Moving to opportunity in Boston: Early results of a randomized mobility experiment. *Q J Econ* 116(2): 604–654.

Lehman JS and Smeeding T (1997). Neighborhood effects and federal policy. In Brooks-Gunn J, Duncan G, Aber JL, eds.: *Neighborhood Poverty: Context and Consequences for Children,* vol. 1. New York: Russell Sage Foundation, pp. 251–278.

Ludwig J, Duncan GJ, Hirschfield P (2001). Urban poverty and juvenile crime: Evidence from a randomized housing-mobility experiment. *Q J Econ* 116(2): 655–679.

Massey DS and Denton N (1993). *American Apartheid: Segregation and the Making of the Underclass.* Cambridge, Mass: Harvard University Press.

McFate K, Smeeding T, Rainwater L (1995). Markets and states: Poverty trends and transfer system effectiveness in the 1980s. In McFate K, Lawson R, Wilson JW, eds.: *Poverty, Inequality, and the Future of Social Policy.* New York: Russell Sage Foundation, pp. 29–66.

Mincy R (1994). The underclass: Concept, controversy, and evidence. In Danziger SH, Sandefur GD, Weinberg DH, eds.: *Confronting Poverty: Prescriptions for Change.* New York: Russell Sage Foundation; Cambridge, Mass: Harvard University Press, pp. 109–146.

National Public Radio, Kaiser Center, John F. Kennedy School of Government (2001). Available online at http://www.npr.org/programs/specials/poll/poverty/staticresults.html

O'Connor A (1999). Swimming against the tide: A brief history of federal policy in poor communities. In Ferguson RF and Dickens WT, eds.: *Urban Problems and Community Development.* Washington, DC: Brookings Institution.

Orfield M (1997). *Metropolitics: A Regional Agenda for Community and Stability.* Washington, DC: Brookings Institution Press; Cambridge, Mass: Lincoln Institute of Land Policy.

Putnam RD (2000). *Bowling Alone: The Collapse and Revival of American Community.* New York: Simon & Schuster.

Rosenbaum JE (1995). Changing the geography of opportunity by expanding residential choice: Lessons from the Gautreaux Program. *Housing Policy Debate* 6: 231–269.

Rusk D (1999). *Inside Game Outside: Winning Strategies for Saving Urban America.* Washington, DC: Brookings Institution.

Schlesinger M and Lee TK (1993). Is health care different? Popular support of federal health and social policies. *J Health Polit Policy Law* 18(3): 551–628.

Spergel IA and Curry GD (1990). Strategies and perceived agency effectiveness in dealing with the youth gang problem. In Huff CR, ed.: *Gangs in America.* Newbury Park, Calif: Sage Publications.

U.S. Department of Commerce, Bureau of Economic Analysis (2000). Date from Table 3.15, Government Consumption Expenditures and Gross Investment by Function, and Table 1.1, Gross Domestic Product.

Wilson WJ (1987). *The Truly Disadvantaged: The Inner City, the Underclass, and Public Policy.* Chicago: University of Chicago Press.

Index